Birth Models That Work

The publisher gratefully acknowledges the generous
support of the General Endowment Fund of the
University of California Press Foundation.

Birth Models That Work

EDITED BY

Robbie Davis-Floyd,
Lesley Barclay, Betty-Anne Daviss,
and Jan Tritten

UNIVERSITY OF CALIFORNIA PRESS

Berkeley   Los Angeles   London

University of California Press, one of the most distinguished
university presses in the United States, enriches lives around the
world by advancing scholarship in the humanities, social sciences,
and natural sciences. Its activities are supported by the UC Press
Foundation and by philanthropic contributions from individuals
and institutions. For more information, visit www.ucpress.edu.

Portions of chapter 3 have previously appeared in Margaret
MacDonald, *At Work in the Field of Birth: Midwifery Narratives of
Nature, Tradition, and Home* (Vanderbilt University Press, 2007), and
her article "Tradition as a Political Symbol in the New Midwifery
in Ontario," in *Reconceiving Midwifery: The New Canadian Model,*
eds. I. L. Bourgeault, C. Benoit, and R. Davis-Floyd (McGill-Queens
University Press, 2004).

University of California Press
Berkeley and Los Angeles, California

University of California Press, Ltd.
London, England

Library of Congress Cataloging-in-Publication Data

Birth models that work / edited by Robbie Davis-Floyd . . . [et al.].
    p.   cm.
Includes bibliographical references and index.
   ISBN 978-0-520-24863-2 (cloth : alk. paper)
   ISBN 978-0-520-25891-4 (pbk. : alk. paper)
   1. Maternal health services—Cross-cultural studies.
2. Childbirth—Cross-cultural studies.   3. Labor (Obstetrics)—
Cross-cultural studies.   4. Midwifery—Cross-cultural studies.
I. Davis-Floyd, Robbie.
[DNLM: 1. Maternal Health Services.   2. Birthing Centers.
3. Cross-cultural Comparison.   4. Delivery, Obstetrics.
5. Midwifery.   6. Models, Organizational.   WA 310.1 B619   2009]
RG940.B55   2009
362.19'82—dc22   2008037220

Manufactured in the United States of America

18   17   16   15   14   13   12   11   10   09

10 9 8 7 6 5 4 3 2 1

This book is printed on Natures Book, which contains 30%
post-consumer waste and meets the minimum requirements of
ANSI/NISO Z39.48–1992 (R 1997) (*Permanence of Paper*).

*To the conceivers, creators, educators, and practitioners of
birth models that work, in the hope that the models you create will coalesce
to set a global standard of excellence in birth and maternity care that
will become the norm for birth, rather than the exception.*

CONTENTS

FIGURES AND TABLES

FIGURES

TABLES

ix

APPENDIX TABLES

Introduction

Robbie Davis-Floyd, Lesley Barclay, Betty-Anne Daviss, and Jan Tritten

> *The humanization of birth does not represent a romantic return to the past, nor a devaluation of technology. Rather, it offers an ecological and sustainable pathway to the future.*
> RICARDO HERBERT JONES, obstetrician

Birth is one of the most powerful of all human experiences, yet it can also be one of the most disempowering. Around the world, there are examples of societies and systems that provide women with true choice, where their desires and wishes and the normal physiology of labor and birth are honored, respected, and trusted. In these places, interventions are applied solely in cases of real need so that their potential misuse does not cause harm. Even though these are only lighthouses in an ocean of over-medicalized care across the globe, their existence shows us that good birth models work—they can combine the best of obstetrical care with the best of contemporary scientific research, ancient wisdom, basic common sense, and compassion to create systems of knowledge, skills, and practice that truly serve mothers, babies, and families. This book is about those lighthouses and their role as beacons for those searching for philosophical and concrete ways to improve maternity care.

BIRTH MODELS THAT DON'T WORK: A BRIEF SYNOPSIS

Characteristics of Birth Models That Don't Work

For years birth activists have been saying it: "That doesn't work; it just doesn't work." By "doesn't work," they mean the contemporary obstetrical treatment of birth around the world. It doesn't work. Yes, babies get born and lives that could have been lost get saved through modern obstetrics, but the price in both money and collateral damage to the mother and baby is increasingly high. This price shouldn't have to be paid, because it is based on misinformation and misunderstanding of the normal physiology of birth and how best to support it. It comes from a system that seeks to avoid mortality through the excess application of interventions while failing to recognize that those very interventions when overused cause unnecessary morbidity—and increasingly, even mortality itself—to the mother or baby. Intervention is now associated with increased maternal and perinatal mortality figures due in part to the excess use of cesarean section in many countries: the increased rate of cesareans has become the unwitting accomplice to the mortality this operation is designed to avoid (see below). As the models described in this volume demonstrate, it is not necessary to "trade off" the morbidity associated with interventions for avoidance of mortality—decreasing intervention and increasing support of normal physiological birth both serve to avoid mortality. Indeed, as we will show in these pages, some low-intervention models of birth can demonstrate lower morbidity and equivalent (or lower) mortality than high-intervention tertiary care.

We have extrapolated the following characteristics of models that don't work from the enormous body of literature written by epidemiologists, midwives, obstetricians, nurses, and social scientists that describes and critiques the scientific, humanistic, and economic deficiencies of contemporary obstetrics in dozens of countries. (See for summaries the Cochrane Library;[1] *Advancing Normal Birth* 2007; Downe 2008; Goer 1999; Kroeger and Smith 2004; Enkin et al. 2000; Rooks 1997; Walsh 2007; the Millbank Report coauthored by Sakala and Corry 2008; and the many resources provided by Childbirth Connection[2] and by the World Health Organization.)

In brief, the characteristics of birth models that don't work include:

- Unnecessary iatrogenic physical, social, and emotional damage resulting from the overuse of drugs and technologies such as labor induction, oxytocin augmentation, electronic fetal monitoring, episiotomy, and cesarean section
- Disregard for the scientific evidence that does not support the routine use of such procedures
- Concomitant disregard for the scientific evidence that demonstrates better outcomes from humanistic, woman-centered, and physiologically effective birth techniques such as labor companionship and upright positions for birth
- Interference with the establishment of breastfeeding through the use of drugs during birth and by separating mother and baby after birth
- The technocratic and patriarchal ideology that assumes women's bodies are dysfunctional machines, and that birth is a problematic and risky process, justifying the overuse of technology in practitioners' minds

- Hospital rules and hierarchies that stifle creative thinking and acceptance of the scientific evidence supporting noninterventionist approaches
- Focus on status or economic gain for institutions and professionals rather than a focus on the mother and baby
- Educational models and programs that socialize professional birth practitioners—physicians, midwives, and obstetrical nurses—into a technocratic approach to birth and allegiances to each other rather than to the women in their care
- Provision of information to women regarding the benefits and harms of obstetrical procedures insufficient to enable them to make fully informed choices, and tacit or overt pressure on laboring women to accept the interventions that are standard in the technocratic approach
- Ignorance of and disrespect for the practices and knowledge systems of indigenous practitioners and the development of culturally insensitive, impractical, and ineffective training programs for traditional midwives
- Ineffective systems of home-to-hospital transport, and inadequate and often inhumane care upon arrival

The writers who have created the body of literature to substantiate these characteristics include ourselves: Robbie Davis-Floyd, a medical anthropologist specializing in the anthropology of reproduction, with special focus on the anthropology of childbirth, obstetrics, and mid-wifery (see www.davis-floyd.com); Lesley Barclay, an Australian midwife, researcher, and professor of health services development; Betty-Anne Daviss, a Canadian midwife, social scientist, and professor, who has carried out extensive epidemiologic research (see www.understandingbirthbetter.com); and Jan Tritten, an American midwife, author, and founder of Mid-wifery Today—a globally known organization that publishes a quarterly magazine by that name and organizes conferences in diverse countries to promote midwifery and normal birth (see www.midwiferytoday.com). As authors, we have published numerous works critiquing the biomedical dehu-manization of birth. In this book, we do not propose to add to the large and growing body of literature about what doesn't work in birth nor to recapitu-late here what has been said elsewhere by so many authors. Rather, we touch briefly on the discussion about negative effects of poor birth models—poor for women, babies, caregivers, and health care systems—in order to establish why it is so very important to seek and replicate birth models that do work.

Effects on Women's Birth Experiences of Models That Don't Work

The most critical concern in childbearing is that mothers in develop-ing countries do not get necessary assistance because their governments and/or ministries of health are dysfunctional, are not motivated to make changes, or do not have the funding to establish or maintain basic and high-risk obstetric care. Inappropriate perinatal and maternal mortality rates therefore occur in sub-Saharan Africa and Southeast Asian countries, but they also occur among the lower socioeconomic and African American/Hispanic sectors in the United States, and in Aboriginal populations of industrialized nations such as Canada and Australia. The eight Millennium Development Goals (MDGs) agreed on at the UN Millennium Summit of 2000 address some of these concerns. The World Health Organization (WHO), the International Federation of Gynecology and Obstetrics (FIGO), and the International Confederation of Midwives (ICM) have launched a campaign to reduce maternal mortality by increasing the number of skilled attendants around the world. Yet the consequences of redirecting funding to increase skills for institutionally trained personnel at the expense of community development and support of practitioners already on the ground have not been well understood and will be addressed in depth in Volume II, *Birth Models That Work: Struggling to Make Models Work.*

We offer the models in this volume as concrete solutions that address the more subtle requirements: skilled care incorporating the knowledge within communities along with respect for privacy and the right to a gentle birth. Besides the horror that every year about a half-million women die from maternity-related conditions that are treatable because they cannot get to facilities or obtain appropriate help, many other women are faced with another dilemma. Thousands of women who do have access to professional care in an institutional setting find themselves bewildered and unsure as to why they feel abnormal because they are fearful and doubtful about the treatment they are receiving. Regardless of whether the setting is impoverished or well equipped, laboring women are not moving around freely, eating to sate their hunger, and drinking to quench their thirst (which they would be doing if their care were evidence-based). Women whose individual needs should be respected, who should be supported to trust the rhythms of labor and to birth their babies through their own power, are lying alone on hospital or clinic beds. Many are confined in this position by the intravenous oxytocics (synthetic forms of oxytocin that interfere with the mother's own production of this essential birth hormone) drip or the electronic fetal monitor belt strapped around their bellies. The baby inside needs the mother to move, change position so that it can receive more blood and oxygen as the contractions squeeze and it works to help itself be born. But its mother lies still because that's what she is told or expected to do, and because were she to rise, there would be no place for her to go. The contractions hurt much more than they should because the synthetic oxytocin, often routinely given even in the poorest clinics, makes the contractions stronger and longer than they need to be, and it's hard for her to cope because she is hungry.

> Once they put me on the pitocin, it was all over for me. The pain was unbearable. I couldn't wait to have a cesarean—at least it would get me out of that misery. (Lisa Smith, quoted in Davis-Floyd 2004: 98)

> I went into labor just after dawn. I called my OB, and he said not to eat, so I skipped breakfast and went on in to the hospital. By that evening, when things were getting really intense, I was so weak from hunger I thought I would die . . . it wasn't till I had the epidural that I started to feel like I could make it. (Charla Lovett, quoted in Davis-Floyd 2004: 91)

If the woman is in a high-resource hospital, she will probably have an epidural so she won't feel the pain of those stronger contractions; she may or may not have a supportive companion to help her feel emotionally secure. If she is in a poor hospital or clinic with no pain-relieving drugs available and no companions allowed, she will writhe in agony when she could be in the arms of someone who would hold her and support her as she cries out her pain. Either way, she will be subject to myriad interventions in her birth process, from IVs to episiotomies, that science has shown to be unnecessary in the vast majority of cases, and often harmful (see *Advancing Normal Birth* 2007). This model doesn't work—it doesn't provide optimal care for either mothers or babies; rather, it makes birth much more difficult, creating problems with technology that then have to be fixed with more technology—a phenomenon that Davis-Floyd (1994) has labeled the One-Two Punch of technocratic birth.

Effects on Women in Low-Resource Countries of Models That Don't Work

In China one of us (Lesley) is undertaking fieldwork in a remote region with an ethnic minority population where around 80% of women give birth at home with traditional midwives, despite well-equipped and staffed Western-style clinics and small hospitals close by. These hospitals are run by the government, which has subsidized costs to try to make hospital birth more attractive because maternal death rates are high. Lesley's research is investigating why women reject these well-meant but often culturally insensitive attempts to improve safety. Clues are provided in multiple anthropological ethnographies, which describe indigenous women in India, Mexico, Tanzania, Haiti, Bangladesh, Thailand, Papua New Guinea, the Congo, and elsewhere saying the same thing about the care they receive in biomedical facilities: "They expose you, they shave you, they cut you, they stick needles in you, they give you nothing to eat or drink, they leave you alone and don't come when you call, they won't allow your relatives to be with you, and when you complain, they yell at you and slap you." Here is a highly representative description from a woman who gave birth in the hospital near her small village in India:

> Before entering the hospital we have first to decide how much money we have to give. We are not admitted unless we first give them money. When the woman enters into the hospital, the doctor behaves rudely with her. Sometimes nurses beat her. They do not let close and affectionate relatives, who came from home with us, stand at our side. They themselves either do not stay near us. We wish that somebody hold us by the waist when pains come, but they do not do it. We have not even to moan, lest they talk sarcastically, make fun of us, which is very hurting, still we have to bear. If we moan too much, they may sometimes slap us. If we happen to say something, they retort by asking us whether they had invited us to come. "Why have you come then? You may go back home!" In hospital we have to lie down on the bed to get delivered. In the hospital they excise the vaginal wall with a blade for enlarging it. The body gets damaged unnecessarily. After delivery we feel terribly hungry, but we consider ourselves lucky if we get a cup of tea. (Quoted in Kolenda 1998: 12)

This woman's experience is echoed in the following description of a hospital birth in rural Papua New Guinea observed by Julia Byford, an Australian nurse-midwife who has become an anthropologist:

> Mispa, a young woman of twenty, was admitted to the hospital this morning. She is seen by the Health Examination Officer, who does a vaginal exam and tells me that she is four to five centimetres dilated . . . and that she may commence a Syntocinon infusion. . . . The labor room is small and the air conditioning unit mounted high on the wall belches cold air at us. When it is on the room gets very cold; when it is off the room gets hot and stuffy. There is a sink but no plumbing to allow it to be operational. There is no water at the hospital today anyway. . . . Mispa asks to sit on the floor and is given permission to do this, but as her labour progresses the nurse says she must stay on the bed so the staff can do their observations. She acquiesces and does not ask for anything else. Most of the time she is left alone. She has not eaten all day and only drunk a small amount of water. Her lips are dry and swollen. The staff do numerous vaginal examinations but none of them are recorded [so when a shift changes, another exam is performed].
>
> During the second stage of labour, every time Mispa has a contraction, the Health Examination Officer inserts a few fingers into Mispa's vagina between the perineum and the baby's head in order to stretch the perineum. Mispa finds this excruciating and tightens her grip on my arm. . . . [After the birth] I am dismayed although not surprised to see that the baby is flat and pale and requires resuscitation. The HEO delivers the placenta by placing one hand on Mispa's abdomen and pulling on the umbilical cord with the other hand. . . . As soon as the placenta is out, Mispa has a large postpartum hemorrhage. The HEO asks me to increase the intravenous infusion rate and then inserts her hand high up into Mispa's vagina and manually removes some retained placental pieces. This is done without explanation or anesthetic. . . .

> Perhaps the hardest thing for me to come to terms with is the lack of care offered to Mispa simply on a human level. She was never consulted, only told what to do and what not to do. . . . No one tended to her basic needs for food or fluids or inquired if she needed to go to the toilet. It was as if Mispa, the embodied person, did not exist. (Byford 1999: 186–90)

Mispa had walked for two days to birth in this rural hospital because nursing aides had insisted to her and others in her village that hospital birth is a safer option than their traditional custom of birthing at home. Kaosar Afsana (2003), a physician studying birth in a low-resource hospital in Bangladesh, describes the frequent reuse of unsterilized needles and gloves, the filthy, overflowing toilets laboring women were expected to use, and the repeated verbal and physical abuse of laboring women. We cannot stress strongly enough that these are not isolated but typical examples, of which we could cite many more (see Chapter 12), which illustrate the dysfunctionality of importing Western biomedical models into developing countries without adequate resources to provide even a semblance of humanized practice.

Women like Mispa do resist. The options of birthing at home or in a freestanding birth center with a traditional or professional midwife are often not available, but when they are, their use is usually a considered decision that women make after weighing the risks and benefits of staying away from the hospital. Anthropologist Soheir Morsy noted: "In villages of the Nile Delta, although modern medical facilities are available, women prefer to deliver at home with the assistance of a local midwife. This choice is not a result of reified 'cultural attitudes' but a measured judgment about the inadequate health care extended to peasants and the urban poor in modern health care settings" (1995: 168).

Anthropologist Denise Roth Allen has described this process of "measured judgment" in detail in *Bodily Risks, Spiritual Risks: Contrasting Discourses on Pregnancy in a Rural Tanzanian Community*. Safe Motherhood policy planners on high decided that each Tanzanian mother should have and be in charge of a card documenting the prenatal care she had received, and her health and pregnancy condition. To make sure each mother carried a card, it was decided that mothers would have to show their cards in order to be admitted into the local clinic for labor and birth. In the city and small town Allen studied, this confronted each pregnant woman with a difficult decision: should she obtain prenatal care, which was costly, time consuming, and often uncaring and inadequate, in case she needed to go to the clinic during labor? Or should she cast her lot with the traditional midwife, who was inexpensive and kind but would be unable to take her to the clinic without the card? Not surprisingly, many women, after careful reflection, chose the latter option; of course, if they then had problems during labor but could not go to the clinic, the traditional midwife would be blamed for the outcome. That approach doesn't work.

Effects on Women in High-Resource Countries of Models That Don't Work

High degrees of dehumanization are now relatively uncommon in high-resource hospitals, where humanism in birth in the form of a respectful, caring attitude has made great inroads in recent decades. Women are generally respectfully treated and have the option of giving birth awake and aware, pain free because of the epidural. In the United States, the 2006 *Listening to Mothers* Harris poll–style survey of 1,600 women conducted by Childbirth Connection showed that although the vast majority of these women experienced high levels of technological intervention, 96% of them also received high levels of emotional or physical support from partners, friends, or caregivers (Declerq et al. 2006), and expressed general satisfaction with their birth experiences. Even so, most of them were not permitted to keep their babies with them during the first hour after birth; although the majority expressed a wish to breastfeed long term, only 51% were still doing so after the first week—a phenomenon that has been shown to be related to the negative impact of birth interventions on breastfeeding success (Kroeger and Smith 2004). Most respondents did not feel that they had enough information to make truly informed decisions about childbirth options, especially the option of natural birth. Since unmedicated, nontechnological birth is increasingly rare in the United States—less than 2% of survey respondents gave birth in this way—most American women have no basis for comparison. In New Zealand, as soon as midwives were widely available, women left their obstetricians and migrated en masse to midwives as their primary care providers (see Chapter 3). In Australia, services that offer natural, midwife-supported birth have long waiting lists and are difficult to access, as is the case in many other Western countries.

The Iatrogenic Cost of Overintervention

The iatrogenic cost to women of technologically controlled birth, even when they choose it, is extremely high. Here we provide a brief summary for readers who might not be familiar with that literature. As we noted above, the primary weaknesses of medical models that don't work is not only mortality but *morbidity*—unnecessary injury to mother or child. Lack of ability to eat or drink at will resulting from hospital policy can lead to weakness from hunger that complicates labor and birth. Overperformance of vaginal exams can lead to infection. Pitocin induction can lead to dysfunctional labor and premature birth, and pitocin augmentation shuts down a mother's own oxytocin production and interferes with her ability to breastfeed. Epidurals can go awry, resulting in intractable headache from puncture of the dura, which can cause spinal fluid to leak afterward. Epidural-induced fevers are indistinguishable from those caused by infection, so a baby whose mother has such a fever will be sent to the neonatal intensive care unit (NICU) "just in case." Epidurals also increase the length of the first and second stages of labor, and they lead to increased use of forceps and vacuum extraction and possibly cesarean section (Klein 2006; Klein et al. 2001).

The increased prophylactic use of antibiotics intrapartum over the last decade and a half is increasing resistant strains of bacteria, as demonstrated in a study showing that infants who contract late-onset strep B infection are more likely to have been exposed to intrapartum antibiotics than noninfected control infants, and their infections were resistant to ampicillin (Glasgow et al. 2005).

WHO's 1985 statement that "there is no justification for any region to have caesarean section (CS) rates higher than 10–15%," has been largely ignored, as evidenced by the increasing cesarean rates around the globe. In 2007 a group of WHO researchers and affiliates made the first attempt to provide a global and regional comparative analysis of national rates of cesarean delivery and their ecologic correlation with other indicators of reproductive health (Betrán et al. 2007). They undertook the task of studying what became evident as the underuse of cesareans in low-resource countries and cesarean overuse in high-resource countries, correlating cesarean rates with maternal, infant, and neonatal mortality. Although very unevenly distributed, 15% of births worldwide were found to occur by CS. Latin America and the Caribbean showed the highest rate (29.2%), and Africa the lowest (3.5%). In developed countries, the average proportion of cesarean births was found to be 21.1%, whereas in least-developed countries, only 2% of deliveries were by CS. Although higher CS rates up to 15% were unambiguously correlated with lower maternal mortality, it was also found to be true that *above this range*, higher CS rates were predominantly correlated with higher maternal mortality. A similar pattern was found for infant and neonatal mortality. The stratified analysis therefore supports the suggestion that "when CS rates rise substantially above 15%, risks to reproductive health outcomes may begin to outweigh benefits" Betrán et al. 2007: 110. (In order to conclusively evaluate the relationship between reproductive mortality and high CS rates, the study authors caution that developed countries will need to reinforce their monitoring strategies, and more detailed individual-level analyses will need to be performed. See also Potter et al. 2001; Villar et al. 2006, 2007.)

Because of the focus on the event of the birth and on perinatal and maternal mortality outcomes, and because both practitioners and women are increasingly familiar with the benefits of cesarean, ignoring the risk, there is a tendency to minimize the negative, long-term consequences of cesareans. These include infection; chronic pain; difficulty with bonding and breastfeeding; maternal and neonatal injury and death; newborn respiratory problems; and problems during future pregnancies, including higher risk of uterine rupture, ectopic pregnancy, preterm delivery, placenta previa, placenta accreta, placental abruption that may necessitate a hysterectomy, and increased incidence of postnatal depression. The cesarean epidemic is transforming the nature of childbirth worldwide, with implications we cannot begin to address here. For us, it serves as a stunning indication of the level at which the biomedical models of birth now dominant in most countries do not work in terms of either morbidity *or* mortality.

One of the most recent and convincing examples of some consequences of overuse of cesarean is a study conducted under the auspices of WHO in Latin America. Jose Villar and colleagues (2006, 2007) analyzed 91% of over 100,000 births from 120 randomly selected Latin American hospitals. The most common rate of cesarean birth was 33%, with much higher rates in private hospitals (many Latin American private hospitals have cesarean rates of 70%–90%) and tertiary care centers, and with first births and women with previous cesareans. An increase in the rate of cesarean delivery was associated with a significantly higher risk for severe maternal morbidity, mortality, and postnatal treatment with antibiotics. These findings also applied to perinatal outcomes: the rate of cesarean delivery was positively associated with an increase in the rates of fetal death, and with the number of infants admitted to the neonatal intensive care unit for seven days and more; it was borderline significant for neonatal death after adjusting for preterm delivery. In most places, risks of preterm delivery and maternal and neonatal death rise when cesarean delivery rates rise beyond 15%. (Preterm delivery is a frequent result of scheduled cesareans.) The overuse of this operation designed to save lives is now costing them.

The long-held myth that Latin American women want cesareans was exploded by Potter et al. (2001), who showed that the majority of Brazilian women who receive cesareans did not in fact want them—in other words, the cesarean epidemic in Latin America is physician driven. In the United States, where cesarean rates have now reached 31%, physicians insist that women are demanding scheduled cesareans, while in fact there is little evidence of maternal request for cesareans and some evidence of physician pressure to have them (Declerq et al. 2006); meanwhile, recent research from Canada is demonstrating excess morbidity from elective cesareans (Liu et al. 2007). This doesn't work.

Effects on Out-of-Hospital Practitioners of Birth Models That Don't Work

In countries like India, where home deliveries have been the norm for centuries, suddenly the policy makers and planners are pushing for institutional deliveries in the Reproductive and Child Health program for the country. Till recently, the Government of India used to conduct training programs supported by WHO for

Traditional Birth Attendants (TBAs) in the art of delivery and care of the newborn at birth. In India, where 25 *million births are taking place every year, out of which about 66% are occurring at home, it is a herculean task to arrange logistics for institutional deliveries of all the babies.*

J.P. DADHICH, neonatologist, member Executive Committee of the National Neonatology Forum of India, Internet communication 2005

Primary keys to safe home birth include effective systems of consultation during pregnancy and the postpartum period, transport to the hospital in cases of need, and effective care on arrival. In rural areas, these often do not exist because there is no transport or communication, or because doctors and hospitals are too far away. When they do exist, their effectiveness is hampered because in many countries biomedicine and home birth (traditional and professional) midwifery exist in separate cultural domains and are based on distinctively different knowledge systems. When a midwife transports a client to the hospital, she brings specific prior knowledge that can be vital to the mother's successful treatment by the hospital system. But the culture of biomedicine in general tends not to understand or recognize as valid the knowledge of midwifery, most especially traditional midwifery, so that midwives often encounter trouble when they transport. Birth models that don't work refuse to take the report of the transporting midwife into serious account, exclude her from staying with the mother, punish the mother either subtly or overtly for having attempted a home birth, and code any bad result of a transport as a "botched home birth" even when the problem that arose was exactly why the midwife transported and regardless of whether she gave good care. Davis-Floyd (2003) describes such experiences as "fractured articulations" between the biomedical and midwifery systems. One effect of such fractured articulations is that both professional and traditional midwives may stay at home with the mother for longer than they should, trying to spare the mother and themselves the harassment they are likely to receive in the hospital. For obvious reasons, that doesn't work.

For professional, out-of-hospital midwives, the greatest effect of birth models that don't work is disrespectful treatment by the medical system; for traditional midwives, it is their demise. In many countries where traditional midwives attended the majority of births a few decades ago, including most Latin American countries, they have been or are being officially phased out and thus are increasingly difficult to find. Ironically, in countries such as Honduras, El Salvador, Nicaragua, the Dominican Republic, and Costa Rica, traditional midwives are forbidden to attend births except in case of emergency—in other words, they can't attend planned home births but can attend women in trouble who can't get to the hospital in time. Thus, they are being de-skilled from lack of experience even while women are still relying on their skills. The skilled attendant clause, created in good faith by the combined forces of the UN Population Fund (UNFPA), ICM, and FIGO, mandating that every woman in the world have access to a "skilled attendant," categorically excludes traditional midwives. The consequence, although thought to be progressive, removes the community traditions on which any good maternity system should be based in the very areas where maternal mortality is high.

In 2005 Betty-Anne took a group of Guatemalan obstetricians into a little town in the Dominican Republic to meet one of the last traditional midwives left there after a major campaign about fifteen years before had moved all births into the hospital. The campaign backfired: in spite of the fact that 97% of births now take place in hospitals, the maternal mortality figures remain high at 110–229 deaths/100,000 births (Miller et al. 2002). Living an hour from a hospital, and afraid of the police coming after her, the traditional midwife they met says she has a new maneuver called *piedra contra la cabeza* (stone against the head). She holds the stone against the head of the baby, hoping it will not come before they reach the hospital, because traditional midwives are not supposed to attend births at all anymore. Similar strategies were reported to Lesley by traditional midwives working in American Samoa; traditional midwives from Nicaragua and Honduras, also prohibited from attending planned home births, described to Robbie and Jan how they often are called to come running because a woman from a rural village, denied access by law to the traditional midwives of her region and trying to reach the hospital, is giving birth in a field or by the side of the road.

The Canadian Association of Midwives, in the face of the joint statement on the "skilled attendant" that prompted removal of funding for traditional midwives, is proposing that the International Confederation of Midwives acknowledge the role that many traditional midwives/traditional birth attendants play in the care of women in certain communities, and support them in gaining the necessary skills and having access to the resources required to provide safe care for childbearing women in their communities.

Often, assumptions about what "people at the top" will and will not support are ill founded. For example, when Betty-Anne worked as the project manager for FIGO's Safe Motherhood Program (2004–5), she noticed that many obstetric societies submitting proposals assumed that the FIGO committee equated the "skilled attendant" with institutional birth. In fact, the FIGO committee was supportive of creative projects that could create safe care in multiple settings, and projects not taking cultural sensitivities into account or categorically expressing zero tolerance for home births were less likely to be accepted. For another example, the Royal College of Midwives (RCM) and the Royal College of Obstetricians and Gynaecologists (RCOG) in the United Kingdom support home birth for women with uncomplicated pregnancies, stating, "There is no reason why home birth should not be offered to women at low risk of complications and it may confer considerable benefits for them and their families" (Royal College of Obstetricians and Gynaecologists and Royal College of Midwives 2007). Some obstetric societies, however, maintain biomedical patterns of power and control, as indicated by the October 2006 statement of the American College of Obstetrics and Gynecology (ACOG) opposing home birth, even after the publication of the largest prospective study on home birth demonstrating its safety (Johnson and Daviss 2005). Such unqualified statements in the face of sound research demonstrate professional territoriality rather than concern for needs, interests, and safety of mothers and babies.

Effects on Hospital Practitioners of Models That Don't Work

A distressing cross-cultural trend is showing up in the growing body of literature about midwifery and birth in the developing world. From Tanzania to Papua New Guinea, anthropologists and others observing professional midwives giving prenatal care and attending births in hospitals or government clinics increasingly note that, far from the midwifery ideal, professional midwives sometimes treat women very badly during birth, ignoring their needs and requests, talking to them disrespectfully, ordering them around, and sometimes even yelling at them and slapping them. For example, Afsana (2003: 119) describes routinely brutal treatment of the laboring women in the hospital she studied in Bangladesh, including insults and spanking: "Prostitute (whore), open up your legs! . . . If you scream one more time, I will hit you again." At the same time, and in direct correlation, the professional midwives are themselves often treated badly by the health care systems in which they work. They are almost always underpaid; are frequently mistreated by physicians, who rank above them in the medical hierarchy; and generally work long hours under stressful conditions that often include inadequate facilities and equipment, and too many women with too few midwives to care for them well. So they take out their own stress and frustration on their patients.

Lesley is frequently asked to advise on educational systems for midwives and nurses in a range of Asian and Pacific countries. Educational systems and opportunities are frequently much poorer for midwives than for nurses and doctors, and their employers rarely take notice of midwives' opinions or needs. The educational programs are very Western in nature; few incorporate studies of traditional birth systems and practices, and if these are mentioned at all, it is mostly in pejorative ways. (Samoa, described in Chapter 4, is an important exception.) In most countries (exceptions include Indonesia, the Netherlands, the United Kingdom, New Zealand, and the countries of Scandinavia), the professional associations representing midwives are not powerful or well positioned with the government, resulting in nonexistent or ineffective systems of advocacy that could improve the conditions under which midwives work. In short, professional, hospital-based midwives are often trapped in the biomedical health care system, a system that is failing to meet the needs of birthing women in both developed and developing countries. As Irish midwife Paula Barry has said (personal communication, 2007),

> I am a midwife currently employed in a busy Irish hospital with over 8,000 births per year. I love midwifery and think women are only fantastic! But unfortunately, like many others, this hospital is medically led with a high rate of cesarean and instrumental deliveries. It makes me so sad to see many normal, low-risk women become high-risk with the unnecessary interventions such as CTG monitors, artificial rupture of membranes, IV infusions, Syntocinon induction, and epidural analgesia (just to mention a few!!). I am delighted when a friend/family member takes my advice and opts for a more normal birth. As a midwife there is nothing more special than to see a woman birth her baby all by herself in a quiet, dim room, with only the midwife and her birthing partner supporting and encouraging her. The flow of love and hormones affects all involved, not just the new mother.

Birth models that don't work are often dysfunctional, hierarchical systems in which the advice or knowledge of those lower down is ignored by those higher up, and those lower down—usually nurses and midwives—have to play manipulative games to help the women they care for or simply to keep from losing their jobs. In order not to "rock the boat," they often give care that they know to be inappropriate because that kind of care is "standard practice" in their hospital. That doesn't work: it makes these practitioners miserable until they become desensitized, and the vicious cycle of unnecessary intervention in birth continues, to the detriment of mothers and babies. Obstetricians often also find it difficult to act as advocates for normal, noninterventionist birth, as such actions often result in sanctions against them, from subtle ostracism to overt punishment.

We repeat: the vast majority of women giving birth in hospitals in both the developed and developing worlds are subjected to many unnecessary interventions that make their births at best more complicated than necessary, and at worst downright dangerous.

In addition, the system or individual is faced with ever accelerating and unsustainable costs directly linked to the cascade of interventions now considered acceptable or necessary for birth (Tracy and Tracy 2003). This situation has opened the way for private medical systems and practitioners to charge higher fees, with each intervention producing additional costs for the hospital and sometimes fees for the women. The pervasiveness of the technocratic model of birth with its supervaluation of technological intervention (Davis-Floyd 2004) provides the rationale for practitioners to apply these unnecessary interventions, believing that they are providing appropriate treatment designed to contain risk and preserve life. Many hospital practitioners rarely see a normal birth and have no training in or understanding of how to practice in ways that keep birth normal. The rarity of normal birth in the United States, for example, is indicated in a profound scene in *The Business of Being Born*, a 2007 documentary film produced by actress Ricki Lake and her associate Abby Epstein. In this scene, Ricki asks a group of white-coated obstetrical residents, "Do you ever see normal birth?" Uneasily shifting their heads and glancing down and sideways at each other, they collectively respond, "Um no, not really—*normal* birth? Um, no, we don't." It is no wonder that "much of the research that purports to be about normal birth is in fact about highly managed obstetric deliveries" (Beech and Phipps 2008: 68)—of course, because this research is conducted in hospitals where birth could theoretically be called "normal" only because it is normal to give birth in hospital and it is normal in hospitals to intervene.

Such practitioners are generally well-intentioned—their training leads them to believe that the interventions they perform are essential to produce a healthy baby (Davis-Floyd 1987: 2004). They are not inhumane— they are simply practicing what their system has created. As a result, many women never experience a normal birth and have no context for understanding or critiquing their biomedical treatment. This global context of technocratic birth ideology makes it enormously difficult to create and sustain birth models that work, as these models go completely against the technocultural grain.

Effects on Health Care System Resources of Birth Models That Don't Work

Birth models that don't work waste enormous amounts of money and resources, including human power, on unnecessary interventions. The cost to the economies of developed countries of technologically controlled birth is enormous; in the United States, for example, maternity care is one of the highest-budget items in the health care system (Perkins 2004), yet birth outcomes in America are not nearly as good as those of the Netherlands, where the cost of maternity care is far lower (see Chapter 1). Anderson and Anderson (1999) demonstrated that the average uncomplicated vaginal birth in the United States cost 68% less in the home than in the hospital. This reduction in fees results from the elimination of hospital fees and the significant reduction in medical intervention (including cesarean section) as shown in the largest home birth study done in the United States (Johnson and Daviss 2005). The Andersons concluded that if all low-risk women in the United States began labor with the intention of giving birth at home with a midwife, there would be an average saving of $3,600 dollars per birth, which would save the United States and private insurers $14 billion per year.

These ever-higher costs were also exposed in Australia by Sally and Mark Tracy. They developed a simple costing formula based on population data that shows the cumulative impact on costs of each intervention. The relative cost of birth increased by up to 50% for women about to become mothers for the first time and up to 36% for low-risk, multiparous women as labor interventions increased. They showed that the initiation of the cascade of interventions for low-risk women is costly to the health system and insurers in Western countries. Using data that had been published previously analyzing over 170,000 births in New South Wales, Australia, they discovered much higher rates of intervention in private hospital births for low-risk, insured women who used private obstetricians than in government-run hospitals with salaried midwives and medical staff (Roberts, Tracy, and Peat 2000).

Increasingly, technocratic birth creates opportunities for economic exploitation of women, escalating costs for hospitals that need to be recouped and creating charges for women that can lead to poverty or avoidance of hospital treatment. In China, for example, we are seeing high cesarean birth rates and multiple ultrasounds at township and county levels, and medical bills are now a major cause of poverty (Liu, Rao, and Hsaio 2003).

All of these negative effects on women, practitioners, and health care systems of birth models that don't work—the vast majority of operating birth models around the world—serve to highlight the necessity for this volume: a book that calls attention to birth models that *do* work. The following pages will present models of both education and practice. The importance of both, and their interlinkages, is emphasized because the type of education practitioners receive strongly influences their practice ideology and style.

BIRTH MODELS THAT WORK: A BRIEF SYNOPSIS OF THE CHAPTERS IN THIS BOOK

How does one define a birth model that works? What are its characteristics? Excellent outcomes are an obvious first answer—excellent not only in terms of low mortality but also of low morbidity, including psychosocial morbidity. *First and foremost, models that work do not cause unnecessary harm to mothers and babies.* We will list other key characteristics in the sections below. Here, we briefly delineate the models presented in this book so that we can draw on them for specific examples when we describe their general characteristics later on.

Each chapter presents a case study of one model that works and describes the impetus for this model's development, the process through which it was developed, its underlying philosophy, and its specific characteristics. How the particular model works is illustrated by examples and stories to make the book accessible to practitioners and policy makers from a wide range of settings and cultures. Some chapter authors are practitioners who have actually developed the model the chapter describes; others are social scientists or midwives who have studied the model; some are both. The settings for the practice models we have chosen to present include hospitals, freestanding birth centers, clinics, midwifery birth services, homes, and in some cases, entire national systems. The education supporting these models is based in universities, vocational programs, and out-of-hospital apprenticeship systems. The models described span the developed and developing worlds, including the Netherlands, the United Kingdom, the United States, Canada, Japan, New Zealand, Australia, Samoa, the Philippines, Mexico, and Brazil. They show how brave and wise pioneers around the world are combining and synthesizing the best knowledge and skills from obstetrics, midwifery, scientific research, and indigenous knowledge systems under a compassionate ideology of care to create exemplary and optimal models of education and practice. We call attention to these successes and urge their replication.

Part One. Large-Scale Systems: National and Regional Models

The Dutch system is known worldwide for its excellent outcomes, low rates of intervention, and high rates of home birth. Deeply rooted in Dutch culture, this obstetrical system is also fully evidence based. In Chapter 1, three sociologists—Raymond DeVries, Therese Wiegers, and Edwin van Teijlingen—team up with Dutch midwife Beatrijs Smulders to describe both the features of the Dutch model unique to the Netherlands and its transportability to other countries. In New Zealand, midwifery came close to disappearing but underwent a full renaissance during the 1990s. A new breed of professional midwives lobbied the government for support, and designed a model and education that works and that is fully incorporated into the national health care system, as is the Dutch model. In Chapter 2, health consultant, midwife, and midwifery educator Chris Hendry describes the mechanisms by which this renaissance was achieved, and the features and characteristics of the New Zealand system, most of which are replicable in developed and many developing countries.

When midwifery was legalized in 1994 in the province of Ontario, midwives benefited from knowledge of midwifery models that were working well (and not working well) in other nations. Thus, the model of midwifery in Ontario today is a product both of local, social, and historical specificity and of transnational networks and knowledge exchange. In Chapter 3, social scientists Margaret MacDonald and Ivy Bourgeault describe the unique structural aspects of Ontario midwifery, which include direct-entry education (standardized academic qualifications combined with learning in an apprenticeship model); autonomous professional status, whereby midwives are primary caregivers with hospital privileges. allowing them to attend women at home or in hospital and to consult with a network of other professionals; a model of clinical care that emphasizes continuity of care, choice of birth place, and informed choice; and public funding that ensures access to all women experiencing normal pregnancy and birth.

In Chapter 4, Lesley Barclay challenges the assumptions, still held in many postcolonial countries, that the migration of Western-style birthing is necessarily a desirable goal. The system of maternity care left behind in the Pacific Rim as New Zealanders, Australians, French, or British moved out leaves much to be desired. The chapter demonstrates how a group of leaders in Samoa has made considerable progress in both reconceptualizing and developing a "postcolonial model" of maternity care. This model integrates social systems and traditional practitioners with professional nurse-midwives in a system of health service delivery that appears to be unique, yet could be replicated in many countries in which traditional and professional practitioners must interact.

Part Two. Local Models in Developed Nations: Hospitals and Birth Centers

In 1993 the British government undertook a careful study of the scientific evidence in favor of out-of-hospital, midwife-attended births and began a national program to support birth's return to the community. To date, this program has resulted in doubling the home birth rate, but it remains at only 2%, in large part because women have been socialized to hospital birth and no longer trust the safety of birth at home. In the early 1990s, the midwives at the Albany Midwifery Practice in the United Kingdom set out to change this situation in their community. By providing excellent care, telling women stories of successful home births they had attended, and helping women gain a sense of trust in their own bodies and their ability to give birth, these midwives have raised the home birth rate in their practice to 48%, with outstanding outcomes for both the home and the hospital births they attend. This is a remarkable achievement, given that the center is in a particularly highly multicultural, low-socioeconomic area, where in other high-resource nations, women in this status often avoid home birth because of stereotypical assumptions about its inferiority to modernity. In Chapter 5, Albany midwives Becky Reed and Cathy Walton recount the development of this practice, its structure and characteristics, and the reasons for its success, stressing its replicability in other developed nations and suggesting concrete ways in which this can be achieved. In Chapter 6, Denis Walsh contrasts conventional U.K. hospital birth with midwifery practice at the Lichfield Maternity Unit, a freestanding birth center that has been in existence since 1993, describing its transformation from a hierarchical to a social model of care based on relationship and a nurturing, physiological approach to birth—a true "birthing community."

A similar transformation occurred at St George Hospital in Sydney, Australia, where the authors of Chapter 7, Pat Brodie and Caroline Homer, helped lead a switch from a traditional, medically dominated culture to one that is flexible, woman centered, and embracing of innovative models of continuity in midwifery care—a process that took the best part of ten years and continues today. Strong, effective leadership from midwives and obstetricians, supported by research, enabled an organizational culture that was forward thinking and inclusive of changes in line with consumer needs, government recommendations, and evidence. The various in-hospital and community-based models of continuous midwifery care developed at St George have influenced policy and practice in Australia, and have become a blueprint for a state-wide maternity service policy and planning for the future. Clinicians and leaders from the hospital are frequently asked to advise and consult for other organizations that are implementing models of continuity of midwifery care.

For decades before World War II, Japanese women gave birth at home, attended by autonomous, professional midwives, who graduated from government-sanctioned midwifery schools. With the American takeover after the war, these independent midwives were largely replaced by nurse-midwives working in hospitals. But a few of them kept right on attending births, opening "maternity homes" in their own houses, where they attended to the reproductive needs of the women of their communities. Today, numbers of younger midwives, disillusioned with the highly interventionist approach to birth in hospitals, are flocking to the birth homes to learn from the few elderly midwives still in practice, and then opening birth homes of their own. These maternity homes of Japan, described by anthropologists Etsuko Matsuoka and midwifery professor Fumiko Hinokuma in Chapter 8, are internationally renowned for their excellent outcomes and outstanding care.

The 20th century saw a tremendous decline in home birth in the United States. Yet now, as in the maternity homes of Japan, the home birth practices of U.S. midwives are internationally recognized as examples of "true" or "real" midwifery (see the Conclusion for a description of the "midwifery model of care"). In Chapter 9, midwife Elizabeth Gilmore describes learning to practice home birth midwifery during the dawn of the American home birth movement in the 1970s, then going on to

open a home- and birth-center birth practice, the Northern New Mexico
Women's Health and Birth Center, an academic program, and finally a
formal midwifery school that teaches the principles and techniques of
out-of-hospital midwifery practice in full integration with the local Taos
community.

*Part Three. Local Models in Developing Nations: Traditional
Midwives, Professional Midwives, and Obstetricians Working Together*

Since 1997, Ricardo Herbert Jones, an obstetrician, gynecologist, and
homeopath, has worked to develop a system of care that brings the
technical work of the obstetrician together with the feminine, holistic
orientation of a nurse-midwife and a doula in the far south of Brazil.
These practitioners offer what they consider to be "the best care":
respecting women's wishes and desires, with full awareness of the most
current scientific evidence, and providing complete continuity of care in
any setting. This simple, three-person model, described in Chapter 10,
has resulted in extremely low intervention rates and highly successful
outcomes.

Founded by American Nadine Goodman, the CASA Hospital provides
full-service care, including maternity care, to the poor of the area in
and around San Miguel, Guanajuato, Mexico. In the late 1990s, Nadine
founded the CASA School for Professional Midwives. In Chapter 11,
anthropologists Lisa Mills and Robbie Davis-Floyd describe the models of
education and practice developed at CASA, a unique feature of which is
the inclusion of a series of apprenticeships with rural Mexican traditional
midwives that foster respect for the traditional midwives and an understanding of the benefits and limitations of their practices. The students
bring this knowledge back into the hospital and to home births they attend
after graduation. This professional midwifery program is the only one of its
kind in Mexico, perhaps in the Americas, and stands as a model that could
work in any developing country.

Chapter 12 describes the creation by a Christian midwife and her family
of a model of birth centers and training programs in the Philippines that
dispel the myth that doctor-attended hospital births would be safer than
midwife-attended births in an out-of-hospital setting for high-risk women
living in poverty. Vicki Penwell's formula for success: avoid interventions
in the normal physiological and social process of birth, be prepared to perform advanced emergency life-saving skills in the event of an emergency,
and be "nice." The beauty of this story is that it takes place in one of the
first countries in the world to be targeted by the World Trade Organization as an experiment in privatization of the health care system—which has
failed miserably to create better health care. This chapter demonstrates

how grassroots work in reforming birth practices can succeed in the midst of and in spite of turmoil around it.

Part Four. Making Models Work

The three chapters in this final section illustrate three efforts in progress to create models that work—the CenteringPregnancy® Group Prenatal Care Model, an outstanding and growing model for prenatal care; a focused effort by the Brazilian Ministry of Health to humanize hospital birth; and a more diffuse social and individual effort by American midwives to develop and practice a midwifery model of care in the face of a partially humanized but still highly technocratic obstetrical system.

The CenteringPregnancy® Group Prenatal Care Model, described in Chapter 13, can be applied anywhere in almost any kind of setting. This model involves collective prenatal care within a group of eight to twelve pregnant women, who meet together with their care provider(s) for extended periods of time that allow them to share questions and answers with each other in a much richer way than short, individual prenatal visits could allow. Centering groups help women gain confidence and agency in managing their own pregnancies, for example, by measuring their own weight and blood pressure. The sense of community and intimacy grows over time and often persists beyond the pregnancy, supporting the mothers after their babies are born.

Brazil has long been cited as an exemplar of extremely high cesarean rates, even though several other Latin American countries have now reached the high rates of Brazil. In Chapter 14, Ministry of Health officials Daphne Rattner, Isa Paula Hamouche Abreu, Maria José de Oliveira Araújo, and Adson Roberto França Santos describe how they have taken on the challenge of humanizing care in order to reduce maternal and neonatal mortality through a national initiative, begun in 2004, involving a series of seminars for hospital staff in every state in the country. These seminars teach evidence-based methods of humanizing birth and improving outcomes, from encouraging women to bring supportive companions to minimizing interventions and facilitating upright positions for birth. (The seminar content is fully described in the chapter.) The initiative includes an evidence-based and culturally appropriate training program for the indigenous midwives of the Amazon region. The data are not yet in on its effects, but there are strong indications that many hospitals and practitioners have altered their practices in favor of humanistic, evidence-based care.

Finally, in Chapter 15, "'Orchestrating Normal': The Conduct of Midwifery in the United States," Holly Powell Kennedy (a nurse-midwife, professor, and researcher) describes the struggles of American midwives as they try to practice the midwifery model of care in the American hospital—walking a fine line between medical and midwifery models of birth and seeking, in the interests of improving care and outcomes, to reform the systems in which they participate without losing their jobs. This chapter describes the multiple ways that midwives "orchestrate" their care to help women achieve birth within the parameters of "normal" in spite of the obstacles they face, blending the science and art of midwifery practice. Kennedy concludes by discussing the barriers to making the midwifery model work and by providing systematic and practical strategies for "orchestrating" normal birth in clinical practice settings.

CHARACTERISTICS OF BIRTH MODELS THAT WORK

In spite of the difficulties, birth models that work exist in hospitals, clinics, birth centers, homes, and villages all around the world. They work because women are either the center of the process or respected partners in a system set up by their society or community to benefit them, their children, and their families. The criteria we use to identify and characterize "birth models that work," exemplified in the models described in this book, include the following:

- A woman-centered ideology internationally known as the midwifery model of care
- Midwives, or practitioners of the midwifery model of care (see Conclusion), as the primary practitioners for normal births (which in midwifery-model practices constitute the vast majority of births)
- Midwifery care based in the community
- Continuity of care (caseload midwifery, one-to-one care)
- Creative use of appropriate technologies and modalities that work to support normal birth
- A focus on avoiding morbidity as well as mortality through providing optimal care
- Cultural appropriateness and sensitivity
- Physicians providing appropriate services for high-risk and emergency births
- Mutually respectful and collaborative relationships among all types of care providers
- "Referring back," meaning that if a woman with a previous risk condition improves and becomes low risk, she can be reclassified as "normal" and referred back to the midwife
- Reflective practice, in which practitioners continually reflect on what they are doing and make efforts at improvement on an ongoing basis
- Viable systems of transport to hospitals for out-of-hospital practices

- Mutual accommodation and cooperation between professional and indigenous practitioners (where relevant)
- Effective and appropriate use of lifesaving interventions like cesarean sections
- Evidence-based practice
- Statistically sound outcomes
- Accessibility to women of all income levels
- Effective systems of communication and referral with other community organizations and services
- Financial viability, including cost-effective mix of skills, technology use, and setting, and sufficient salaries for staff
- Sustainability
- Replicability within similar cultural and economic settings
- Practitioner education that encourages and facilitates all of the above
- Regional and national organizations and communication networks that support this work, which include major consumer components that can generate political support and facilitate practitioners in their abilities to humanize care

All the chapters that follow illustrate these characteristics in action, showing how each one becomes essential to the whole. Most of these characteristics can best be exemplified through a detailed examination of the first one, the ideology internationally known as "the midwifery model of care." In the Conclusion to this volume, we will fully explicate that model in relation to our above list of characteristics of models that work, drawing on the specific models we present to illustrate its myriad yet cohesive, woman-empowering components.

None of the models described in this book is perfect, but all of them work well for mothers and babies. Chapter authors show us to what extent each model meets these criteria, pointing out what "getting there" takes and what obstacles and limitations each model faces in attempting to do so. Perfection is not the issue; functional (as opposed to dysfunctional) maternity care is. These functional models deserve international attention; this book is designed to help them achieve it and to encourage the creation of many other such models around the world.

ACKNOWLEDGMENTS

We express our deep appreciation to our chapter authors for their enormous contributions to the health and welfare of mothers and babies, and for their hard work in writing the chapters that describe those contributions in clear and concrete ways so that others can use them as guidelines for the development of many more models that work.

NOTES

1. The *Cochrane Database of Systematic Reviews*, one of the databases in the *Cochrane Library*, http://www.thecochranelibrary.com, provides at no charge all abstracts/current citations and plain-language summaries. You can search in many ways. Especially helpful is to go to the "topic" button, choose Pregnancy and Childbirth, and then use the topical outline.

2. The U.S.-based organization Childbirth Connection has identified the need to organize in a database all of the systematic reviews that are available in the field of birth, which number in the hundreds; most are not from the Cochrane Collection, and more are coming at an exponential rate. As a result, Childbirth Connection is looking for the resources to accomplish this goal. Epidemiologist Carol Sakala of Childbirth Connection has highlighted many of the more relevant reviews in her quarterly columns since January 2003. All columns are collected together and freely available at www.childbirthconnection.org. See also Childbirth Connection's "Current Resources for Evidence-Based Practice" columns and *Harms of Caesarean versus Vaginal Birth* (www.childbirthconnection.org/article.asp?ck=10271), *What Every Pregnant Woman Needs to Know About Caesarean Section* and *Why Does the National U.S. Cesarean Section Rate Keep Going Up?* (www.childbirthconnection.org/article.asp?ck=10456 and www.childbirthconnection.org/article.asp?ck=10164). There are also important summaries in DARE (abstracts that assess quality of systematic reviews, free at http://www.york.ac.uk/inst/crd/crddatabases.htm), and clinical evidence at www.clinicalevevidence.com.

REFERENCES

Advancing Normal Birth. 2007. Supplement to the *Journal of Perinatal Education* 16.1. The Coalition for Improving Maternity Services: Evidence Basis for the Ten Steps of Mother-Friendly Care. Washington, DC: Lamaze International.

Afsana, K. 2003. "Power, Knowledge, and Childbirth Practices: An Ethnographic Exploration in Bangladesh." Ph.D. dissertation, Edith Cowan University, Perth, Western Australia.

Allen, D.R. 2000. *Bodily Risks, Spiritual Risks: Contrasting Discourses on Pregnancy in a Rural Tanzanian Community.* Ann Arbor: University of Michigan Press.

Anderson, R., and D. Anderson. 1999. "The Cost-Effectiveness of Home Birth." *Journal of Midwifery and Women's Health* 4.1:30–35.

Beech, B., and M. Phipps. 2008. "Normal Birth: Women's Stories." In *Normal Childbirth: Evidence and Debate*, 2nd ed., edited by Soo Downe, 67–79. Edinburgh: Churchill Livingstone.

Betrán, A., M. Merialdi, J.A. Lauer, W. Bing-shun, J. Thomas, P. Van Look, and M. Wagner. 2007. "Rates of Caesarean Section: Analysis of Global, Regional and National Estimates." *Paediatric and Perinatal Epidemiology* 21:98–113. http://www3.interscience.wiley.com/journal/118486257/abstract.

Byford, J. 1999. "Dealing with Death Beginning with Birth: Women's Health and Childbirth on Misima Island, Papua New Guinea." Ph.D. dissertation, Australian National University, Canberra.

Cochrane Collaboration. http://www.cochrane.org/.

Cochrane Library. http://www3.interscience.wiley.com/cgi-bin/mrwhome/106568753/ HOME?CRETRY=1&SRETRY=0.

Davis-Floyd, R. 1987. "Obstetric Training as a Rite of Passage." *Medical Anthropology Quarterly* 1.3:288–318.

———. 1994. "The Technocratic Body: American Childbirth as Cultural Expression." *Social Science and Medicine* 38.8:1125–40.

———. 2003. "Home Birth Emergencies in the U.S. and Mexico: The Trouble with Transport." *Social Science and Medicine* 56.9:1913–31.

———. 2004. *Birth as an American Rite of Passage*, 2nd ed. Berkeley and London: University of California Press.

Declerq, E., C. Sakala, M. Corry, and S. Appelbaum. 2006. *Listening to Mothers II: Report of the Second National U.S. Survey of Women's Childbearing Experiences, Executive Summary*. New York: Childbirth Connection. www.childbirthconnection.org.

Downe, S. (ed.). 2008. *Normal Childbirth: Evidence and Debate*, 2nd ed. Oxford, UK: Churchill Livingstone.

Enkin, M., M. Keirse, J. Neilson, C. Crowther, L. Duley, E. Hodnett, and J. Hofmeyr. 2000. *A Guide to Effective Care in Pregnancy and Childbirth*, 3rd ed. New York: Oxford University Press. Freely available at http://www.childbirthconnection.org.

Glasgow, T. S., P. C. Young, J. Wallin, C. Kwok, G. Stoddard, S. Firth, M. Samore, and C. L. Byington. 2005. "Association of Intrapartum Antibiotic Exposure and Late-Onset Serious Bacterial Infections in Infants." *Pediatrics* 116.3:696–702.

Goer, H. 1999. *The Thinking Woman's Guide to a Better Birth*. New York: Penguin Putnam/Perigree.

Hodnett, E., S. Gates, G. J. Hofmeyr, and C. Sakala. 2004. "Continuous Support for Women during Childbirth." *Cochrane Database Syst. Reviews*, 2007, Issue 2. Art. No.: CD003766. DOI: 10.1002/14651858.CD003766.pub2.

Johnson, K. C., and Daviss, B.-A. 2005. "Outcomes of Planned Home Births with Certified Professional Midwives: Large Prospective Study in North America. *British Medical Journal* 330:1416.

Klein, M. C. 2006. "Does Epidural Analgesia Increase Rate of Cesarean Section?" *Canadian Family Physician* 52:419–21, 426–28.

Klein, M. C., S. Grzybowski, S. Harris, R. Liston, A. Spence, G. Le, D. Brummendorf, S. Kim, and J. Kaczorowski. 2001. "Epidural Analgesia Use as a Marker for Physician Approach to Birth: Implications for Maternal and Newborn Outcomes." *Birth* 28:243–48.

Kolenda, P. 1998. "Fewer Deaths, Fewer Births." *Manushi* 105:5–13.

Kroeger, M. 2004. *The Impact of Birth Practices on Breastfeeding: Protecting the Mother and Baby Continuum*. With L. Smith. Sudbury, MA: Jones and Bartlett.

Liu, S., R. Liston, K. Joseph, M. Heaman, R. Sauve, and M. Kramer. 2007. "Maternal Mortality and Severe Morbidity Associated with Low-Risk Planned Cesarean Delivery versus Planned Vaginal Delivery at Term." *Canadian Medical Association Journal* 176:455–60.

Liu, Y., K. Rao, and W. C. Hsiao. 2003. "Medical Expenditure and Rural Impoverishment in China." *Journal of Health, Population and Nutrition* 21.3:216–22.

Miller, S., A. Tejada, P. Murgueytio, J. Diaz, R. Dabash, P. Putney, S. Bjegovic, and G. Caraballo. 2002. *Strategic Assessment of Reproductive Health in the Dominican Republic*. New York: Population Council.

Morsy, S. 1995. "Deadly Reproduction among Egyptian Women: Maternal Mortality and the Medicalization of Population Control." In *Conceiving the New World Order: The Global Politics of Reproduction,* edited by F. Ginsburg and R. Rapp, 162–76. Berkeley: University of California Press.

Perkins, B. 2004. *The Medical Delivery Business: Health Reform, Childbirth, and the Economic Order.* New Brunswick, NJ: Rutgers University Press.

Potter, J. E., E. Berquó, I. Perpétuo, O. Leal, K. Hopkins, M. Souza, and M. Formiga. 2001. "Unwanted Caesarean Sections among Public and Private Patients in Brazil: Prospective Study." *British Medical Journal* 323:1155–58.

Roberts, C. L., S. Tracy, and B. Peat. 2000. "Rates for Obstetric Intervention among Private and Public Patients in Australia: Population-Based Descriptive Study." *British Medical Journal* 321.7254:137–41.

Rooks, J. 1997. *Midwifery and Childbirth in America.* Philadelphia: Temple University Press.

Royal College of Obstetricians and Gynecologists and Royal College of Midwives. *Joint Statement No. 2* [Home Births]. April 2007.

Sakala, Carol, and Maureen P. Corry. 2008. *Evidence-Based Maternity Care: What It Is and What It Can Achieve.* New York: co-published by Childbirth Connection, the Reforming States Group, and the Millbank Memorial Fund. www.milbank .org/reports/0809MaternityCare/0809MaternityCare.html.

Tracy, S. K., and M. B. Tracy. 2003. "Costing the Cascade: Estimating the Cost of Increased Obstetric Intervention in Childbirth Using Population Data." *British Journal of Obstetrics and Gynaecology,* 110:717–24.

Villar, J., G. C. Carroli, N. Zavaleta, A. Donner, D. Wojdyla, A. Faundes, A. Velazco, et al. 2007. "Maternal and Neonatal Individual Risks and Benefits Associated with Caesarean Delivery: Multicentre Prospective Study." *British Medical Journal,* www.bmj.com, published online Oct. 30, DOI: 10.1136/bmj.39363.706956.55. www.bmj.com/cgi/content/abstract/335/7628/1025.

Villar J., E. Valladares, D. Wojdyla, N. Zavaleta, G. Carroli, A. Velazco, A. Shah, et al. 2006. "Caesarean Delivery Rates and Pregnancy Outcomes: The 2005 WHO Global Survey on Maternal and Perinatal Health in Latin America." *Lancet* 367.9525:1819–29. www.thelancet.com.

Walsh, Denis. 2007. *Evidence-Based Care for Normal Labour and Birth: A Guide for Midwives.* UK: Routledge.

WHO/FIGO/ICM. 2004. *Making Pregnancy Safer: The Critical Role of the Skilled Birth Attendant: A Joint Statement.* Geneva: World Health Organization.

World Health Organization. http://www.who.int/en/; see also http://www.who.int/ library/en/.

FURTHER RESOURCES

Childbirth Connection. This website provides outstanding summaries of available scientific and practical information for mothers and practitioners. www .childbirthconnection.org.

International Alliance of Midwives (IAM) is an online organization with a quarterly electronic newsletter, directory of practitioner members, and country contacts for over fifty countries. There are flags from each country with a country contact with Web references on midwifery and childbirth from each country. www.midwiferytoday.com/iam.

International Confederation of Midwives (ICM) works to educate the world about midwives and holds regional conferences, with a global conference every three years. www.internationalmidwives.org.

International MotherBaby Childbirth Organization (IMBCO)—formerly known as CIMS International. Developed the *International MotherBaby Childbirth Initiative: 10 Steps to Optimal Maternity Care*, which includes the 10 Steps of the Baby-friendly Hospital Initiative (BFHI). www.imbci.org.

Red Latinoamericana y del Caribe para la Humanización del Parto y el Nacimiento (RELACAHUPAN). In English, the Network of Latin American and Caribbean for the Humanization of Labor and Birth. Sends an electronic newsletter in Spanish and maintains country contacts for each of the Latin American and Caribbean countries. www.relacahupan.org.

PART ONE

Large-Scale Systems

National and Regional Models

Chapter 1

The Dutch Obstetrical System

Vanguard of the Future in Maternity Care

Raymond De Vries, Therese A. Wiegers, Beatrijs Smulders, and Edwin van Teijlingen

INTRODUCTION

The German poet Heinrich Heine is reported to have said, "When the world comes to an end, I shall go to Holland, for everything there happens fifty years later." For some, this Dutch "quaintness" explains the unusual system of obstetric care found in the Netherlands, a system where nearly one-third of births occur at home and where midwives have a degree of professional independence unrivaled by midwives in any other country.[1] Heine's observation about the Netherlands suggests that the unique Dutch way of birth is a vestige from a bygone era—a credible conclusion if you believe that humans are helpless in the face of technology. But the stubborn persistence of midwifery and home birth in the Netherlands, in spite of the declaration of medical professionals elsewhere that midwife-attended birth at home is a dangerous anachronism, forces us to conclude that Dutch obstetrics can be the vanguard of the future.

The singularity of the Dutch maternity care system has made it a model for all those who seek to slow or reverse the march toward the medicalization of birth found in the developed world (Van Teijlingen et al. 2004). For birth activists, the Netherlands has become *the* destination for inspiration and for instruction on how to reorganize birth in their home countries. The uniqueness of the system, coupled with the desire of short-term visitors to find what they are looking for, has resulted in mischaracterizations of the Dutch way of birth. For example, Mehl-Madrona and Mehl-Madrona (1993: 1) claimed that "over 70% of births [in the Netherlands] are still attended by midwives." In *fact*, in the early 1990s midwives accompanied about half of all births in the Netherlands (see Table 1.1). As far back as 1910, the first year a breakdown by caregiver is available, midwives in the

TABLE 1.1 Births in the United States and the Netherlands, 1940–2002
(percent of all births)

	Births Supervised by Midwives		Home Births	
	United States	The Netherlands	United States	The Netherlands
1940	8.7	47.7		
1945	6.1	36.1		
1950	4.5	41.1		
1955	2.9	40.9	5.6	76.1
1960	2	36.6	3.4	72.6
1965	1.5	35.3	2.6	68.5
1970	0.4	36.7	0.6	57.3
1975	0.9	38.6	0.9	44.4
1980	1.7	39.4	1	35.4
1985	2.7	41.7	1	36.6
1990	3.9	44.4	1.1	32.1
1995	5.9	36.3	1	31.6
2000	7.7	33.9	1	30.3
2001	8	33.9	1	28.9
2002	8.1	33.4	1	29.4

SOURCE: NCHS (www.cdc.gov/nchs), CBS (www.cbs.nl), TNO (Anthony et al. 2005).

Netherlands attended 57.7 percent of all births, and at no point since did they attend more than 60 percent of births. Midwives *do* attend over 70 percent of the births that occur at home. It is likely the authors heard this statistic and somehow assumed that the 70 percent figure applied to *all* Dutch births. In her ethnographically based discussion of the lessons of Dutch obstetrics for Americans, Rothman (1993: 201) sets the scene by discussing windmills, tulips, bicycles, and Rembrandt, giving an over-romanticized picture of Dutch midwifery and society. Her description of the Netherlands as a "Mecca for midwives" and the home of noninterventive obstetrics makes it difficult to believe that Dutch midwives once argued for the right to wield forceps (see Marland 1995: 328) or that they are beginning to outfit their offices with the apparatus for sonograms (see Pasveer and Akrich 2001).

Even the Dutch misrepresent their obstetric system. For example, *Expecting*, an annual special issue on pregnancy and birth of a Dutch parenting magazine, states that "in the Netherlands about 70% of babies are born at home, without complication or unusual interventions" (Schiet 1994: 112). In the early 1960s, this *was* the case (72.6 percent of births were at home in 1960), but throughout the last decades of the twentieth century, the percent of births at home continued to decline. By 1994, the date of the article in *Expecting*, the home birth rate was just over 30 percent.

Although we count ourselves among the champions of the way obstetrics is organized and accomplished in the Netherlands, we believe that the Dutch system can serve as a model *only* if we see it clearly, with its strengths and its flaws, and with its ties to the structure and culture of Dutch society. To that end, we offer a description of the Dutch way of birth that includes (1) stories and statistics that paint a picture of the players and outcomes of the system; (2) accounts of the history of midwifery and its place in the organization of medical care; and (3) explanations of the ways obstetrics in the Netherlands expresses the culture of that country.

SEEING MATERNITY CARE IN THE NETHERLANDS

Too often descriptions of the Dutch way of birth are limited to statistical portrayals of caregivers and outcomes; even though these are clearly necessary, they exclude the voices of midwives and the women and families they serve, and they fail to convey what occurs in the homes, polyclinics,[2] and hospitals of the Netherlands. In the following pages, we provide a statistical picture of the Dutch way of birth, interspersed with stories of births that reveal what birth in the Netherlands feels like and how it is valued.

We open with a story told by a Dutch mother that illustrates the features of maternity care in the Netherlands much admired by non-Netherlanders:

My second pregnancy was not as exciting as my first. I was often tired and had many colds. [My labor began when] I felt a weak contraction, and then a while later, another small one. I decided to go to bed nice and early. If I could get to sleep, maybe the contractions would stop. That did not work. I was definitely having contractions, so I went with my big bare belly and stood in front of the gas heater. That felt great! The contractions became stronger and more regular, and we called the midwife.

First came the assistant and then the midwife. My friend Jetske came with a big bouquet of fragrant lilies. My neighbor, Otto, happened to come by and asked if he could stay. Sure, why not? Between contractions I was able to relax, and when another came, I was able to handle it easily. I felt like an old hand at this. Gradually the contractions became more frequent and intense, and I suddenly recalled how vicious some contractions can be.

I began to feel irritated and impatient. I had had enough of this; I wanted no more. Soon came the urge to push, but I had to keep these strong contractions at a distance, I had to puff them away. But they were so powerful I had to go along with them, and when I did I found that I enjoyed them. The midwife broke the membranes. And then, an enormous relief, my second child arrived, a beautiful little girl with dark hair, Rosa.

She lay next to me safe and warm, softly groaning as if gradually recovering from her journey. When everyone had gone and Frans, my husband, was sleeping on the sofa and Swaan, my little daughter, was in her bed, and Rosa [was] in my arms, the room changed into an island of rest, the center of the universe. [3]

From the point of view of the midwife, the Dutch way of birth has additional advantages. One of us, Beatrijs Smulders, is a practicing midwife in the Netherlands, and in this chapter she reflects on her work to complete our picture of midwifery in her home country. In this story Beatrijs describes the "deep feeling of emancipation" that accompanies birth at home:

A good birth strengthens the self-image of the birthing woman at a deep, non-rational level. A system in which women do the delivery themselves emancipates women. Often women say after the delivery, "After this I can do anything!" or "Because I was forced to rely on myself during the delivery, I learned all of a sudden to trust myself."

This is well illustrated by the story of a professor, whose pregnancy at the age of 43 was unexpected and unwanted. She never had the desire to have children. She had, in fact, achieved everything that a woman could achieve in a "man's world." She was a university professor, had written bestsellers, and was on several important policy committees. And then this, totally unexpected! At her prenatal visits she was often confused, not knowing whether to be happy or grief stricken. She worked harder than ever, and she wanted to return to work as soon as possible after the delivery. She was not looking forward to the birth. This cool-headed woman preferred to go to hospital with plenty of pain relief. She questioned why we midwives were so keen on the use of water—being under the shower or in the bath during contractions. To her that seemed totally ridiculous. Her mind was made up and I promised to respect her wishes.

But during the pregnancy she changed—she followed a parent-craft course, attended an antenatal education evening and during the last check-up she suggested that "the first few centimeters dilation I'll stay at home, and well, the pain relief can come at the end."

Her delivery started slowly. She found it extremely difficult to put aside the troubling thoughts that filled her head and to give in to her contractions, to her body. When she finally let go, the delivery went unbelievably fast. She insisted on staying at home, and even hopped into the "damned" bath. She dilated fully and within an hour she had a beautiful son in her arms.

Six weeks later she came for her postpartum check-up. She was a very different person: in one arm her son breastfeeding, in the other a big bunch of roses. When I asked her to reflect on her birth she glowed and said: "For years I have fought to make it in a man's world. Even though I succeeded something essential was missing. Now that I have had a baby, I know what that is. At a very deep level I was always unsure about myself; now something fundamental has changed. Rationally I can't put my finger on it, but bodily, intuitively, I have a new self-esteem that I had never experienced before, and as a result I am certain that everything will become easier for me."

TABLE 1.2 Birth in the Netherlands by place, 1995–2002
(percent)

	Polyclinic (midwife or GP)	Home (midwife or GP)	Clinic (gynecologist)
1995	11.7	31.6	56.6
1996	11.1	30.3	58.5
1997	10.5	29.6	59.8
1998	10.7	29.1	60.1
1999	10.6	30.8	58.6
2000	10.2	30.3	59.4
2001	10.5	28.9	60.4
2002	11.2	29.4	59.4

SOURCE: TNO (Anthony et al. 2005).

This is the kind of reason that makes it so crucial that we in the Netherlands must hold onto a maternity care system that allows women, as much as possible, to make their own decisions and take control over pregnancy and birth, a system where women can choose their own midwife and take things into their own hands.

These narrative pictures of birth naturally lead to questions about the broader dimensions and the trends in the Dutch way of birth. Here is where statistics can help. Tables 1.1 and 1.2 present the most-requested information about midwifery and birth in the Netherlands: the extent of home birth and the role of midwives in birth.

These tables are unsurprising and surprising at the same time. We are unsurprised to learn that the rates of home birth and midwifery involvement in birth are much, much higher than those found in the United States. In the United States there are very few births at home, and midwives are involved in less than 10 percent of births (Martin et al. 2005). But many will be surprised to see that the percentage of births at home in the Netherlands has dropped dramatically in the past four decades, and that—compared to Scandinavian countries where midwives attend nearly all births—Dutch midwives accompany fewer than half of all births.

Of course, the inevitable question that arises in the minds of those first learning about the Dutch way of birth is, is it safe? The answer to this question is found by looking at infant mortality rates in several countries.[4] Table 1.3 shows that the Netherlands has rates lower than those in the United States, similar to those in the United Kingdom and Canada, and higher than those found in Sweden.

TABLE 1.3 Infant mortality rates for various countries, 1960–2005

	The Netherlands	Canada	Sweden	United Kingdom	United States
1960	17.9	27.3	16.6	22.5	26
1965	14.4	23.6	13.3	19.6	24.7
1970	12.7	18.8	11	18.5	20
1975	10.6	14.3	8.6	16	16.1
1980	8.6	10.4	6.9	12.1	12.6
1985	8	8	6.8	9.4	10.6
1990	7.1	6.8	6	7.9	9.2
1995	5.5	6	4.1	6	8
2000	5.1	5.3	3.4	5.6	6.9
2001	5.4	5.2	3.7	5.5	6.8
2002	5	5.4	3.3	5.2	7
2003	4.8	5.3	3.1	5.3	6.9
2004	4.4	5.3	3.1	5.0	6.8
2005	4.9	5.4	2.4	5.1	

NOTE: Infant mortality rate is defined as the number of deaths in the first year of life per 1,000 live births.

SOURCE: Eurostat (epp.eurostat.cec.eu.int), StatCan (www.statcan.ca), NCHS (www.cdc.gov/nchs), OECD Health Data.

Another measure of the outcome of maternity care is the proportion of births that are accomplished surgically. The cesarean section (CS) rates for the United States show a gradual increase from 23.5 percent in 1995 to 29.1 percent in 2004, a steady increase over the past fifteen years: in 2004 nearly one in three women in the United States was delivered surgically. The CS rate in the Netherlands nearly doubled in the same period, from 7.5 percent in 1990 to 13.8 percent in 2004, but it is still less than half the rate in the United States.

Maternity care in the Netherlands is remarkable for its degree of cooperation between caregivers at different levels and locations in the system. Those who attend home births in other nations often find that hospital-based caregivers are reluctant to offer support to home birth mothers and are prone to scolding women whose care is transferred to the hospital (De Vries 1996; Davis-Floyd 2003). In the Netherlands the transition from home to hospital is much smoother—so smooth that some worry about overreliance on backup care and consequent overuse of the hospital.

Rothman describes a typical transfer from home to hospital. She is an American sociologist who went to the Netherlands to take a look at its much-discussed maternity care system; as she says, "It is kind of a rite of passage for the childbirth aficionado." But instead of witnessing a calm and cozy affair, she got to see what happens when a home birth mom is transferred to the care of a gynecologist:

> The labor was not progressing, and the midwife became concerned. Perhaps bladder pressure was a problem. She tried a catheter, change of position, more time, more changes. Then the decision to move to the hospital: helping the woman slip some clothes on, all of us helping her maneuver down [the] stairs, placing her in the car next to her boyfriend, waving goodbye to the worried grandmother-to-be, jumping in the car with the midwife, and the two cars going off to the hospital. I remember holding the hospital door open for the midwife, carrying one of her bags while she carried another, with the birth stool tucked under her arm. There was a friendly welcome at the entrance, and a warmer welcome from the nurse on duty. A brief exchange of information, and the nurse set things up the way the midwife liked them—an experienced team comfortably working together. More time, more changes of position. I found myself alone with the laboring woman, who was stretched out on a padded table, crying in a Dutch that even I could understand, "I want to go to sleep, let me sleep." Reassuring her (in English—who knows what a laboring woman understands of a language she studied in high school?), but aiming for the right tone of compassion and assurance, I said the midwife would be right back, "She's coming, she'll be right here." Then finally the consultation . . . the obstetrician coming in, conferring with the midwife, briefly examining the woman, and agreeing to do a Caesarean section . . . the goodbyes, and the midwife assuring the woman and the boyfriend that things were now okay. She said she would see them tomorrow, and off we went. (Rothman 1993: 206)

Rothman was both surprised and pleased with the easy transfer of care from midwife to specialist, which is unlike the situation she observed in the United States, where women transferred from home to hospital are often subject to lectures and harsh treatment from obstetricians and nursing staff (see Davis-Floyd 2003 for examples).

Beatrijs reflects on how the setting of birth influences the midwife's attitude toward the event:

> The midwife knows two kinds of fear: the fear of making a mistake and the fear of the immensity of the occasion. The first fear is not something to really worry about. If you have the skills, you will know exactly what to do in each situation, and when you should or should not intervene. The rules are clear, and with increasing experience, you learn to trust your judgment.
>
> The second fear is much more present at home than in the hospital. In the hospital, equipment helps you to allay fear. You can hide behind the technology. Listening with a big imposing CTG [cardiotocograph, electronic fetal monitor] machine is no more efficient than listening with a little wooden Pinard, but the former mystifies. It impresses your audience, and it seems to remove the fear in the midwife. The institution radiates the

ultimate control. At home there is nothing to mystify. The woman does it
herself, with your support. You try to disturb this process as little as possible,
so you listen with your Pinard or Doppler. Strange as it may sound, at home
you feel much more that the baby floats between heaven and earth, that a
new life is on its way.

The art of the midwife is to never act on the basis of fear. You must learn
not to identify with fear. You experience your feelings and let them pass over
like clouds, until the sky is blue again. That's when you act. When you act out
of fear, there is the risk that you medicalize. Before you know it, you have sent
a woman to an obstetrician or to hospital unnecessarily.

Beatrijs's comments are instructive for those who would like to understand
the shift of birth from hospital to home. She notes that fear of birth leads
to its medicalization, but it is also true that medicalization leads to fear:
as birth becomes defined as a medical event, both mothers and midwives
begin to fear that birth requires all the accoutrements of medicine, creating a spiral toward complete hospitalization.

What do statistics reveal about the transfer of care from midwife to
gynecologist and from home to hospital in the Netherlands? Interestingly,
more women are choosing to *start* their care with midwives or general
practitioners (GPs). The number of women receiving care from a gynecologist at the start of pregnancy dropped from 18.7 percent in 1995
to 14.3 percent in 2002, and over the past decade, nearly 60 percent of
women *started their labor* under the care of either a midwife or a general
practitioner at home or in the polyclinic. At the same time, however, referrals during antenatal care increased from 23.8 percent of all pregnant
women in 1995 to 28.3 percent in 2002 (Anthony et al. 2005).

It is also noteworthy that in recent years, the rate of transfers from
home to hospital has been remarkably stable: referrals during labor
and birth increased from 14.1 percent of all birthing women in 1995 to
16.8 percent in 2002. Less than 10 percent of women who start labor at
home are transferred to hospital, and 6 percent to 7 percent of women
who start labor in a clinic with a midwife or GP are transferred to the
care of an obstetrician.

THE STRUCTURE OF MATERNITY CARE
IN THE NETHERLANDS AND HOW IT GOT THAT WAY

Birth stories from the Netherlands—including the ones we have retold
here—present cozy pictures that can lull us into assuming that Dutch caregivers simply know how to get along, and that mothers instinctively know
how to give birth. But in reality, the coziness of Dutch birth is the product

of a system of rules, regulations, educational programs, and arrangements between professionals. And as we will see, the elements in this system are constantly reviewed, argued over, and negotiated.

Indeed, most explanations of the persistence of home birth and independent midwifery in the Netherlands look to the structure of maternity care and health care (e.g., Van Teijlingen 2003: 124). The unique features that combine to produce the Dutch way of birth include

1. A state-organized health care system that mixes public oversight with a (commercial) health insurance industry. The Obstetrics Indications List carefully distinguishes "physiological" and "pathological" pregnancies and births, and women in the first category are reimbursed only for care provided by midwives and GPs.[5] As a result, almost 80 percent of Dutch women begin their prenatal care with a midwife, and an additional 6.5 percent begin with a GP. As a result of referrals to secondary care during the course of prenatal care and labor, midwives are independently caring for over 37 percent of women at the time of birth, GPs an additional 3.2 percent, and gynecologists just under 60 percent (some of which are, in fact, accompanied by midwives). Of the women remaining in the care of the first line (those accompanied by midwives and GPs), the majority (71 percent) give birth at home, resulting in a total home birth rate of just under 30 percent (Wiegers 2006).

2. Well-educated midwives, GPs, and specialists who—thanks to guidelines developed by government, insurance companies, and professional organizations—know how to work with each other. The midwives and GPs are trained to select those women who are at increased risk during pregnancy, birth, and the postpartum period. Like most European countries, the Netherlands has many more midwives and GPs than it does specialists in gynecology and obstetrics, a structural decision that reflects the attitude that birth is normal and requires specialist attention only in those rare cases where something goes wrong (see Table 1.4).

3. A system for postpartum care provided by *kraamverzorgenden*— maternity home care assistants. This feature of Dutch obstetrics is the provision of postpartum care by specially trained caregivers, who come to the home of the new parents and do everything from watching the condition of mom and baby, offering instruction in baby care and feeding, to household chores and shopping, and if necessary, cooking (Van Teijlingen et al. 2004). Expectant parents must register for these services early in the pregnancy; unfortunately, because of a shortage of *kraamverzorgenden* in recent years, the average number of hours of

TABLE 1.4 Practicing gynecologists, midwives, and family
doctors in the Netherlands, 1980–2007

	Gynecologists	Midwives	Family Doctors
1980	545	814	5,522
1985	673	945	6,212
1990	604	1,122	6,800
1995	592	1,332	7,125
2000	655	1,578	7,706
2001	675	1,627	7,763
2002	699	1,731	7,945
2003	NA	1,825	8,107
2004	NA	1,955	8,209
2005	NA	2,080	8,408
2006	NA	2,197	8,495
2007	833	2,265	8,673

SOURCE: NIVEL (Hingstman and Kenens 2007a, 2007b; Van der Velden,
Vugts, and Hingstman 2004; Van der Velden et al. 2008).

maternity care assistance spread over the first eight days postpartum has
been reduced from sixty-four to forty-four hours after normal childbirth
(Wiegers 2006).

4. "Polyclinic" settings in hospitals organized to provide low-tech, high-touch
   birth.
5. A system for well-child visits.
6. Strong political support for midwifery and home birth across the political agenda (see De Vries 2005: 93–137).
7. A network of roads and hospitals that allows easy access to specialist
   care.[6]

Two of the above features—the Obstetrics Indications List and the unique,
protected position of the midwife—are especially distinctive and require
further explanation.

Indications for Cooperation

Pregnant women in the Netherlands move freely between care settings
and caregivers. Without some sort of organization and control, these back-
and-forth referrals would quickly become confusing, if not dangerous. If
there were no rules governing the comings and goings of obstetric clients,
some gynecologists might "hold on" to the women referred to them, reluctant to send them back to midwives and GPs, who in turn would be slow

to send clients to specialists, preferring to manage even complicated cases at home or in the polyclinic.

From the point of view of health policy, this management of interprofessional rivalry in the Dutch system is remarkable. The system does more than simply control the competition for clients between midwives, GPs, and gynecologists; it also generates an unusual degree of cooperation between midwives and physicians. The Obstetric Indications List, a set of guidelines that specifies the conditions for referrals between primary and secondary care, facilitates this cooperation. The Obstetric Indications List defines what "healthy" means, distinguishing between normal ("physiological") and high-risk ("pathological") pregnancies and births. These definitions are then used to identify the conditions that require midwives and general practitioners to refer their clients to (obstetric) specialists. Without such a list, the preference for primary care in Dutch obstetrics would not be possible. The Obstetric Indications List is a critical part of the unique Dutch way of birth. Having a screening system for identifying "physiological" and "pathological"—rather than "high-risk" and "low-risk"—pregnancies allows the Dutch to avoid the assumption, made in other industrialized countries, that all births should be defined in terms of "risk." When a woman with a healthy pregnancy is labeled "low risk," it puts her on a continuum that ends in "high risk," justifying the need for the monitoring of her pregnancy, and indeed all pregnancies, by a specialist.[7]

Midwives

Midwives in many other countries admire, if not envy, the autonomy of their sisters in the Netherlands (Van Teijlingen et al. 2004: 163). When they see the relative freedom enjoyed by Dutch midwives, they are often eager to know how this happened. Elsewhere in Europe, the rise of modern obstetric technology relegated midwives to the position of doctor's assistant. How did Dutch midwives escape this fate? It is clear that *current* regulations favor midwives, but how did those regulations come to be?

Intrigued by these questions, historians have explored the events that allowed Dutch midwifery to arrive in its present position.[8] The consensus of these histories is that midwives in the Netherlands benefited from the early arrival of municipally sponsored education and regulation. Unlike their European neighbors, the Dutch believed that if midwives had the proper training and regulatory oversight, they could be important figures in securing safe childbirth and promoting population growth. Rather than marginalizing midwives—a strategy used by municipal and regional authorities elsewhere in Europe—city leaders in the Netherlands sought to educate these women and put them to work in service of the townspeople.

As early as 1463, the town of Leiden appointed a municipal midwife, who was given a small salary to see to the care of all parturient women. Her services were provided without charge to the poor; the rich were instructed to make a contribution for care received (Van der Borg 1992: 44–45). She was required to call a physician for help in complicated cases and to train aspiring midwives. These fifteenth-century rules foreshadow the development of midwifery in the Netherlands: the "work terrain" of midwives was limited to "normal" births (physician assistance was required in difficult cases), and midwifery was recognized as a distinct field of practice (student midwives should train with midwives). By the eighteenth century, most towns in the Netherlands had appointed municipal midwives.[9]

In the nineteenth century, municipal regulations and training programs were gradually replaced by national laws and state-funded education. The first national law regulating midwifery was the 1818 Health Act that gave midwives a clear and defined sphere of practice. Midwifery was specifically included among the several *medical* professions regulated by the Act, and the competencies and duties of midwives were distinguished from those of others providing birth care: men-midwives (trained by apprenticeship) and obstetric doctors (academically trained). Additionally, the Act confined midwives' practices to those births "which were natural processes or could be delivered manually, so that the midwife may never use any instruments for this purpose" (quoted in Lieburg and Marland 1989: 299).

Reviewing the early efforts to regulate midwifery in countries outside the Netherlands, Van der Borg (1992: 144) points out that the Dutch system of educating and regulating midwives gave the profession another advantage. Less regulated and less educated, "midwives in other Western European countries lacked the necessary protection from the competition of physicians and men-midwives who were becoming skilled in obstetrics."

The introduction of state examinations and schools for midwifery was part of the government intervention in the organization of maternity care. The first state school for midwives was established in Amsterdam in 1861, and a second one in Rotterdam in 1882; a Roman Catholic school was opened in Heerlen in 1912, and a fourth school was established in Groningen in 2002. The training program in these state schools lasted two years. Topics included general anatomy and physiology, special knowledge of the female parts, the care of infants and sick women, and both theoretical and practical midwifery. In 1920, a third year was added to midwifery training, allowing further competence in infant and prenatal care.

TABLE 1.5 Distribution of primary-care midwives working in different types of practices, 1980–2007

	Solo Practice		Duo-Practice		Group Practice		Total	
	n	%	n	%	n	%	n	%
1980	391	67.6	136	23.5	51	8.8	578	100.0
1985	322	46.8	269	39.1	97	14.1	688	100.0
1990	235	27.6	326	38.3	291	34.2	852	100.0
1995	135	13.2	316	30.8	575	56.0	1,026	100.0
2000	88	7.2	243	19.9	889	72.9	1,220	100.0
2005	63	4.3	189	12.8	1,222	82.9	1,474	100.0
2006	70	4.6	174	11.4	1,282	84.0	1,526	100.0
2007	76	4.8	169	10.7	1,332	84.5	1,577	100.0

SOURCE: Hingstman and Kenens 2007a.

Dutch midwives continue to be among the best-educated midwives in the world, a fact that is made more striking to many because midwifery education in the Netherlands remains *outside* the university. The number of students admitted to the four schools of midwifery is deliberately limited in order to guarantee every trained midwife a job (Van Teijlingen 1994: 146). In the late 1990s, approximately 1,000 applicants applied for the combined 120 openings for first-year students (Rooks 1997: 14). The schools use a modified lottery system to select those to be admitted: candidates are screened, and those who are approved are put into a pool from which names are drawn.

In 1994, a fourth year was added to the midwifery curriculum. During their four years of midwifery school, students are trained in antenatal and postnatal care; the management of normal, physiological births both at home and in the polyclinic; the identification of high-risk situations in the antepartum, intrapartum, and postpartum periods; and techniques of scientific research. Midwifery students spend about half of their education learning in the classroom and at the "bedside" (i.e., in clinical settings) and the other half apprenticing with a qualified midwife. Skills training is an important part of the curriculum, with particular emphasis on (1) diagnostic, (2) therapeutic, (3) laboratory, and (4) social skills, as well as (5) skills needed to manage pregnancies.

The way midwives work is also changing (see Table 1.5). Until the 1980s, less than 10 percent of midwives worked in group practices; most worked single-handedly and were on call 24/7. This way of working offered a high level of career continuity. The pregnant woman could be fairly certain that her own midwife would attend all antepartum care, attend the birth, and provide the postpartum checkups. Just two and a half decades later, the overwhelming majority of Dutch midwives work in group practices of three or more midwives. The move to group practice is a reasonable strategy for midwives who want to create a more balanced life, but it subtly alters the relationship between midwives and mothers.

BUT WHY? THE CULTURAL FOUNDATIONS OF DUTCH MATERNITY CARE

These structural features provide a fine, sociological explanation of Dutch maternity care, but they cannot tell the whole story. We still must ask, Why did the Dutch create these structures to support home birth when, everywhere else in the world of modern obstetrics, birth at home was largely abandoned? To answer *that* question we must look beyond structures to the culture of the Netherlands. There is simply no other way to explain the Dutch way of birth. The foundations of Dutch maternity care rest in cultural ideas that are peculiar to the Dutch: ideas about the family, about women, about home, about bodies and the efficacy of medical treatment, about thriftiness, about heroes, about solidarity. We consider each of these in turn.

The Dutch were the first among modern nations to experience the "nuclearization" of the family. The Dutch family nuclearized in the late seventeenth and early eighteenth centuries, earlier than the rest of continental Europe, a peculiarity that is confirmed in the language. Dutch is the only Germanic language with a unique word for the nuclear family: *gezin*. Furthermore, as the wives of farmers, fishers, and traders—the primary occupations in the Netherlands—Dutch women have been tied, both economically and ideologically, to home and family. The strong identification of femininity with home and with the *gezin* is reflected in their historically high fertility rates and their low rates of participation in paid employment. How has this fact affected birth practices?

According to Dutch sociologist Van Daalen (1988, 1993), the unique features of Dutch family life created and maintain a preference for home birth. She points out that in other European countries, the nuclearization of the family occurred simultaneously with industrialization and was marked by the increasing use of professional help for events once attended by family members: birth, sickness, and death. Having nuclearized earlier, the Dutch family resisted the institutionalization of birth and death. An effort in the early nineteenth century to establish maternity clinics in Rotterdam was deemed by the city council to be inappropriate because the very idea of giving birth outside of the home was in opposition to the "national character." Incidentally, these distinctive Dutch ideas about the family also explain a few present-day oddities of family life in the Netherlands, including the limited use of professional childcare by Dutch parents and the less-than-generous policies for maternity leave of an otherwise progressive government. The care of children is work that is to be done within the family, not farmed out to childcare professionals.

Domestic confinements also fit well with Dutch ideas about home. According to Rybcinski (1986), the Dutch are responsible for our current notions of "home" as a place of retreat for the nuclear family. For a variety of social, economic, and geographic reasons, the Dutch were the first to develop single-family residences—small, tidy, well-lit homes—ideally suited for the *gezin*. The importance of the nuclear family, coupled with the domestic role of women and the tidiness of their homes, made home the logical place for birth. When Dutch women and men are asked why they prefer birth at home to birth in the hospital, they will often reply that home birth is more *gezellig*. *Gezelligheid* is often translated as "coziness," but in fact there is no single English word that captures the full meaning of the term. *Cozy* comes close, but *gezellig* also implies warmth, affection, contentment, enjoyment, happiness, sociability, snugness, and security. For the Dutch, birth at home is *gezellig* in a way birth in the hospital never can be.

Home birth fits well with Dutch ideas about medicine and science and with Dutch notions of "thriftiness." The Dutch are not quick to seek medical solutions to bodily problems, a fact evidenced by their low use of medications. Compared to their European neighbors, the Dutch go to the doctor less and use fewer prescribed and over-the-counter medications. Furthermore, Dutch public policy is characterized by rationalist ideas about the use of science in the formation of public policy, leading to the avoidance of moralistic stances and to an institutionalized willingness to experiment with new approaches to health (and social) policy that test their efficacy and efficiency. This frame of mind shapes Dutch policy on soft drugs, prostitution, euthanasia, *and* the location of births. The government has funded many studies to examine the safety, cost, and desirability of home births, and has made policy decisions based on those studies.

Dutch ideas about heroes also seep into maternity care policies. The Dutch are disinclined to celebrate the heroic, a fact that is evidenced by the absence of large monuments in their cities. Dutch children are still reminded, "Doe maar gewoon, dan doe je al gek genoeg" ("Just behave normally, that is crazy enough"), and "Kom niet boven het maaiveld" ("Don't stick out above the mown field," implying that if you do, you might get your head cut off). Gynecology in the Netherlands reflects this Dutch tendency to downplay the heroic. In marked contrast to U.S. obstetricians—who are *inclined* to heroic interventions, rescuing a laboring woman from protracted pain and life-threatening complications with surgery (episiotomies, forceps, and cesarean sections) or medications—gynecologists in the Netherlands shun the role of hero. During interviews, De Vries noticed that several Dutch gynecologists went out of their way to mention that they do not take a heroic approach to birth. The following is typical:

Q: *De Vries: Why is the Dutch maternity system so different?*

A: Gynecologist: I think maybe it has a lot to do with the history of our country. We always have been very individual, self-assured, emancipated people; a little bit mistrusting anyone . . . including doctors. I always say hospitals are dangerous. . . . And maybe it has to do with the character of the people, that the doctors think with a little bit of relativity about their own duties and possibilities. We are not so much heroes, we do our best. That's the difference. [When you play the hero] you don't let [your patients] grow. [You should] just play your role in a very simple way. . . . You're there, like a tiger sleeping in the sun, I sometimes say. With just one eye open to do the correct thing in the right time. Just a moment, and then you sleep again.

This cultural disinclination toward obstetric heroism is sustained by a system that minimizes competition among gynecologists and between gynecologists and midwives. In market systems, obstetrician/gynecologists have an incentive to sell their "superiority" as the heroes of birth.

Finally, like many other European nations, the Dutch value "solidarity," the responsibility of all for each other. The idea of a guaranteed basic package of benefits, of controls on the price/cost of services, and of limited access to certain services works in the Netherlands in a way that is impossible to imagine in the more individualistic, market-driven United States. Some say that European notions of solidarity are the product of two world wars that required cooperation for daily survival. Dutch solidarity is often linked to the "polder model" of economic and social organization—a model that takes its name from the kind of cooperation needed to keep the polders[10] from flooding. The polder model is characterized by ongoing and constructive dialogue between employers, trade unions, and the government, and it is credited with reducing government debt, lowering the overall tax burden, and strengthening the market economy. This attitude of solidarity allows the Dutch to see their own health care in the context of the larger system ("If I demand specialist care for my normal birth, it will drive the cost of health care up and reduce access for others") and promotes cooperation between different caregivers in the health care (and maternity care) system.

THE FUTURE OF MIDWIFERY AND HOME BIRTH IN THE NETHERLANDS

In November 1999 one of us (De Vries) had a conversation about the future of midwifery and home birth in the Netherlands with a well-known Dutch health researcher. His comments reflected a level of concern, indeed of pessimism, shared by many at that time. He is a strong supporter of the Dutch obstetric system and an advocate for home birth, yet he said: "Heine was right. Other nations abandoned home birth fifty years ago and now the Dutch are finally following their lead. In five years it is over . . . there will be no home birth in the Netherlands." Time has proven him wrong, but are his worries about the future of birth in the Netherlands legitimate? Given the favorable geographic, structural, political, and cultural climate for midwifery and home birth in the Netherlands, and given the fact that the percentage of births occurring at home seems to have stabilized at around 30 percent, should supporters of the Dutch model be concerned?

Having looked at the factors that helped sustain the system, let us briefly consider the developments that are pushing the Dutch to seek maternity care in hospitals: lessons learned here are particularly pertinent for those who want to make their obstetric/midwifery systems less medical. The steepest decline in home births occurred in the 1970s (see Table 1.1); some suggest this move to the hospital was largely the result of a government decision to allow healthy women the option of a short-stay hospital birth (i.e., a polyclinic birth).[11] But this policy decision alone cannot account for the decreased popularity of midwife-assisted birth at home: other trends in society encouraged women and midwives to choose this option. For example, increased use of hospital birth is associated with Dutch women's increased level of participation in paid labor. It is true that Dutch women participate in the paid labor force at lower rates than do women in other industrialized countries; however, it is also true that their participation rates have risen rapidly over the past twenty years (see Pott-Buter 1993; Henkens, Grift, and Siegers 2002). This upward trend has resulted in an increase in older mothers (who have a greater likelihood of being diagnosed with a "complication" than do younger mothers), a decrease in fertility, and changing notions of the family and the woman's place in it. For many working women, the hospital seems a convenient choice, a respite from the duties of their job and the chores of housekeeping.

Interviews with expectant parents show that Dutch attitudes toward birth are becoming more like those in other countries. When asked why they chose a polyclinic birth, parents who had done so expressed attitudes toward home and technology similar to those expressed in surrounding lands. The most common reasons for not staying home for birth are *te veel rommel* (too much mess) and the desire to have *alles bij de hand* (emergency equipment readily available) (see Wiegers 1997). Dutch women are increasingly choosing the "convenience" of institutionalized birth over the *gezelligheid* of home birth. These developments suggest that there may be a further decline in midwife-assisted home birth.

The Dutch response to these changes suggests what must be done to export the Dutch way of birth to other countries. Today, all the forces that have shaped midwifery in other countries exist in the Netherlands: medical technology and hospital efficiency are being used to achieve the (professional) goals of medical specialists and to meet the needs of a new generation of clients. The Dutch government, midwives, and consumer groups have responded by calling on the unique cultural and structural features of Dutch society described above to create policy and organize consumer campaigns. Government support for midwifery and home birth remains strong, as evidenced by recent decisions to train more midwives, to increase their salaries, and to reduce the *normpraktijk* (i.e., the number of births a midwife is expected to attend each year).[12] In these efforts to protect midwives and birth at home, the Dutch show the way forward for midwives elsewhere, offering a model of how to weather social change and social conditions that seem incompatible with a strong profession of midwifery.

It is for us to discover features of our societies and our cultures that favor midwives and the healthier, more satisfying births they offer. In the United States, for example, advocates of home birth and midwives can build on the American obsession with health and fitness: it is a cultural contradiction that pregnant women in the United States will do so much to ensure the health of the fetus and then, at the moment of birth, subject the baby to all the dangers of the drugs and devices of modern medicine. Birth activists should seize on this contradiction and use it as a wedge to open a policy conversation about the costly, impersonal, and dangerous way of birth in the United States. Those in other countries must look for similar cracks in the system, places where cultural values and policy objectives can be used to promote the safe, sane approach to birth offered by midwives. This kind of activism will help midwifery regain its rightful place as the standard of care for pregnancy and birth.

Vanguard or vestige? There are those—both outside and inside the Netherlands—who are convinced that the Dutch way of birth is nothing more than a vestige, a remnant from an earlier period in history. We believe

Information for Foreigners

The following list of sites is adapted from the English website
for the Royal Dutch Organisation of Midwives (KNOV):
http://www.verloskundigeninnederland.nl/home/%5Fservice/
information%5Ffor%5Fforeigners/.

Registratie en Informatie Beroepsgroepen in de Zorg
   (http://www.ribiz.nl/): Helps people with foreign health care qualifications who wish to practice their profession in the Netherlands
   by directing them to the right institutions. This site informs you
   about the available possibilities.

The Verloskunde Academie Amsterdam
   (http://www.verloskunde-academie.nl/default.aspx): Helps people
   with foreign midwifery qualifications with assessments and education.

Midwives Information and Resource Centre (MIDIRS)
   (http://www.midirs.org/): An educational not-for-profit organization that aims to be the central source of information relating to
   childbirth.

International Confederation of Midwives
   (http://www.internationalmidwives.org/): An international
   non-governmental organization that unites eighty-five national
   midwives' associations from over seventy-five countries.

European Midwives Association (EMA)
   (http://www.europeanmidwives.org/): An association that aims to
   represent all midwives in the EU and the wider European area.

Parenting in Holland
   (http://www.parentinginholland.com/): Information in English,
   for people living in the Netherlands, about pregnancy, birth,
   and parenting issues. (This site is not related to the Royal Dutch
   Organisation of Midwives, which takes no responsibility for the
   content in this site.)

that midwifery in the Netherlands is *not* just another quaint feature of the
lowlands, akin to wooden shoes, destined to disappear from everyday practice. It is a way of birth that is closely tied to both cultural and structural
features of Dutch society, a way of birth that can serve as a vanguard for
midwives elsewhere, if midwives and their supporters will connect midwifery
to features of their own local and national cultures.

ACKNOWLEDGMENTS

This work was supported by grants from the Fogarty Center of the National Institutes of Health (Grant number Fo6-TWo1954), the Netherlands Institute for Health Services Research (NIVEL), the Catharina Schrader Stichting (Utrecht, the Netherlands), and several faculty development grants from St. Olaf College.

NOTES

1. Midwives in several Scandinavian countries have a great deal of independence, but nothing like the independence associated with attending births at home, away from the watchful eyes of obstetrician/gynecologists.

2. In Dutch, the term "polyclinic birth" (*poliklinische bevalling*) refers to a short-stay birth (fewer than twenty-four hours) that occurs in a hospital and is attended by a midwife or a general practitioner. A polyclinic birth takes place in a birthing room at the hospital, without referral to specialist care and therefore without formal admission to the hospital. Midwives (and GPs) can use the hospital birthing rooms for their clients, but they do not have admitting privileges. By way of a contrast, a "hospital birth" occurs after referral by a gynecologist: the birthing woman is formally admitted to hospital and gives birth in the clinic under specialist supervision. A curious fact of the Dutch system is that a polyclinic birth and a hospital birth may occur in the same bed—the difference is in the caregiver who accompanies the birth, and in fact, a hospital birth without complications can be counted as a polyclinic birth if the woman returns home within a few hours.

3. From *Bevallen en Opstaan*, Spanjer et al. 1994: 366–67.

4. Infant mortality rates offer an admittedly rough measure of the quality of a perinatal care system including pre- and postnatal care. Neonatal mortality rates are a measure of care at and before birth, but are less available for comparison (see Declercq and Viisainen 2001).

5. This contrasts strongly with countries where obstetricians are reimbursed for care of healthy women, a structural condition that immediately creates competition between specialists and midwives.

6. The closing of smaller hospitals in the last few years has made access to backup care more difficult, causing some to worry about the future of home birth in the Netherlands (see Wiegers, Hingstman, and Van der Zee 2000; Bleker 2000).

7. See Bleker et al. 2005 and De Vries 2005: 116–37 for more detail. An English-language version of the new list, the *Verloskundig Vademecu*, is available at http://www.jiscmail.ac.uk/files/MIDWIFERY-RESEARCH/official_dutch_obstetric_guidelines or http://europe.obgyn.net/nederland/default.asp?page=/nederland/richtlijnen/vademecum_eng.

8. For more complete accounts of the fascinating history of Dutch midwives, see Lieburg and Marland 1989; Marland 1987, 1993a, 1993b, 1995; Van der Borg 1992; Drenth 1998; and Schama 1988: 481–562.

9. In Sweden, where contemporary midwives have a great deal of autonomy in the clinic, municipal regulation and training began in the seventeenth century (see Romlid 1997).

10. A polder is a large area of land below sea level, protected by dikes and kept dry by pumping the water out.

11. Ironically, the government made this decision in an effort to forestall the decline of births at home. Government officials believed that the growing popularity of gynecologist-assisted hospital births was the result of women "inventing" complications because they wanted to be in a hospital. These officials reasoned that if women with no complications were allowed to choose a hospital birth, then more of them would stay under the care of midwives and general practitioners.

12. The *normpraktijk* is a hypothetical number on which fees for service are based. The fees for an equivalent of 120 births will provide a midwife with an income that is regarded as proper for a full-time working professional.

REFERENCES

Anthony S., M.P. Amelink-Verburg, G.W. Jacobusse, and K.M. van der Pal-de Bruin. 2005. *De thuisbevalling in Nederland, 1995–2002. Rapportage over de jaren 2001–2002.* Bilthoven/Leiden: SPRN/TNO.

Benoit, C., S. Wrede, I. Bourgeault, J. Sandall, R. De Vries, and E. van Teijlingen. 2005. "Understanding the Social Organisation of Maternity Care Systems: Midwifery as a Touchstone." *Sociology of Health and Illness* 27.6:722–37.

Bleker, O.P. 2000. "Verloskundige zorg" [Midwife Care]. *Medisch Contact* 55.35: 1206–1208.

Bleker, O., L.A. m. van der Hulst, M. Eskes, and. G.J. Bonsel. 2005. "Place of Birth: Evidence for Best Practice." In *Recent Advances in Obstetrics and Gynaecology,* vol. 23, edited by J. Bonnar and W. Dunlop, 77–100. London: Royal Society of Medicine Press.

Davis-Floyd, R. 2003. "Home Birth Emergencies in the U.S. and Mexico: The Trouble with Transport." *Social Science and Medicine* 56.9:1913–31.

Declercq, E., and K. Viisainen. 2001. "The Politics of Numbers: The Promise and Frustration of Cross-National Analysis." In *Birth by Design: Pregnancy, Maternity Care, and Midwifery in North America and Europe,* edited by R. De Vries, C. Benoit, E. van Teijlingen, and S. Wrede New York: Routledge.

De Vries, R. 1996. *Making Midwives Legal.* Columbus: Ohio State University Press.

———. 2005. *A Pleasing Birth: Midwives and Maternity Care in the Netherlands.* Philadelphia: Temple University Press.

De Vries, R., C. Benoit, E. van Teijlingen, and S. Wrede (eds). 2001. *Birth by Design: Pregnancy, Maternity Care, and Midwifery in North America and Europe.* New York: Routledge.

De Vries, R., S. Wrede, E. van Teijlingen, C. Benoit, and E. Declercq. 2004. "Making Maternity Care: The Consequences of Culture for Health Care Systems." In *Comparing Cultures: Dimensions of Culture in a Comparative Perspective,* edited by H. Vinken, J. Soeters, and P. Ester, 209–231. Leiden: Brill Academic Publishers.

Drenth, P. 1998. *1898/1998: 100 jaar vroedvrouwen verenigd* [1989/1998: 100 Years of Midwives United]. Bilthoven: Nederlandse Organsatie van Verloskundigen.

Henkens, K., Y. Grift, and J. Siegers. 2002. "Changes in Female Labour Supply in the Netherlands, 1989–1998: The Case of Married and Cohabiting Women." *European Journal of Population* 18:139–57.

Hingstman, L., and R.J. Kenens. 2007a. *Cijfers uit de Registratie van Verloskundige: Peiling 2007.* Utrecht: NIVEL.

———. 2007b. *Cijfers uit de Registratie van Huisartsen: Peiling 2007.* Utrecht: NIVEL.

Lieburg, M., and H. Marland. 1989. "Midwife Regulation, Education and Practice in the Netherlands during the Nineteenth Century." *Medical History* 33:296–317.

Marland, H. (ed.). 1987. *Mother and Child Were Saved: The Memoirs (1693–1740) of the Frisian Midwife Catharina Schrader.* Amsterdam: Roldopi.

———. 1993a. "The Guardians of Normal Birth: The Debate on the Standard and Status of the Midwife in the Netherlands around 1900." In *Successful Home Birth and Midwifery: The Dutch Model*, edited by E. Abraham-Van der Mark, 21–44. Westport, CT: Bergin and Garvey.

———. 1993b. "The '*burgerlijke*' Midwife: The *stadsvroedvrouw* of Eighteenth-Century Holland." In *The Art of Midwifery Early Modern Midwives in Europe*, edited by H. Marland, 192–213. New York: Routledge.

———. 1995. "Questions of Competence: The Midwife Debate in the Netherlands in the Early Twentieth Century." *Medical History* 39:317–37.

Martin, J.A., B.E. Hamilton, P.D. Sutton, S.J. Ventura, F. Menacker, and M.L. Munson. 2005. "Births: Final Data for 2003." *National Vital Statistics Reports* 54.2. Hyattsville, MD: National Center for Health Statistics.

Mehl-Madrona, M., and L. Mehl-Madrona. 1993. "The Future of Midwifery in the United States." *NAPSAC News* 18.3–4:1–32.

Pasveer, B., and M. Akrich. 2001. "Obstetrical Trajectories: On Training Women/ Bodies for (Home) Birth." In *Birth by Design: Pregnancy, Maternity Care, and Midwifery in North America and Europe*, edited by R. De Vries, C. Benoit, E. van Teijlingen, and S. Wrede, 229–42. New York: Routledge.

Pott-Buter, H. 1993. *Facts and Fairy Tales about Female Labor, Family and Fertility.* Amsterdam: University of Amsterdam Press.

Romlid, C. 1997. "Swedish Midwives and Their Instruments in Eighteenth and Nineteenth Centuries." In *Midwives, Society and Childbirth: Debates and Controversies in the Modern Period*, edited by H. Marland and S. Rafferty, 38–60. London: Routledge.

Rooks, J. 1997. *Midwifery and Childbirth in America.* Philadelphia: Temple University Press.

Rothman, B. K. 1993. "Going Dutch: Lessons for Americans." In *Successful Home Birth and Midwifery: The Dutch Model*, edited by E. Abraham-Van der Mark, 201–11. Westport, CT: Bergin and Garvey.

Rybczynksi, W. 1986. *Home.* New York: Penguin.

Schama, S. 1988. *The Embarrassment of Riches: An Interpretation of Dutch Culture in the Golden Age.* Berkeley: University of California Press.

Schiet, M. 1994. "Bevallen in het buitenland" [Birthing in Other Countries]. *In Verwachting* [Expecting] 1:112–113.

Spanjer, J., E. de Haan, H. Dijk, L. Poortman, A. Gorter, M. de Waal, M. de Jong, and H. Hagens. 1994. *Bevallen en Opstaan* [Birthing and Uprising]. Amsterdam: Uitgeverij Contact.

Van Daalen, R. 1988. "De groei van de ziekenhuisbevalling: Nederland en het buitenland" [The Growth of Hospital Birth: The Netherlands and Elsewhere]. *Amsterdams Sociologisch Tijdschrift* 15.3:414–45.

————. 1993. "Family Change and Continuity in the Netherlands: Birth and Child-bed in Text and Art." In *Successful Home Birth and Midwifery: The Dutch Model*, edited by E. Abraham-Van der Mark, 77–94. Westport, CT: Bergin and Garvey.

Van der Borg, H. A. 1992. *Vroedvrouwen: Beeld en Beroep* [Midwives: Image and Profession]. Wageningen: Wageningen Academic Press.

Van der Velden, L.F.J., L. Hingstman, W. van der Windt, and E.J.E. Arnold. 2008. *Raming benodigde instroom per medische en tandheelkundige vervolgopleiding 2009–2019/2015*. Utrecht: NIVEL.

Van der Velden, L.F.J., C.J. Vugts, and L. Hingstman. 2004. *Monitor arbeidsmarkt gynaecologe, Behoefteraming, 2001–2015: Tussenbalans 2003*. [Monitor Labor Market Gynecologists, Needs Assessment, 2001–2015: Intern Assessment 2003]. Utrecht: NIVEL.

Van Teijlingen, E. 1994. "A Social or Medical Model of Childbirth? Comparing the Arguments in Grampian (Scotland) and the Netherlands." Ph.D. thesis, University of Aberdeen.

————. 2003. "Dutch Midwives: The Difference between Image and Reality." In *Gender, Identity and Reproduction: Social Perspectives*, edited by S. Earle and G. Letherby, 120–34. London: Palgrave.

Van Teijlingen, E., G. Lowis, P. McCaffery, and M. Porter (eds.). 2004. *Midwifery and the Medicalization of Childbirth: Comparative Perspectives*. Hauppauge, NY: Nova Science.

Wiegers, T.A. 1997 "Home or Hospital Birth: A Prospective Study of Midwifery Care in the Netherlands." Ph.D. thesis, Leiden University. Utrecht: NIVEL.

————. 2006. "Adjusting to Motherhood: Maternity Care Assistance during the Postpartum Period: How to Help New Mothers Cope." *Journal of Neonatal Nursing* 12:163–71.

Wiegers, T.A., L. Hingstman, and J. van der Zee. 2000. "Thuisbevalling in gevaar" [Home Birth in Danger]. *Medisch Contact* 55.19:701–04.

Wiegers, T. A., and Janssen, B. M. 2006. *Monitor Verloskundige Zorgverlening; Eindrapport* [Monitor Maternity Care: Final Report]. Utrecht: NIVEL.

Chapter 2

The New Zealand Maternity System
A *Midwifery Renaissance*

Chris Hendry

INTRODUCTION

New Zealand is a small country with a population of just over 4 million people. We live in relative geographic isolation on two main islands (with a combined land mass greater than the United Kingdom) in the Southern Pacific Ocean, three hours flight time from Australia, which is our nearest neighbor. As a nation, we see ourselves as fiercely independent, yet we have a critical dependence on the vagaries of international markets for income from the sale of our products, mainly consumables, manufacturing, and increasingly, tourism. Politically, we tend toward the center left and pride ourselves on our anti-nuclear stance and our affinity with nature and ecology. We have a long history of government-funded social services such as the provision of health care and education, including that of health professionals such as doctors and midwives. Over the years, these combined features have supported the development of many social and political innovations that have been viewed as revolutionary by other nations. Our maternity service is no exception.

The main objective of this chapter is to present the development of the New Zealand model of maternity care, which has been predominantly midwifery led. This model of care has evolved over the past eighteen years and continues to evolve. Had it not been for initial legislation in 1990 enabling midwives to access government funding independently from the medical profession for the provision of maternity care, it is unlikely that such a model would have developed and been sustained. In the 1970s and 1980s, a group of consumers and activist midwives, dissatisfied with the increasing medicalization of maternity care, were the catalysts for change. Many of the midwives and a number of the consumers have remained active in political and professional leadership of women's health and midwifery since that time.

Midwifery in this country has continued to "push the boundaries" of women-centered maternity care, mainly, I believe, because of the home- and community-based nature of the services and because women have increasingly chosen midwives over medical practitioners as the preferred providers of primary (uncomplicated) maternity care. Over time, almost all general medical practitioners other than obstetric medical specialists have opted out of the direct provision of maternity care, and midwives have enthusiastically taken over the service.

At this point, it would be useful to introduce myself and declare my ongoing interest in the provision of maternity services by midwives. I have lived in the South Island of New Zealand all my life. In my thirty-year midwifery career, I have had many experiences in this country's maternity services, from consumer through to practitioner and midwife manager. In 1994 I worked with midwifery colleagues in the New Zealand College of Midwives (NZCOM) to set up one of the first hospital-funded continuity of midwifery care teams. This small unit within a general hospital in Christchurch has maintained its delivery of midwife-led services to the present day.

I have also been involved in midwifery education over the years, and combined my practice with my own study, ultimately completing a doctorate in 2003 with a thesis on the provision of maternity services by midwives in New Zealand. I am currently involved in the midwifery profession in a number of leadership roles centered on the logistics of maternity service provision, including as part-time Executive Director of the national Midwifery and Maternity Providers Organization (MMPO), which provides practice management support to about 80% of New Zealand's caseload midwives.

In case others are thinking of replicating the New Zealand model, it is important to understand the context of maternity service provision in this country. It is unique. Our maternity service is not provided in isolation from other health services, nor without a history that has had a profound impact on service development and relationships with other professions. Understanding the drivers of change that produced the various aspects of this model may be more important than obtaining a recipe for transplanting this model to "foreign" soil. Crucial factors in the development and success of the New Zealand midwifery model include (1) the groundwork of legislative and/or regulative change; (2) the political astuteness and determination of midwife leaders and home birth consumers presenting a united front; (3) the desire and ability of midwives to embrace change and work differently. [Editors' note: These factors have also proven critical to success in other regional models described in this book, including those in the Netherlands (Chapter 1) and Ontario (Chapter 3), and in the recent success of midwives in various U.S. states and other Canadian provinces in achieving legalization and licensure (Chapter 9; Davis-Floyd and Johnson 2006; Bourgeault, Benoit, and Davis-Floyd 2004).]

THE NEW ZEALAND CONTEXT

Much of the uniqueness of New Zealand maternity service provision stems from a number of features of New Zealand's culture and environment that have both required and enabled unique health service developments to occur. Our geographic isolation along with the sparse and widely spread population provide real challenges to traditional notions of health service provision, particularly that of a tertiary service centered around a large hospital/university complex. For example, as part of my research, I worked with midwives in small rural settings who, even in the best of weather, would take two to three hours to complete an ambulance ride to reach a hospital and who cannot transfer women to a hospital easily in winter because of low clouds, snow, and road closures. These geographic realities, which favor the development of alternative health service delivery, coupled with our small population, enable us to get to know and influence politicians—an ability that has enabled deep-seated and universal change to occur within a relatively short space of time.

To understand the potential for change, it is useful to gain a little insight into the political system. In New Zealand, political power is centralized within a one-house national parliament—a feature that makes possible rapid and comprehensive legislative changes (Blank 1994). Health services are predominantly publicly funded, and have been shaped over the years by the philosophy of the political party in power at the time. We have a long history of government-subsidized health care (Cheyne, O'Brien, and Belgrave 1997), with most health care providers (including midwives) dependent on the government for the bulk of their income.

Over the years, consumer expectations of free or low-cost health care have been fostered, and accordingly, private health insurance has not been a popular option for citizens who believe that "the state will provide." This contrasts strongly with our near neighbor, Australia, where private health insurance has fueled obstetric inroads into normal, healthy birth.

From an economic perspective, the situation of public dependence on the state for health care became an increasing burden on the government.

The Role of Midwives in the Decades Leading Up to the 1990 Changes

From the mid 1930s until 1990, almost all birthing women in New Zealand maternity hospitals had midwives care for them during labor and childbirth. The women generally received their antenatal care from the local family doctor (GP) or in an antenatal clinic, which was run by the local maternity hospital. The doctor (either an obstetrician or GP) would see a woman periodically during pregnancy. Midwives carried out "booking" visits antenatally, in which they assessed women for risk in relation to choice of birth place (primary low-risk unit or obstetric hospital). The doctor would instruct the woman to go to the hospital when labor began, and a midwife would meet the woman at the door; take her to a prep room for a pubic shave and enema; carry out an assessment, including abdominal palpation and vaginal examination; and then call the doctor with a progress report. The doctor might or might not call in, depending on the woman's progress and his comfort with the midwife's skills.

Following this first contact with the doctor, midwives or student midwives cared for women intrapartally, generally only calling the doctor again when birth was imminent or progress was delayed for some reason. Often the doctor would instruct the midwife over the phone. Thus, in a sense, midwives worked relatively autonomously, particularly in primary (low-risk) birthing units. And the doctors were on to a financial winner: the midwives generally did all the work, with the doctors coming in at the last minute so they could clock in and earn their (publicly funded) fee. It was my experience, both personally as a birthing woman and as a midwife in the 1970s, that many women thought this was a "rip-off," and actually asked the midwife *not* to call the doctor, just to carry on and assist them to birth the baby. Midwives were obliged to call the doctor in for the birth, but depending on the woman's wishes, could choose not to be in a rush to do it so that the mother could give birth before the doctor arrived. So when the law changed, women naturally wanted a midwife because they knew the midwife would be with them for the long haul, but the doctor would not.

Obstetricians really worked only in the base obstetric hospitals, not in the eighty or so primary maternity units where most healthy women birthed. GPs provided the medical cover in these facilities, doing forceps births and (often routine) episiotomies, and suturing perinea.

A shift in economic stability that occurred for New Zealand in the early 1980s prompted the government of the day to plan for a severe reduction in public expenditure. One area targeted was the heavily subsidized health service. Attempts were made and elections were lost trying to dilute the dependence on the state for health and social services that had been nurtured over the previous fifty years.

It was within this environment that the government promoted "managed competition" (Cheyne, O'Brien, and Belgrave 1997: 227) as a model for health service provision in New Zealand. Maternity services were to provide a very clear demonstration of this model in action. From 1990 on, when women had the choice of either a doctor or midwife as the main clinician providing maternity care, free of charge, women quickly chose midwives over doctors. Most midwives, because of their familiarity with hospital systems, also continued as advocate and midwifery care provider even if a woman developed complications. General practitioners (GPs) were not generally able to offer this service. By 2003 (Ministry of Health 2006), the majority of pregnant women in New Zealand, 78.1%, chose a midwife as their Lead Maternity Carer.

In 1990 "consumer choice" was the marketing strategy that sold the notion of "competition" to the public. As a result, midwives became the dominant providers of primary maternity care and increasingly continued providing the midwifery component of care even when their clients experienced complications in pregnancy or birth, requiring specialist medical care. Thus, women began to experience a greater degree of continuity of care from midwives than from GPs, who handed over care of the woman to the obstetric specialist service if complications arose (in the obstetric specialist service, women were cared for by the midwife on duty at the time).

A greater proportion of Maori, New Zealand's indigenous group, had birthed in rural and primary maternity units and thus generally managed to avoid the level of medicalization experienced by non-Maori. In other words, Maori were predominantly attended by midwives, with doctors popping in to be present at the birth. Following the 1990 legislative changes, Maori could more legitimately birth closer to home with a midwife. Maori midwives are few in number and thus have tended to be overwhelmed by providing services for Maori women and *whanau* (family), who have twice the birth rate of non-Maori. For some midwives, this has led to burnout and a short working life, something that Maori, through Nga Maia, the national Maori midwives' group, with support from the New Zealand College of Midwives, are trying to address. The issue of the impact of the midwifery renaissance on Maori midwives is a story more appropriately told by Maori midwives themselves.

Home Birth as a Rallying Point

There were few incentives to provide home birth midwifery services in New Zealand pre-1990. Consumers within this subsidized health service environment did not expect to pay directly for services, and midwives were prevented from charging for services if they received any public funding. Midwives were entitled to some funding for "domiciliary confinements" (home births), but the income they were entitled to was significantly lower than that paid to midwives employed within hospitals. To birth a woman at home, a registered midwife was also required by law to have a doctor in attendance. Over time, the number of midwives available to birth women at home and doctors willing to "supervise" diminished.

By 1977 there were estimated to be only 176 planned home births in the country, equating to about 0.3% of all births (Donley 1998a). This situation prompted a group of Auckland parents to form the Home Birth Association in 1978, with a vision toward making home birth a viable choice for women. Within two years, there were branches of this organization throughout the country, and the first national Home Birth Association conference was held. Beginning in 1980, this organization began to form close links with other women's consumer groups and became a major force behind the establishment of the New Zealand College of Midwives.

Joan Donley was an early midwife leader who, through her involvement in home birth, formed an active partnership with the consumers. Joan provided one of the earliest examples of the power of a midwifery partnership with women. Her connections with the community also enabled her to influence local politicians, one of whom was later to become the Minister of Health and shepherd through the 1990 legislative changes that paved the way for midwifery autonomy from both nursing and medicine.

THE HISTORY OF MIDWIFERY IN NEW ZEALAND

Midwives were first registered in this country in 1904, initially as a community-based profession. But the transition of birthing from home to hospital in the 1920s and 1930s quickly saw the profession become institutionalized and dominated by medicine and later by nursing. The 1970s and 1980s were particularly hard times for those identifying themselves as midwives. In 1971 a Nurses Amendment Act required all births to be supervised by a doctor—a requirement with the potential to effectively eliminate the need to have a midwife at all. In 1976 the Maternity Services Committee set up by the Board of Health published a document condemning home birth as endangering the safety of babies (Health Funding Authority 2000).

By the 1980s midwifery in New Zealand had literally and practically been subsumed under nursing, following the Nurses Act in 1977 that implicitly defined midwifery as "obstetric nursing" (Pairman 1998). The underpinning philosophy supporting this move was acceptance of institutionalized childbearing and the "technical assistant" role (Donley 1998a) expected of the midwife/nurse in the running of an efficient maternity hospital.

In 1982 a Board of Health report called for domiciliary midwives to be certified by a senior obstetrician in the hospitals (Health Funding Authority 2000). In 1983 further erosions to the scope and practice of midwifery occurred through amendments to the Nurses Act, preventing midwives who were not also registered nurses from attending births in any place other than a hospital. This legislation also enabled registered nurses to practice within areas that were previously the domain of the midwife. These actions were viewed as a direct response to a midwifery workforce crisis, exacerbated by a rising birth rate and the lack of nurses choosing to enter the one-year, polytechnic-based midwifery registration program (Guilliland 1998).

Nurses were not used to paying for their education, so most refused to take time away from their employment to complete midwifery training. At the time, midwifery training was a fee-paying, full-time course of study. This refusal by the nurses had a profound effect on resources available for midwifery education, which further reduced the attractiveness of the programs. Few midwives registered in New Zealand out of these nursing/midwifery education programs during the 1980s.

Although the 1983 Nurses Amendment Act posed a huge threat to the continued existence of midwifery in New Zealand, it ultimately served as a catalyst in the reemergence of midwifery as a profession separate from nursing (Donley 1998b; Pairman 1998; Abel 1997). Midwife members of the New Zealand Nurses Association (NZNA), the only recognized voice of the profession, were feeling betrayed by nurses as a result of the 1983 legislation, and were becoming more active and vocal in supporting midwifery.

Later that year, a consumer pressure group was formed out of the Homebirth Association, called Save the Midwives. In 1986 the coordinator of this group, Judi Strid, was instrumental in establishing a thirteen-member taskforce with a view to getting a direct-entry midwifery course[1]

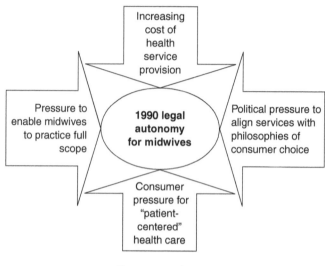

Figure 2.1. Pressures supporting the emancipation of the midwifery profession in New Zealand.

established within two years, thereby eliminating the ties between midwifery and nursing. Strid was later to reflect (Tully 1999) that at the time, there was no public awareness of midwifery at all. While running publicity campaigns as a home birth consumer at shopping malls, Strid found that although most women knew they had the option of home birth, few knew what a midwife was (see Figure 2.1).

Meantime, members of the midwives' section of the NZNA were becoming more frustrated with continued road blocks to the recognition of midwifery as a profession separate from nursing. At the 1988 Midwifery Conference in Auckland, Joan Donley, midwife and activist, challenged her colleagues to form their own professional body (Pairman 1998). The challenge was accepted, and fifty midwives and other women paid NZ$50 each to set up a task force to draft a constitution. The New Zealand College of Midwives had its inaugural annual general meeting in Christchurch in April 1989. The constitution recognized women (midwifery consumers who are not midwives) as equal members at every level of the organization—a thoroughly unique feature.

Sally Pairman, midwife educator and activist for the profession, viewed this inclusion of women within the professional body as a social

The Consumer Voice

Consumerism became an important factor in shaping political direction in New Zealand during the 1980s. The feminist movement began to critique the nature and quality of health services provided to women in the country, expressing concern that society was becoming increasingly medicalized and that too much power and responsibility were being given to the medical profession (Tulley 1999).

Mistrust of the medical profession was heightened in 1988 following a judicial inquiry into a research program that involved conservative treatment of women with cervical cancer by a professor of gynecology and obstetrics at New Zealand's largest women's hospital. It was discovered that over a period of twenty years, women were followed up but left untreated to determine whether carcinoma in situ led to invasive cancer. The women were uninformed participants in the research. The resulting national outrage and major overhaul of medical ethics processes heralded the beginning of active consumerism and an opportunity for "complementary" or "alternative" therapies to challenge the hegemony of the biomedical model (Tulley 1999).

These events fed into pressures from health service strategists, home birth groups, and increasing midwife activism to contribute to successful mobilization and to profound changes around birthing services, particularly impacting the notion of choices for heath care consumers.

mandate that carried with it "a moral obligation for the midwifery profession to provide the kind of service women want" (Pairman 1998: 11). Karen Guilliland, Pariman's friend and colleague, was elected the first chairperson of the new College, which quickly formed an effective political lobby group during a period of rapid legislative changes. These changes were aimed at increasing the autonomy of individuals and freeing up publicly funded organizations to deliver more responsive services to the community.

Within this environment of a growing midwifery voice and the acknowledgement of midwives and birthing women as political consumers, an amendment to the Nurses Act was put before Parliament in 1990, preceding the triennial political elections, by Minister of Health Helen Clark (a longtime supporter of midwifery, later to become Prime Minister). This amendment seemed fairly innocuous, for it only required three simple words—"or registered midwife"—to be added to the 1977 Nurses Act. The amendment was passed by the House, and these three words had "a profound effect on the scope of midwifery practice, payment and status" (Abel 1997: 106). The word preceding the "or registered midwife" was "doctor," thereby enabling midwives to have access to the same level of funding and resources for the provision of maternity care as doctors.

Midwives at last had a legal mandate to provide maternity care to women in any setting without requiring medical supervision. They also gained hospital and prescribing privileges previously afforded only to doctors. This new status for midwives immediately presented maternity hospitals with a unique set of challenges and potential opportunities. At the same time, the medical profession was caught unaware of the implications of this change and the profound effects it would have on them as well as on maternity services of the future. Women now had the choice of a midwife rather than a doctor to provide their personal maternity care needs.

Midwifery Emancipation

Karen Guilliland, the inaugural chairperson of the College, recalls that in the first year of legislated autonomy, fifty midwives became self-employed by moving into independent practice and claimed public funding through the Maternity Benefit (Guilliland 1998). Most of these midwives had recently been or were still currently employed by maternity hospitals. Midwives argued that if doctors could maintain public employment and privately take on clients, so could midwives. These emergent signs of competition, actively stimulated by government legislation, finally triggered action from the medical profession, which to this point had been relatively subdued (Abel 1997). Abel contends that physicians "did not anticipate the extent of the change to the midwifery scope of practice" (105).

Prior to that time, doctors had only seen midwives providing nursing-type care to women in labor and assisting with baby care and breastfeeding postnatally. They had not envisioned midwives providing complete care from early pregnancy through six weeks following the birth, and they certainly had not anticipated the popularity of this service with women. Within a very short time, the impact of the midwifery care option was demonstrated by a clear trend of women choosing midwives rather than doctors for their care in childbirth (Ministry of Health 2003).

The Midwifery Care Option

In her thesis "Doing Professionalism Differently: Negotiating Midwifery Autonomy in Aotearoa/New Zealand" (1999), Liz Tully provides insight into midwives' first attempts at establishing themselves as a community-based maternity care option. The Wellington Midwifery practice was formed by four midwives in March 1990. These midwives offered women both home birth as well as a hospital birth option, which included early discharge following the birth with midwifery care given in the home. In fact, the hospital birth option proved to be the most common choice of both women and midwives (and continues to be so to the present day).

The midwives worked in pairs, covering each other for days off and leave. They initially negotiated a contract with the local hospital to use beds (as did the doctors), and even managed to obtain some seed money from the hospital to set up their practice. The midwives note that growth in their client base was gained purely by word of mouth. For example, one described caring for a woman who worked in a bank, and before long, her practice was providing care to a continuous stream of women from that same bank: "It's when others see how wonderful the service is," said the midwife. "I have had the same thing with air traffic controllers. I had two women whose partners were air traffic controllers and have just booked a third" (Tully 1999: 150).

Health Reforms of the 1990s

Soon after the passage of the Nurses Amendment Act in 1990, there was a change of government from Labor (Left) to National (Conservative). The new government was quick to focus on health as a means of reducing public spending. In line with this philosophy and in an effort to make sense of maternity service provision within the new health climate as a whole, a key report entitled *First Steps towards an Integrated Maternity Services Framework* (New Zealand Regional Health Authorities 1993) was produced for the government and presented to the health funding agencies of the day. It emerged from a consultative process involving consumer groups and key health providers, and it recommended that childbearing should be funded publicly. The report supported a continuation of public funding (free to the consumer) for all maternity services, including the provision of maternity care by individual health practitioners, as an integrated package for women.

The new government also recognized midwives as legitimate providers of health care to childbearing women. This document was followed by

Hospital-Employed Midwives Also Embraced Change

These were exciting times for midwives, with many opportunities available to break away from traditional ways of working within the health sector. The next challenge was to change the way services were provided within the hospital for both midwives and women. In 1994, having been enthusiastically involved in the College of Midwives since its establishment five years previously, I chose to make the transition from my role as Course Supervisor and teacher in the one-year Diploma in Midwifery program for registered nurses, and return to practice.

As a consequence of a recent round of health service contracting, a fifteen-bed, suburban maternity ward situated within a suburban rehabilitation hospital became isolated from the influence and guidance of the main base obstetric hospital, thirty minutes away within the central city. The hospital management, following advice from NZCOM, decided to convert the GP-based maternity unit, which had about 500 births per year, into a fully functioning midwifery unit, with some of the employed midwives taking on caseloads and providing continuity of care for local pregnant women.

I successfully applied for the role of managing this project and worked with the midwives at great haste to make changes, in case hospital management changed their minds! Within a period of ten weeks, the ward was redesigned and refurbished, and staffing was reconfigured to start offering a new service to local women. We reduced the number of midwives per shift to one, giving others the option of managing their own caseloads of pregnant women and working more flexibly on call.

We also developed the new role of birthing unit assistant. We employed four local women to work on shifts alongside the midwife on duty in the hospital. These women took charge of the "hotel maintenance" side of the service, with complete responsibility for the food, cleaning, and linen budget. They were also charged with communications maintenance and the general smooth running of the ward, leaving the midwife time to provide collegial backup and support for the caseload midwives, particularly when women were birthing. The midwives were also more available to give midwifery advice to women in the unit, particularly on breastfeeding.

The whole way the service was provided changed. Although the ward remained our base for birthing women, the caseloading midwives provided most of the antenatal and postnatal care in the women's own homes. They got to know the women and their families. They attended women at home in early labor and came in with them into the hospital to birth. Often the whole family came. We negotiated to convert the birthing theater, which was unused because of the lack of operative births in the hospital, into a large water birthing room with a beautiful birth pool. The whole atmosphere of the ward changed over this time, with women taking charge of themselves and their care, and midwives dispensing with their uniforms—it took on a whole new look.

Even though I left in 1997 to take on other project management roles, the ward still functions in a similar way. Over the years, it has been the building ground for a number of future midwifery leaders and educators.

another, which provided more detail on how this service should be constructed, and established the philosophical framework for a major shift in the nature of maternity services in this country. The College of Midwives formed a small but effective negotiating team, including Sally Pairman and Karen Guilliland, who were informed and buoyed by strong regional networks of midwives who were already out in the community, staking their claim to this new way of working. By 1994 it is estimated that about 23% (450) of the midwifery workforce identified themselves as "independent"/ self-employed midwives (Guilliland 1998).

Our midwife leaders were becoming politically savvy and worked hard to stay well connected to government and senior bureaucrats. This was one of NZCOM's key strengths—recognizing the need for midwives and midwifery to be visible, strong, and strategic at such crucial times. The relationships these midwife leaders and the profession as a whole formed with consumers and consumer groups added strength to their cause, which was a shared vision for the provision of a woman-centered maternity service fully funded by the state.

The health reforms of the 1990s preoccupied medical practitioners, particularly those in general practice, who at the time were the main providers of community-based maternity services through to the mid-1990s. Funding for the non-maternity components of general practice came under significant review and change at this time. As the monetary value of maternity funding was significantly less than that for all other GP services, the medical practitioners put more energy into negotiating other components of the GP income than in fighting to retain maternity care. They also found it too difficult to compete with the midwife's personalized, home-based service.

Midwifery Becomes a Dominant Influence in Maternity Service Changes

Apart from a decline in birthing numbers in 2002 and 2003, there had been consistently around 57,000 births per year for the past ten years in New Zealand (Ministry of Health 2004, 2006). The maternity service is made up of obstetric and specialist medical services and around eighty maternity hospitals, forming a relatively small and very discrete component of the publicly funded health service. It served midwifery well, early on, to distinguish itself strategically from nursing and to compartmentalize maternity care as wellness-focused, home-based, and primary (uncomplicated) care, because anything related to nursing, medicine, and hospitals was (and still is) generally viewed by the government as large, costly, and complex.

By the mid 1990s, however, it became clear that there needed to be a more structured way for the state to directly fund the individual maternity practitioners (midwives and doctors). The flood of midwives out of the hospitals and into community-based self-employment, where they could access the same level of payment as doctors for providing care to pregnant and birthing women, was alleged to have pushed up the cost to the government for this service, which was paid on a hourly basis. Since midwives spend more time with women in labor and birth than doctors, for the first few years of their access to medical funding for childbirth, independent midwives earned very good money (which could relate to about ten times the hourly rate received by hospital-employed midwives). This difference created some resentment between hospital-employed and independent midwives, an issue that has required targeted work by the NZCOM to rectify. The hospital midwives provided midwifery care for women who chose to have a doctor manage their labor and birth. Hospital midwives, then, were providing the same level of midwifery care for doctors' women when they were in the hospital as the self-employed midwives did for their own women. In fact, when a doctor was the maternity carer, the government paid twice—once for the hospital midwife and again for the doctor.

Development of a National Model of Maternity Care

In 1994 the health funding bodies of the day set up a Joint Maternity Project to negotiate a more equitable maternity funding arrangement than the model that was based on an hourly rate, which had enabled midwives to earn more than doctors. NZCOM and the New Zealand Medical Association (NZMA) were the only parties involved in the direct negotiations.

These negotiations became very protracted and complex. The NZCOM negotiating team included practicing midwives. These midwives were able to work through the logistics of payment models very clearly, and obviously influenced the government negotiators. The combined political acumen and midwifery knowledge of Karen Guilliland, then national manager of the New Zealand College of Midwives, and her friend and colleague, Sally Pairman, a midwifery educator and practitioner at the time, proved formidable. In a small country, knowledge of political systems and people of influence, combined with the ability to demonstrate alignment of public (health) service development initiatives with current government policy, enable potentially long-reaching changes to be implemented.

Subsequently, a new section (Section 88) was added to the original Health and Disability Services Act in 1996, changing the payment framework into a series of modular payments for each woman. In total, a midwife or doctor receives about NZ$2,000 per completed "case" (woman and baby), which is broken down into first and second trimester, third trimester, labor and birth, and postnatal payment modules. In order to claim the payments, the midwife or doctor has to register with the woman as the Lead Maternity Carer (LMC), and submit the claim for payment following each module of care provided. If the LMC ceases to provide the care at any point, the woman needs to register with another LMC before this new LMC is entitled to any payments (and from that point on, the previous LMC cannot make any claims for payment). This process is designed to encourage continuity of care by one LMC for all modules of care. The LMC registers with the woman to provide and manage access for this woman to maternity care for the duration of her pregnancy and up to six weeks following the birth.

Ultimately a clear and explicit framework for the provision of maternity services to individual pregnant women and their babies by individual health practitioners was developed. The full and detailed Maternity Services Notice Section 88 document is available at www.moh.govt.nz under "publications—Maternity Services notice." A key objective of this framework is to provide the woman with one main health practitioner, who is paid on a modular basis per case (woman and baby) per year, for the duration of her childbearing experience. Access to Section 88 funding is only available to "authorized practitioners, either a midwife or a doctor with a current practising certificate" (Ministry of Health 2002).

Although some midwives with large caseloads (and correspondingly long hours of work) experienced a reduction in income (owing to the capped payment per case regardless of how long the episodes of care were), this model did provide a more substantial and prescriptive framework around maternity service provision than had been in existence before. It also provided more direction for midwives new to community maternity service provision. This legislation introduced the concept of one named LMC for a pregnant women. This practitioner, either a doctor or midwife, was responsible for the provision of care (24/7) for the entire pregnancy, birth, and up to six weeks following the birth. There was no restriction placed on the number of women a midwife or doctor could provide care for, but the specifications describing the level of care expected per case would

TABLE 2.1 Proportion of births managed by maternity provider type

Births (n) Managed by LMCs	1999	2000	2001	2002	2003	2004
Registered live births in NZ[a]	57,421	56,994	56,224	54,021	56,134	58,723
LMC profession unidentified	—	—	—	—	—	2,463
Midwives[b]	23,197	24,140	24,062	23,761	33,531	33,715
General Practitioners[b]	6,902	5,699	3,851	3,185	3,376	2,005
Obstetricians[b]	5,085	4,694	4,846	3,827	3,342	2,680
Total births managed by LMCs[c]	35,184	34,533	32,759	30,773	40,249	44,430

SOURCE: *Report on Maternity, 1999* (Ministry of Health 2001); *Report on Maternity, 2000 and 2001* (Ministry of Health 2003); *Report on Maternity, 2002* (Ministry of Health 2004); *Report on Maternity, 2003* (Ministry of Health 2006); *Report on Maternity, 2004* (Ministry of Health, 2007).
[a]These are registered as living babies with Births, Deaths, and Marriages (government department).
[b]These data are based on data captured by the Section 88 maternity payment schedule (Ministry of Health 2002).
[c]The remaining births will have been managed by maternity hospital teams of doctors and midwives, not LMCs.

restrict most practitioners, particularly those with family commitments. The NZCOM recommended a full-time caseload of about fifty completed cases per year; however, many midwives managed sixty to eighty women per year, particularly if these were uncomplicated, multiparous women. Competition for cases among midwives also acted as a disincentive to overbook, as women did compare how much time their midwives gave them per visit and how available they were when called.

Table 2.1 indicates that by 2003, the majority (72.5%) of births were being managed within the LMC model. It also demonstrates that midwives provided the bulk of this service, with 83% of these births managed by midwives in 2003. Section 88 (Ministry of Health 2002) which specifies the LMC model and payment schedule, is a complex piece of legislation, and the payments for the LMC are broken into modules of care. To illustrate the concepts, I have used the experience of my daughter's pregnancy and birth to demonstrate the process.

In the LMC model, the service is paid for following the completion of modules of care. Apart from during the first trimester of pregnancy, where an unlimited number of claims for care can be submitted, there is only one payment allowed per woman for each subsequent module of care. After the

The Maternity System Experience for Women

In 1999 my daughter, Sarah, became pregnant with her first child. We both agreed that although I was a midwife, I was also her mother and wanted to be in that role, so she decided to find herself another midwife. Sarah knew through her network of friends that she had to choose a midwife early on in her pregnancy because they get booked up fast, and she might miss out on her first choice.

Sarah wanted a home birth since she is not keen on hospitals, believing they should only be used as backup, so she contacted a midwife in the local home birth practice. Contact details for midwives are available in local telephone books, in libraries, on websites such as www.nzcom.org.nz, and in midwifery practice rooms dotted throughout the city and towns.

Sarah made an appointment for the midwife to visit her at home for her first visit at eight weeks, when she had a preliminary checkup and discussion about their future working relationship: how often the visits would occur, where and for how long, whom else would Sarah like involved in the visits, and what would be involved at the visits; they also discussed the fact that Sarah had the option of changing midwives if she did not feel the relationship would work. Sarah was also presented with her own set of maternity notes and information on pregnancy in preparation for her registration visit at fourteen weeks.

Following this visit, Sarah conferred with her partner, family, and friends, and decided that she was happy with the midwife, would book with the practice, and would register the midwife as her Lead Maternity Carer (LMC) at the next visit. Sarah had miserable first and early second trimesters, with nausea and vomiting. She contacted the midwife a number of times for ideas. She was not becoming dehydrated, though, and she asked for advice from me, the midwife, family, and friends on how to survive this period.

At fourteen weeks, Sarah had her "big" appointment with the midwife. She chose to visit the midwife at a clinic attached to the local midwifery resource center. Sarah's partner, Nick, also attended. This hour-long visit included an in-depth physical examination, blood tests, discussion on planning for the pregnancy and birth, and questions associated with the process. The maternity notes were filled out with all the details of the examination and beginning plan of care was documented. The midwife retained a carbon copy of the notes, and Sarah had the full set, which she also wrote in as she felt necessary between visits. For Sarah and Nick, these notes also formed a story of the pregnancy and the birth for them to pass on to their baby later in life.

As the pregnancy progressed, Sarah met with the midwife at pre-arranged dates, with weekly visits toward the end. Sometimes Sarah was visited at home by the midwife; other times, Sarah visited the clinic rooms. As the visits progressed, Sarah built up her knowledge of the birth process and what would be required of her as a new mother. She learned about her body and the signs she should be looking for to let her know she might be in labor. Because the pregnancy had been unexpected, and she had irregular periods, Sarah was happy to have no specific due date, other than "sometime at the end of April/early May." She also met two of the other midwives who were to back up her midwife, so that she would feel comfortable with them when they were needed. The home birth midwives always had two midwives at a home birth.

Because Sarah was well and healthy, she did not see a doctor during her pregnancy. She did have 24/7 access to her midwife or the backup. Sarah called them occasionally, usually when she was concerned about slowed fetal movements toward the end of pregnancy and a couple of times when she thought she was going into labor. Each time she was reassured over the phone, and only once did the midwife need to visit to reassure her and carry out a quick check.

When Sarah did go into labor, late one afternoon, she was encouraged to have a small snack, tuck up in her bed, and rest as much as possible in preparation for the more active phase of labor. Sure enough, at 3 A.M. she called me to come around, which I did. When I arrived, we called the midwife, and she came about two hours later. Nick was doing such a good job supporting Sarah that we made coffee in the kitchen and caught up on news. Sarah and Nick managed well without us interfering, but we were handy when needed.

Following a lengthy labor, going through to the end of the following day, Sarah decided, even though the baby was fine, to go to the hospital for a consultation with an obstetrician. She managed to get into the car for the short ride to the hospital, where she had a cesarean birth. Emily was born at 5 A.M. on the fifth day of the fifth month 2000—my mother's seventy-fifth birthday! Emily weighed in at nine pounds, three ounces.

Following the birth, the midwife negotiated the care plan for the stay with the hospital staff. She became the advocate for Sarah and Nick. Sarah wanted the baby and herself attended by a family member at all times. The hospital respected this wish. After thirty-six hours, I received a call at home from Sarah to come immediately with the baby car seat: she was going home. She had informed the midwife, who would meet her at home.

Sarah's postnatal adaptation was very smooth; the baby latched onto the breast with no problems. Sarah was a new woman! She took charge of her baby and her life with great enthusiasm. The midwife visited at home daily for the first week, then twice weekly, then weekly until the sixth week following the birth. At this stage, the midwife carried out her last full physical assessment of Sarah and the baby, and wrote a referral letter to Sarah's GP. This was the midwife's final visit. Sarah went on to breastfeed Emily for over two years. Sarah did not have to pay for either the midwifery or the hospital care.

first trimester, the pregnant woman needs to choose an authorized practitioner, then officially register (sign an agreement) with that authorized practitioner in order for the practitioner to receive any public funding. That practitioner, the LMC, is the only practitioner who can claim government payment for care of the woman during her pregnancy and birth, and up to six weeks postnatally.[2] The NZCOM recommends a caseload of about fifty women per year, which equates to a net income of about NZ$100,000 (US$61,000 or EUR 45,712) for a full-time LMC midwife. Midwives, being self-employed, need to supply all their own equipment and meet business costs, of which communications and transport form a large part, which equates to about 30% of their income. They are not permitted to charge the women directly for any services. In New Zealand, pregnant and birthing women are entitled to subsidized laboratory, radiology, tests and pharmacology products. Legislation enables midwives to prescribe and order these as appropriate.

Maternity Specialists and Maternity Hospital Services

Midwives providing caseload practice are viewed politically and practically as providing "primary health services" because they primarily practice within the community (e.g., in offices within communities) other than when providing labor and birth care in hospital, and they need to refer to specialist services if their women are classified as high risk and develop complications. Hospital-based maternity specialist services are viewed as "secondary" and "tertiary" health services. The Ministry of Health issues specifications for these services, but the actual configuration and level of funding that actually reaches the maternity service is determined locally. There is no clear policy around how the LMC should hand over care to hospital-based specialist service midwives, which means that many LMC midwives continue to provide the midwifery component of maternity care even if the responsibility for the women's overall care is transferred to an obstetric specialist. This confuses the definition of LMC midwives as "primary health care providers," because they do continue to provide care within the secondary and tertiary hospital setting if they choose to.

There are fifty-nine primary (low-risk, midwifery-run, community-located) maternity hospitals in the country. These small hospitals are required to have a midwife available twenty-four hours a day. Most are located in rural towns and often consist of two to three beds in a community hospital with no on-site medical coverage and no operative births available. Women encountering complications during birth are transferred out to the nearest secondary or tertiary facility by helicopter or ambulance. All of these small hospitals are under threat of closure because of the low number of women using them and the increase in rural home birth.

There are eighteen secondary maternity hospitals. These have round-the-clock obstetric and neonatal medical services. They are located in provincial towns and manage all but complex obstetric care, which is managed by one of the country's six tertiary maternity facilities. All hospital-based maternity care is free to the consumer, and each facility is expected to allow the woman's LMC midwife or doctor to provide care on the premises and access referral services directly at no cost.

From 1999 on, the Ministry of Health has published an annual *Report on Maternity* (see, for example, Ministry of Health 2006), each of which provides the mothers' demographics and an overview of birth numbers and outcomes. These reports demonstrate a very slow increase in birth interventions. Because these reports rely on hospital data, home births are not included. Therefore, the cesarean rates are not calculated on the total live registered birth numbers. Of interest in these reports is the huge variability (up to 8%) between regions of the country.

The most recent Report on Maternity 2004 (Ministry of Health 2007) indicated that 66.5% of women birthing in that year had spontaneous vaginal births, 23.7% had cesareans (9.2% of them elective), 9.9% had spontaneous vaginal breeches, and 9.9% had assisted births (ventose or forceps).

Because data on home births are not consistently captured, the only way the number of home births can be calculated currently is by subtracting the hospital births from the total live registered birth numbers, but the

Ministry of Health (2001, 2004, 2006, 2007) cautions that not all hospital births may have been captured. It is estimated that between 5% and 7% of births in this country occur at home (conversation with NZCOM Midwifery Advisor, 2006). If true, the rate has increased significantly since the mid-1970s, when it was estimated at 0.3%. Even though midwives who carry out home births are paid a "home birth supplement" to cover the costs of equipment and supplies, the Ministry of Health payment department seems unable to identify the actual number because if a midwife and woman plan to birth at home, but have to transfer to hospital during labor, the midwife can still claim the supplement. Plans are currently underway to have these data recorded from January through July 2007.

Midwives in the MidCentral District Health Board (DHB) region, where I have been acting as Midwifery Advisor, conducted an informal tally among colleagues of home birth numbers in their region for the previous year. There were 103 known home births out of a total of 2,293 births in that region, which gave a home birth rate of about 4.5% in 2006. MidCentral DHB, situated in the lower half of the North Island, is one of twenty-one DHBs in New Zealand.

My experience over the years leads me to believe that there are three key reasons why home birth numbers are so low in this country, even with midwifery autonomy:

1. *Home birth is no longer a "cause."* Because midwives in New Zealand can choose to work in any setting, home birth is not seen as the only environment where midwives can work autonomously, so there is no need to develop a "home birth culture" to protect midwifery.
2. *There is a focus on saving primary (community) maternity hospitals from extinction.* In many quarters, including the College of Midwives, there is a real focus on encouraging both midwives and women to birth in the primary units. If these community-based, primary maternity hospitals are not used, they will be closed. The number of births within these primary hospital births has risen slowly from a low point of 12% (6,488 births) in 1999 to 15.6% (8,628 births) in 2004. If the 5% or so of home births is added to this number, we could state with confidence that at least one in five women (20.6%) in New Zealand birthed babies in venues that did not have any form of obstetric intervention such as anesthetics, operating theaters, or even forceps and ventose. Nor do they have obstetric specialists on-site for emergencies. Services in the primary units are provided by midwives, and home birth midwives use a colleague as a backup during the birth.
3. *Birth is "risky."* An increasing number of women (and many midwives) do not feel confident enough to birth in a low-tech environment. This fear is exacerbated by the media and the general cultural ethos.

STAFFING MATERNITY HOSPITAL SERVICES

The staffing in maternity hospitals in this country is regulated, which enables maternity wards and hospitals to remain primarily the domain of the registered midwife, even though most midwives were initially trained as nurses. Fortunately, the midwifery renaissance occurred before the wholesale introduction of nurses into maternity wards was seen as the answer to the midwifery workforce shortage in the late 1980s. In fact the shortage provided an added impetus for unshackling midwifery from the constraints of nursing, which in turn did much to increase the numbers of nurses wanting to become midwives.

Only registered midwives are allowed to attend women in labor, and an LMC midwife birthing a woman in a hospital has the right to expect the hospital to provide a registered midwife as backup. Medical cover in maternity hospitals ranges from none in most primary maternity hospitals—where midwives communicate directly with referral obstetric hospitals in case of need to consult or transfer—to full coverage with obstetric, anaesthetic, and pediatric medical coverage in all secondary and tertiary obstetric hospitals. The numbers of both midwifery and medical staff employed within each hospital are governed by the number of patients that used the service in the previous year, and by the availability of qualified staff. Currently, New Zealand has a shortage of hospital-employed midwives.

The New Zealand College of Midwives

A parallel thread in the development of the New Zealand model of maternity care was the ongoing evolution of the New Zealand College of Midwives (NZCOM). Established in 1989, just preceding the passage of the Nurses Amendment Act (1990), the organization initially consisted of a breakaway group of midwives from the nurses' organization, combined with activists from consumer groups such as the Homebirth Association. Many of these women had already been working within women's groups and related political movements, so the organization really got off to a flying start. It needed to, because as soon as the doctors realized the threat midwives posed to their livelihood, they took action to undermine consumers' confidence in midwives as "safe" practitioners (Hendry 2003).

This issue provided a focus and priorities for the newly established College. Very early on, we developed a set of Standards for Practice. These standards outlined and documented agreed-upon expectations for the nature, timing, and quality of midwifery care, framed within the full scope of midwifery practice as described by the International Confederation of Midwives (ICM). We also developed processes for monitoring the quality of midwifery care and receiving feedback directly from consumers on midwifery care issues.

The NZCOM set itself up based on the notion that it had the responsibility and mandate to work with women to develop and maintain maternity services that would best suit the women of this country. Many midwives had also been consumers of the country's maternity services in the 1970s and 1980s, and were committed to supporting a better experience for future mothers, including their own daughters. We could not rest on our laurels after the achievements of the early 1990s. The NZCOM has not only had to manage the complexity of midwifery development required in this country to establish and maintain the woman-centered maternity service we fought so hard for, but continually has had to reposition or strategize to retain this model.

Consumers have always played active roles in all levels of the College and continue to do so; they have representatives on the National Committee and are involved in annual reviews of midwives' practice. Consumers advise and represent consumer groups in a variety of midwifery- and maternity-related College activities. This willingness to collaborate with consumers seems to reflect the partnership model that underpins most policy and legislation in New Zealand—a model that emanated from the Treaty of Waitangi signed in 1840 between the Maori and the Queen of England shortly before planned settlement of this country by immigrants from Great Britain. This Treaty provides a guide for relationship development between Maori and non-Maori in this country. Maori have managed to retain significant portions of their land and continue to negotiate with the government for compensation in recognition of land that was taken in the past by the Crown. Maori have become active in establishing health services for their communities, particularly in rural localities. Increasingly, midwives have either become employed by these services, or have worked in collaboration with them.

The Treaty also formed the conceptual basis of the midwifery partnership model that was created by Karen Guilliland and Sally Pairman in 1995, and continues to guide midwifery practice in this country. Consumers provide a valuable resource of knowledge and common sense as well as strength in numbers when required.

Over the years, the NZCOM has increasingly become the first point of contact for midwives, maternity managers, policy analysts, and consumers with queries, issues, and concerns about midwifery and maternity care. In order to manage these contacts, the College established the role of Midwifery Advisor. Although this position was initially held by one experienced midwife, the existing networks established within the College enabled her to quickly contact others around the country who had expert or specialist knowledge for advice or opinions.

Subsequently, the College now has a number of midwifery advisors, some in part-time employment, with specific areas of interest, such as rural midwifery, professional development, and legal and employment relationships. In support of these advisors, the College also ensures that networks are maintained with groups of midwives who have specific areas of interest, such as midwifery educators, hospital-based midwifery advisors, midwifery researchers, midwives who provide expert opinions at legal proceedings, and those who provide mentorship for other midwives. The College holds regular forums for these midwives to meet and network with each other.

NZCOM also recognized the need to support self-employed midwives to remain in business. To manage this, in 1996 the College established the Midwifery and Maternity Provider Organisation (MMPO) as a registered company focusing on the business needs of midwives (for information, see www.mmpo.org.nz). Because midwives were new to self-employment, there were no immediately useful electronic practice management systems (PMS) developed, other than medical systems, which were focused more on appointment scheduling and invoicing rather than gathering the care activity and outcome information required by midwives.

Claiming for payment under Section 88 requires practitioners to submit to the government payment arm significant amounts of data on care activities and outcomes. In 1996 midwives did not have the history or experience of submitting claims for payments that doctors had, and many did not have the infrastructure to manage these processes well. From its inception, the MMPO was determined to develop an electronic claiming and payment system that matched the maternity payment schedule while simultaneously building up a national database of midwifery activities and outcomes from midwives who were working in different parts of the country.

The first step involved the development of a multifunctional set of maternity notes that the midwife could use in any setting. At the time the MMPO was being established, Karen Guilliland, the NZCOM National Manager, was undertaking her postgraduate studies. She used this opportunity to focus on the development of a set of midwifery maternity notes that would chronicle the woman's experience and care activities throughout the entire childbearing experience. Following an international and national search for existing sets of notes, Guilliland, along with a number of midwife colleagues, constructed this set of maternity notes. These also contained the required data to be submitted to the government payment agency to meet payment claiming requirements.

The notes were to become the linchpin in the midwifery practice management system. They were comprehensive, portable, and reliable—they could work anywhere, even with candle power. Midwives had to enter clinical data only once into the maternity notes for each woman to meet the requirements for payment claiming and recording pertinent clinical information. Each page of the notes is carboned (uses carbon paper), allowing the data to be captured in triplicate: one copy for the midwife, one for the woman, and one to be sent to the MMPO for entry into the database of midwifery outcomes and to be sent electronically for payment. (Membership in the MMPO is not compulsory, and thus this database does not contain all home births.)

From small beginnings in Christchurch in 1996, with fewer than 50 midwives collecting and sending in these data for the first year or so, the MMPO has been built up into a national organization with a membership of around 700 midwives and an annual turnover of NZ$60 million worth of claims. I joined the organization in 2002 as Executive Director, working two days per week (I was still working as a midwifery lecturer and health service advisor at the time). Changes in how the government paid midwives and others at the time allowed for national expansion of the MMPO. Following significant growth since that time, we are now the largest maternity provider organization in the country.

Regulation of the Profession

In 2004 the regulation of midwifery ceased to be the responsibility of the Nursing Council. The Health Practitioner's Competence Assurance Act (2003) established the Midwifery Council, which from 2004 on undertook both regulatory and disciplinary processes for the profession. The Council, with membership consisting of consumers and health professionals, is appointed directly by the government. More information can be obtained through www.midwiferycouncil.org.nz.

Midwifery Education

Midwifery education in this country represents yet another co-developing strand of the midwifery renaissance. Because midwifery education is also publicly funded, lobbying at the national level by the combined voices of midwifery educators and practitioners, orchestrated by NZCOM, has been essential. In the late 1980s, an increase in the birth rate coupled with a decreasing number of graduates from the mainly nursing-based, tertiary midwifery training programs placed a timely focus on the programs that were being delivered by the polytechnics of the day. At the time, there were four programs available in the country, most consisting of one-year advanced nursing courses. Midwifery clinical practice experience was restricted to hours allotted to a "special project," and registration was achieved by meeting specific clinical experience hour (which required much out-of-school time) and task requirements, capped off by a state examination set by Nursing Council.

Most courses had minimal midwifery input in the classroom components of the program, and pressure was successfully applied to separate midwifery from nursing courses. The small number of midwifery students was a key reason why swift changes were able to be instituted at very little cost to the educational institutions. The few available, educated midwifery lecturers worked hard, and institutions got value for their money. Incensed by the lack of interest in developing midwifery into a three-year degree program, as had happened in nursing, the few midwifery lecturers in the country formed an effective lobbying group. Nurses were in charge of the schools where midwifery programs were run. Although it seemed an uphill battle, education was also working within a competitive environment. By demonstrating the potential student growth associated with the expansion of the one-year diploma in midwifery program into a three-year, undergraduate degree program, midwives were able to convince both the government and the educational institutions to make the changes. The nurses were not happy: this constituted yet another signal of midwifery's autonomy from nursing.

By 1992 most midwifery programs had already moved to a three-year, direct-entry structure. This appealed to the tertiary institutions because it offered another course option to attract students. The initial programs were inundated with applicants, many of whom were non-nurse consumers who had been active participants in the early struggles of the College. Currently, there are five schools of midwifery in New Zealand situated within universities or polytechnics, each offering a three-year degree program with a curriculum framework that requires approval from the Midwifery Council. Midwives also now have the option of postgraduate study up to the doctorate level.

Starting Out in Practice as an LMC Midwife

Starting out as a new, self-employed midwife can be daunting for a new graduate. The following story illustrates the process, including the role of the NZCOM and the MMPO.

Most self-employed midwives work within a practice with a number of colleagues who share their philosophy and provide backup and time out when necessary. There are hundreds of midwifery practices throughout the country: some operate from shared premises and others work out of midwives' cars and meet at each other's houses. Midwives advertise their practices in newspapers, on the radio, and in the phone book under Health Practitioners, and also produce colorful brochures for woman to read. Many midwives' "rooms" are well signposted, with advertising boards now a common sight. Midwives in New Zealand provide almost 80% of all Lead Maternity Care services in the country (New Zealand Health Information Service 2006).

Profile of a Midwife Starting Out in Practice

Sandra received her results from Midwifery Council just before Christmas. She was now a registered midwife and had received a temporary practicing certificate in the mail with the results from her national examination. After three years of hard work as a student, she was legally able to practice as a midwife.

During her last year in the program, she had been encouraged to think about joining a midwifery practice in her home town. Two women in the local midwifery practice of three had recently had babies, and they were only available to provide short-term relief and backup for the remaining midwife. The midwives really needed another full-time midwife and were excited at Sandra's decision to join. Sandra had spent the past four months as a third-year student in the practice and had come to know the midwives and the women well, so she felt quite confident she would receive good support as a new graduate.

In preparation for Sandra joining the practice, the two relieving midwives had started to build up a small caseload of women for Sandra to take on once she was registered. Sandra had contacted the Midwifery and Maternity Provider Organisation (MMPO) for a "new practitioner" joining pack, which included information on getting set up in self-employment, a sample set of maternity notes, an MMPO joining form, and tax-related information. Sandra had also contacted the New Zealand College of Midwives, which had sent her information on her professional responsibilities as a self-employed midwife and a form to change her membership from student to "self-employed." She knew the College was just a phone call away if she had any questions about her start-up.

Following receipt of her practicing certificate, Sandra sent off her MMPO joining form, including her Nursing Council registration number, which enabled her to start sending claims to the government for payment. There were also a number of other business-related expenses for her at this stage, including the purchase of all her clinical supplies, including Sonicaid, stethoscope, sphygmomanometer, baby scales, and other related equipment. She also needed to announce her new position and contact information within the community through brochures and business cards, and invest in a mobile phone and pager.

Because she was joining an established practice, Sandra did not need to find her own clinic rooms: the money she paid into the practice on a monthly basis covered the cost of using the rooms in the building on the main street, which was rented by her new practice. She did have to apply to the local hospital for an access agreement to enable her to birth women there. This was a formality because, as a registered midwife with a current practicing certificate, she was entitled to have access. She had also joined the New Zealand College of Midwives as a self-employed midwife, which provided her with indemnity insurance cover—a requirement for access.

Sandra's family had been prepared for the commitment she would be required to put into establishing herself in practice. Her children were eight and ten years old; her partner, a teacher, had happily managed the household around Sandra's unpredictable hours when she had been a midwifery student and was prepared to continue this while Sandra worked as a registered midwife. In fact, Sandra was looking forward to working her visits around her family and believed, as other midwives had found, that she would see more of her children during the day than when working regular hours. Many midwives have found that labor and birth frequently occur at night. With a full-time caseload of five birthing women per month, this was likely to represent only five or six periods of lengthy unavailability per month.

With support and advice from her new colleagues in the practice, Sandra was able to register with her first pregnant woman as the Lead maternity Carer (LMC) by early January. This meant that from then on, she had to be available to this woman 24/7 and arrange for another midwife to be available when she took her regular two days off a month. Because she had been on call as a student, Sandra adapted to this well. Her children and partner also knew how to contact her if local women rang her home number.

To raise her profile as a new member of the midwifery practice, Sandra arranged to meet all the local general practitioners, the child health nurses, and the members of the women's health network in town. However, it did not take long before most people knew she had joined the practice, and she was stopped in the supermarket a number of times by women with questions about pregnancy and childbirth. This would become a more common occurrence for Sandra as her role in the community became more established.

Early in the new year, Sandra's permanent practicing certificate arrived, and this reminded her of her professional obligations to plan and keep a record of all her midwifery activities and care outcomes, for these data would contribute to her annual Midwifery Standards Review,[1] a compulsory requirement for her maintaining her annual midwifery practicing certificate. Sandra would also need to make sure she booked in time for attendance at a series of compulsory professional development activities (outlined in www.midwiferycouncil.org.nz).

By the beginning of April the next year, Sandra will have completed her first home birth as a registered midwife, with her colleague in the same practice as backup. She will have about twenty women in various stages of pregnancy, for whom she serves as LMC, and by the end of her first year of practice, she will have birthed about twenty-five women. As her caseload builds up, by the end of her second year, she will have birthed about fifty women.

[1]The annual Midwifery Standards Review (MSR) process requires a midwife to analyze and present her annual care outcomes (statistics) to a small group of colleagues and a consumer. She is also required to present a plan of learning (professional development activities) to challenge herself for the next year.

The Interface with Employed Midwives

Fortunately in New Zealand, we still have sufficient midwives to provide care to women within maternity hospitals, but this is becoming more of a struggle as a large number of midwives are reaching retirement age. It is estimated that almost 60% of midwives in the country are employed working in maternity hospitals. More recently, midwives have distanced themselves further from nursing and joined a midwifery union, MERAS (Midwifery Employee Representation and Advisory Service), which was set up by the NZCOM. This union promotes far more midwifery-oriented employment conditions, recognizing the increased responsibility expected of midwives in hospitals in New Zealand compared with that of nurses, who do not have the same level of access to diagnostic testing or prescribing (see www.midwife.org.nz).

Because most women enter the hospital with their own midwives, employed midwives in secondary and tertiary obstetric hospitals are increasingly being used to care for complex cases, to provide backup, and to offer advice and consultation to the primary midwife. This is a very sophisticated role, so new graduate midwives are generally encouraged to begin their working life in the community, rather than obtaining hospital employment as their first postregistration experience. New graduates are generally viewed as being best suited to work as community-based midwives, with the knowledgeable, experienced midwife on hand as a resource in the hospital when needed. However, most hospitals have begun to develop comprehensive, "first year of practice" programs for new graduates who, for whatever reason, choose to start practicing in the hospital environment.

CHALLENGES TO THIS MIDWIFERY MODEL

The maintenance of this national maternity model is an ongoing challenge for midwives and for women. There will always be the need to adapt and change to meet environmental conditions. Maternity services in New Zealand were one of the first to undergo such dramatic changes, particularly with regard to the notion of continuity of care and the focus on primary care that midwives have given the service. These are now fashionable within the health sector as a whole. Other sectors are moving (some are being dragged) toward the goals of client-centered care, continuity of care, and an emphasis on the importance of community-based primary health care. Nurses are attempting to move out from under the constraints of the medical model. Midwifery offers a model to aspire to for nonmedical health professionals.

In all these efforts to achieve the utopian health service model, midwifery has had to be vigilant in case processes are set in place by others that could destabilize the present midwifery/maternity model. This need for vigilance has required the College of Midwives, in conjunction with equally interested parties such as midwifery educators, maternity service providers, and the Midwifery Council, to work closely and attempt to manage the future. New Zealand has also experienced the international trend of increasing intervention in childbirth. Lack of reliable and accessible national data on birth outcomes had obscured the extent of this phenomenon until 2001, when the first *Report on Maternity* was published. The most interesting aspect of this issue is the large disparity between regions. There appears to be up to a 12% difference in cesarean section rates across regions (Ministry of Health 2004). The reasons for these differences have yet to be explored, and the New Zealand College of Midwives is working closely with the College of Obstetricians and Gynaecologists in an attempt to address the issues surrounding the rising rates of intervention in childbirth.

CONCLUSION

Midwifery in New Zealand has come a long way in the last eighteen years. Initially, the occupation was barely distinguishable from nursing, and now it has become a fully autonomous profession with its own regulatory body, the Midwifery Council, and direct access to publicly funded health resources denied to most other nonmedical health professionals. The level of lobbying and planning undertaken by the College of Midwives and consumer groups to achieve this woman-centered maternity service has often been understated. Midwives and women worked opportunistically with the social and political structures of the day. They formed an amazing network throughout the country that not only warned of potential risks to the service and profession, but also enabled fast communication of strategies for managing difficult situations.

The underlying philosophy of the College, one of partnership with women/ consumers, has been the mainstay of the network over the years. As more midwives have been promoted to positions of authority and into advisory roles, and as more women have experienced the service, the underlying framework of the system has been cemented into the health system as a whole. The question now most commonly asked of women following news of a pregnancy is, "Who is your midwife?" Women seem to be taking a much more active role in their pregnancies, with their midwives working as partners on the journey. They work together through choices and options, with the midwife advocating when required if referral to specialist services is needed.

The maternity service will continue to undergo change; however, strategies set in place by midwives and women should enable the major concepts of the service to remain. Advancement in midwives' postgraduate education and research, the continued adaptation of the College of Midwives to meet new challenges, and the establishment of a separate Midwifery Council, have significantly contributed to the maintaining and thriving of a woman-centered, midwife-provided maternity service.

ACKNOWLEDGMENTS

I would like to acknowledge the midwives of New Zealand who have inspired me to continue working for the profession throughout the years. I have particular respect for those midwives who early on just went out and provided their services to women in an exceptionally professional way, lighting the path for those who had been waiting to join the profession as soon as they did not have to first become nurses.

NOTES

1. One that permitted the education of a midwife who was not previously a nurse.

2. Payment for the hospitalization phase of the pregnancy, birth, and postnatal period is covered by another contract, which is managed by the District Health Boards directly with the hospital in which the woman has care.

REFERENCES

Abel, Sally. 1997. "Midwifery and Maternity Services in Transition: An Examination of Change Following the Nurses Amendment Act 1990." Ph.D. thesis, University of Auckland, New Zealand.

Blank, Robert. 1994. *New Zealand and Health Policy*. Oxford Readings in New Zealand Politics. Auckland, NZ: Oxford University Press.

Bourgeault, Ivy, Cecilia Benoit, and Robbie Davis-Floyd (eds.). 2004. *Reconceiving Midwifery: The New Canadian Model of Care*. Toronto: McGill/Queen's University Press.

Cheyne, Christine, Mike O'Brien, and Michael Belgrave. 1997. *Social Policy in Aotearoa New Zealand: A Critical Introduction*. Auckland, NZ: Oxford University Press.

Davis-Floyd, Robbie, and Christine Barbara Johnson (eds.). 2006. *Mainstreaming Midwives: The Politics of Change*. New York: Routledge.

Donley, Joan. 1998a. *Birthrites: Natural vs. Unnatural Childbirth in New Zealand*. Auckland, NZ: Full Court Press.

————. 1998b. "A Response to the New Zealand Nursing Organisation." *New Zealand College of Midwives Journal* 19:18–21

Guilliland, Karen. 1998. "A Demographic Profile of Independent (Self-Employed) Midwives in New Zealand Aotearoa." M.A. thesis, Victoria University of Wellington, New Zealand.

Guilliland, Karen, and Sally Pairman. 1995. *The Midwifery Partnership: A Model for Practice*. Monograph Series. Victoria University of Wellington, NZ.

Health Funding Authority. 1998. *Notice Issued Pursuant to Section 51 of the Health and Disability Act 1993 Concerning the Provision of Maternity Services*. Wellington, NZ.

————. 2000. *Maternity Services: A Reference Document*. Wellington, NZ.

Hendry, Christine. 2003. "Midwifery in New Zealand, 1990–2003: The Complexities of Service Provision." Ph.D. thesis, University of Technology, Sydney, Australia.

Ministry of Health. 2001. *Report on Maternity, 1999*. Wellington: New Zealand Health Information Service.

————. 2002. *Maternity Services: Notice Pursuant to Section 88 of the Public Health and Disability Act 2000*. Wellington: New Zealand Ministry of Health.

————. 2003. *Report on Maternity, 2000 and 2001*. Wellington: New Zealand Health Information Service.

————. 2004. *Report on Maternity, 2002*. Wellington: New Zealand Health Information Service.

————. 2006. *Report on Maternity, 2003*. Wellington: New Zealand Health Information Service.

————. 2007. *Report on Maternity, 2004*. Wellington: New Zealand Health Information Service.

New Zealand Government. 1990. *Nurses Amendment Act: Information for Health Providers*. Wellington: New Zealand Department of Health.

New Zealand Health Information Service. 2006. *2005 Health Workforce Statistics*. Wellington: New Zealand Health Information Service.

New Zealand Regional Health Authorities. 1993. *First Steps towards an Integrated Maternity Services Framework.* Report by Coopers and Lybrand. Wellington: New Zealand Regional Health Authorities.

Pairman, Sally. 1998. "The Midwifery Partnership: An Exploration of the Midwife/ Woman Relationship." M.A. thesis, Victoria University of Wellington, New Zealand.

———. 2000. "New Zealand College of Midwives Education Framework 1999." *NZCOM Journal* 22:5–14.

Tully, Elizabeth. 1999. "Doing Professionalism Differently: Negotiating Midwifery Autonomy in Aotearoa/New Zealand." Ph.D. thesis, University of Canterbury, New Zealand.

Chapter 3

The Ontario Midwifery Model of Care

Margaret E. MacDonald and Ivy Lynn Bourgeault

As a profession, Canadian midwifery is a latecomer of sorts, only having been officially integrated into several provincial health care systems beginning as recently as 1994. Prior to this time, Canada had no formally recognized profession of midwifery. Midwives in most Canadian provinces are now autonomous professionals who provide primary, continuous care at home and in the hospital. Midwifery is legally accessible to women in these provinces experiencing normal, uncomplicated pregnancy and birth, and in all but one province where services are provided, it is publicly funded.

Drawing on ethnographic, historical, and sociological data, in this chapter we describe the integration of midwifery in the province of Ontario from its days as a grassroots social movement to its present status as a full profession.[1] We begin by outlining the history of midwifery in Canada and the ways in which it has influenced the profession's contemporary form. We then go on to detail the structural aspects of midwifery in Ontario that make it unique, including midwives' autonomous, professional status; their model of care, including home birth and public funding; and their direct-entry education program. We show how these aspects of the Ontario midwifery profession work to support women to "give birth safely with power and with dignity" (College of Midwives of Ontario 1994: 1) in their choice of birth setting. In building a case for Ontario midwifery as a birth model that works, we also include data on client satisfaction and clinical outcomes. Finally, we reflect on several challenges and questions still facing midwifery in Ontario and Canada as it continues to grow.

HISTORICAL FORCES SHAPING CANADIAN
MIDWIFERY: A PIONEERING SPIRIT AND A HISTORY OF ERASURE

Canadian midwifery's contemporary philosophy and form has been shaped significantly by its unique history, including the pioneering spirit of traditional midwives in the 18th and 19th centuries, and the history of their subsequent denigration and erasure. In the 20th century, the most significant shaping forces included the central values and goals of midwifery as a social movement as it emerged in the 1970s and 1980s, the role of the state, and the influences of professional midwifery in other jurisdictions.

Historically, the nature of midwifery practice varied across Canada. Neighbor networks, in which women were assisted in childbirth by local women respected for their expertise, were common in Ontario and in some western provinces, while established midwifery professions existed in Nova Scotia, Quebec, Newfoundland, and in certain ethnic and aboriginal communities (Benoit 1991; Biggs 1983; Kaufert and O'Neil 1993; Laforce 1990; Mason 1988; Mitchenson 2002). Historical accounts of midwifery in Canada tend to represent it largely as a set of social practices embedded in women's domestic culture in which continuity of care was central: midwives stayed with the mother throughout the labor; guided and comforted her; offered gifts of food, clothing, and housework; and ensured a postpartum rest period. As in many places in the world, such forms of traditional midwifery either were stamped out or faded away. Starting in the mid-19th century, physicians in Canada, concerned with establishing their authority and obtaining a reliable clientele, engaged in a successful campaign to discredit traditional midwives as incompetent, unclean, and outdated (Ehrenreich and English 1973; Mason 1988; Mitchenson 1991). At the same time, childbirth was being redefined as a medical event for which women were considered essentially unsuited as attendants and too frail to attempt unaided by male experts. Thus, prevailing gender ideals—especially among the middle and upper classes—also contributed to the demise of midwifery (James-Chetalet 1989). Hospital-based, physician-attended childbirth grew steadily through the late 19th and early 20th centuries in Canada, and by the 1940s, traditional forms of midwifery virtually had ceased to exist.[2] In the United Kingdom and the United States, the maternity care gap opened up by the elimination of traditional forms of midwifery was to some extent filled by the introduction of professional nurse-midwifery, but this was not the case in Canada. Consequently, Canada had the dubious distinction of being one of the only industrialized nations without a midwifery profession for more than a century.

This social and legal void was significant in that it left open a space for midwifery to emerge as a social movement because "midwife" was not a protected title in Canada. The space left open was an imaginative one as well. Lesley Biggs has pointed out that the demise of traditional forms of midwifery in Canada was, in fact, variable and "uneven," yet the image of the traditional neighbor came to be the "dominant motif" in both popular and scholarly histories of midwifery in Canada (2004). This form of midwifery was characterized by the social equality of the participants, the absence of biomedical (and for some, male) control, and the presence of the knowledge and skills of the midwife as well as the capable body of the birthing woman in a home setting. Thus, the traditional neighbor midwife and the natural birth that she attended became central to the "recovery project" of professional midwifery in the late 20th century (Biggs 2004: 17; MacDonald 2004).[3] Sociologist Cecilia Benoit suggests that while a certain critical nostalgia "can be helpful in challenging the many negative aspects of medically dominated maternity care, the accompanying bias towards pre-modern midwifery remains problematic" (1991: 92). Indeed, many contemporary midwives themselves are critical of such a romanticized version of midwifery history, citing the harsh reality of maternal and infant suffering and death on the Canadian frontier during that time (MacDonald 2004). Yet even as the vision of a new midwifery was forged that involved access to biomedicine and emergency services, many midwives still express a sense of kinship with traditional midwifery and its pioneering spirit. Certainly the traditional midwife has been put to important and effective strategic and symbolic purposes in reading Canadian midwifery as a renaissance (Biggs 2004; MacDonald 2004). Further, the rhetorically powerful symbols of tradition and nature help to construct biomedicine as the "other" against which midwifery identity has, in part, been formulated.

MIDWIFERY AS A SOCIAL MOVEMENT AND A PROFESSIONALIZATION PROJECT

Midwifery reemerged in several pockets across Canada in the 1970s. In Ontario it took the form of a grassroots social movement devoted to offering women-centered, low-tech alternatives to mainstream obstetrical care. In addition to the shaping forces of history—and nostalgic contemporary readings of it—midwifery at this time was influenced by the Women's Health Movement and its philosophy of self-knowledge and choice for women in health matters. It was also influenced by feminist ideologies that identified reproduction as a site of women's oppression and, therefore, potential liberation. New middle-class notions about togetherness in marriage, and the positive re-evaluation of motherhood, contributed as well (Michaelson 1988: 4; Daviss 1999). Thus, the midwifery movement in Ontario reflected diverse political alliances (Rushing 1993). Overall, this new midwifery sought to counter and critique dominant medical models of birth by supporting women as competent birthers and attendants, and offering them home birth as an option.

Midwifery at this time was relatively informal, and training was eclectic. Some midwives had nursing or nurse-midwifery credentials from the United Kingdom or the United States. Many participants, however, began by simply attending one another's births at home, developing their skills as they went through a combination of self-teaching, participation in study groups, apprenticeship with more experienced midwives, and formal education. Some aspiring community midwives in Ontario went for short-term, intensive training at privately run midwifery clinics in El Paso, Texas, and Kingston, Jamaica.[4] Apprenticeship training—to learn by watching and doing—was considered ideal. Practicing midwives were not recognized nor regulated by the state, and yet, because they worked within the standards and expectations of the communities they served, they may be seen as "regulated" and "accredited" in this way (Barrington 1985; Bourgeault 2006: 91–92).

Throughout the 1970s and 1980s, what came to be known in Canada as community midwifery flourished in its own way almost completely outside the health care system.[5] A small number of supportive physicians provided informal collaboration and backup services to midwives and their clients; other times, midwives were linked to the formal health care system when they needed it only through walk-in emergency services, where they and their clients were often treated with hostility by disapproving medical personnel. As midwifery grew in popularity, so did its sense of vulnerability vis-à-vis the legal and medical systems. Community midwives in Ontario formed the Ontario Association of Midwives (OAM) in 1981 which, like the other provincial midwifery associations also emerging around time, sought to strengthen and legitimize the movement by setting voluntary standards for clinical practice and encouraging record keeping among their members (Bourgeault 2006; Van Wagner 1988). The OAM membership at that time included not only midwives but also consumers and other midwifery supporters. Together, they made up a small but politically active lobby striving for more choice and control in childbirth. By the mid-1980s, an estimated fifty midwives were providing care to about 1,500 birthing women a year in Ontario (Van Wagner 1988: 115; Tyson 1991). The Ottawa Valley, downtown Toronto, and the Kitchener–Waterloo region were three key areas for this grassroots midwifery activity. Beyond their clinical work, the midwifery movement at this time was also striving to increase the visibility of midwifery outside of the health care system, while working toward the goal of legislation that would bring professional autonomy and government funding for midwives as well as access for all women to their services (Van Wagner 1988: 115).

The goal of professionalization for midwifery was also, in part, a response to external forces (Bourgeault 2006: 104). A coroner's inquest into the death of an infant in Kitchener, Ontario, after a transfer from

Becoming a Midwife

Like many community midwives in Ontario, Maya (a pseudonym) began as an apprentice midwife learning her skills from "hands-on work" with several more experienced midwives in her community, including a British-trained nurse-midwife and a self-trained community midwife. Maya's interest in becoming a midwife was first sparked by her work as a childbirth educator and her personal experience of having community midwives attend the birth of her second child. She became further politicized about birth when she became involved in a support group for women who had had c-sections. After a time in this group, she was asked to do labor coaching by some of the other members. "One thing led to another," she said, "and the next thing I knew I was attending births with other midwives." Maya combined her clinical apprenticeship with studying textbooks on her own for several years, and then undertook a four-month clinical midwifery program in El Paso, Texas, at Maternidad La Luz, receiving her permit to practice in that state. It was only then (1987) that she set up her own practice in her home and began to call herself a midwife.

Maya was one of the community midwives who became registered in Ontario through the Michener Institute of Health Sciences Pre-Registration Program in 1993, on the eve of the official declaration of midwifery as a profession—the process that assessed the qualifications of community midwives and brought them into the system (described in more detail in the text). Of her route to becoming a midwife she says: "I am an apprentice midwife, and I'm proud of it because I believe it was a very hard thing to do. I really had to apply myself. I had to go out there and get involved" (MacDonald 2007).

a midwife-attended home birth in 1982, was the first such important, though tragic, turning point. This inquest rallied public support for midwifery and set the stage for midwives to become more politically focused. Significantly, the jury recommended the regulation of midwifery. That same year the College of Physicians and Surgeons of Ontario (CPSO) issued a statement strongly discouraging its members from attending home births (CPSO 1982: 2). As a result, midwives across the province who had been working with home birth physicians now found themselves on their own. Another coroner's inquest following the death of another infant at a midwife-attended birth on Toronto Island in 1985 generated even more publicity and controversy. This inquest became a public forum to debate the legitimacy of midwifery in general when midwives called their own expert witnesses to testify. They also deliberately engaged the media to promote public awareness about the benefits and legitimacy of midwifery. This inquest, too, resulted in the jury's recommendations that midwifery be regulated and integrated into the provincial health care system.[6]

Another external force in the professionalization of midwifery in Ontario was the Health Professions Legislation Review (HPLR). The HPLR contacted both the OAM and the Ontario Nurse-Midwives Association (ONMA)[7] in 1982 to make submissions. At this critical juncture, "the midwifery movement realized that if it did not take up the issue of regulation and seek to define its own standards of practice and training, midwives would be defined by others" (Van Wagner 1988: 116). The protection of home birth was especially important. In response to the HPLR, community midwives, alongside a group of supportive nurse-midwives, came together to have their say in defining this new midwifery as a profession within the formal health care system. The OAM and the ONMA collaborated on a single submission to the HPLR as the Midwifery Coalition and eventually merged to form the Association of Ontario Midwives (AOM). The Province of Ontario—responding to the jury recommendations, the growing public support for midwifery, and the timing of the HPLR process—declared its intention to regulate midwifery in 1986. Though many influential politicians and health critics were supportive of midwifery, it is safe to say that the province was primarily concerned with public safety rather than issues of women's choice and autonomy in maternity care.

The goal of professionalization was not held by all midwives in Ontario, and divisions within the community intensified as the process unfolded. Those who favored professionalization were tired of working on the fringes and being poorly remunerated, and they were also committed to greater access to midwifery care that legitimacy and public funding would provide. Many midwives in the province, however, were concerned about the exclusion that formal education and training would entail and feared that the medicalization of midwifery would inevitably follow its move into the mainstream health care system. One midwifery advocate, Jutta Mason, warned in an essay, "The Trouble with Licensing Midwives" (1990), that midwives and clients would be drawn back into a system of knowledge and authority from which they had deliberately opted out. Mason feared that professionalizing midwifery would ultimately reduce women's choices in childbirth by circumscribing midwives' autonomy.

Whether midwifery at this time is best described as a social movement or as a professionalization project is debatable. Certainly the prospect of legislation to legitimate midwifery contributed to the growth of midwifery in the 1980s. In fact, midwifery as a social movement and midwifery as a professionalization movement were inseparable (MacDonald 2007). Issues that arose at this time—concerns about medicalization and loss of autonomy for midwives, concerns about loss of true choice for women—remain salient more than a decade after midwifery made its transition from the margins to the mainstream. We will look at some of these issues in more detail below in our section on the challenges and innovations in contemporary midwifery.

International Influences

As midwives in the province of Ontario pursued integration, they had the benefit not only of a strong social movement with a vision for a new kind of maternity care in Canada, but also the knowledge of professional midwifery models that were working well—or not working well—in other jurisdictions. In shaping their vision for the new profession of midwifery in Ontario, community midwives drew on the scholarly and professional literature available on midwifery models abroad and on their own international networks. Though Canadian midwifery shares much in common ideologically with independent midwifery in the United States and radical midwifery in the United Kingdom, Canadian midwives have read some of the challenges faced by American and British midwives as "cautionary tales" (Davis-Floyd 2006). For example, it was well known that "independent (lay) midwives" in the United States (who worked much like community midwives in Canada prior to legislation) were vulnerable to prosecution and were left out of the loop of third-party health insurance. U.S. certified nurse-midwives (CNMs) meanwhile, worked without much autonomy and were largely restricted to hospitals. Furthermore, U.S. lay and nurse-midwives were engaged in sometimes bitter battles over educational routes, with the lay/direct-entry home birth midwives insisting on the value of apprenticeship and vocational schools, and the CNMs insisting on university-based education (Davis-Floyd 2006). Some members of the OAM (before it became the AOM) were involved with the Midwives Alliance of North America (MANA), an organization founded primarily by lay midwives in 1982, which still advocates multiple routes to becoming a midwife and strives to uphold ideals and practice models similar to those Ontario midwives envisioned. To support the Ontario process, MANA held its 1984 annual meeting in Toronto at the same time as a Private Members Bill arguing for the integration of midwifery was presented in the provincial legislature. On that day, midwives, mothers, and babies from across the United States and Canada who were attending the MANA conference filled the visitors' gallery at Queen's Park in a great show of support for the bill (Betty-Anne Daviss, personal communication 2006).

International influences were also salient in the way various aspects of midwifery were implemented in the province. The government-appointed Task Force on the Implementation of Midwifery in Ontario looked specifically to the Netherlands while investigating and making recommendations on how to build upon community midwifery for a regulated model of midwifery that would work in Ontario. The Dutch midwifery model is characterized by professional autonomy, choice of birthplace, and the assumption that normal birth is the domain of midwives, while abnormality is the domain of obstetricians (see Chapter 1). Low rates of intervention, high rates of patient satisfaction, and among the best infant and maternal outcome statistics in the world also recommended the Dutch model to Ontario midwives. Preference for the Dutch model was the case even for the francophone province of Quebec, where a stronger influence from France might have been expected if not for that country's highly medicalized form of midwifery (Vadeboncoeur 2004). In addition, the Michener Institute of Health Sciences (the site of the preregistration program whereby midwives already practicing in the community and those with midwifery credentials from other jurisdictions applied to be "grandmothered" into the new profession) recruited an international faculty from the Netherlands, Denmark, Britain, and New Zealand to test the applicants' clinical knowledge and skills. Thus, the model of midwifery in Ontario today is a product of both local social and historical specificity as well as international networks and knowledge exchange—a fact that lends weight to one of the purposes of this book: to support midwifery internationally by sharing models that work.

UNIQUE STRUCTURAL CHARACTERISTICS OF ONTARIO MIDWIFERY

On January 1, 1994, midwifery became officially recognized as a profession and as part of the provincial health care system in Ontario. The College of Midwives of Ontario (CMO) is the governing body for midwifery in Ontario; its mandate is to administer the Midwifery Act in the public interest. Meanwhile the Association of Ontario Midwives (AOM) continues to be the professional body representing midwives and the practice of midwifery in Ontario. The number of midwives and the number of births attended by midwives in Ontario has grown steadily since 1994. In 2006 there were sixty-three practice groups including 380 midwives licensed to practice in Ontario. They attended approximately 8%

of all births in the province, and 20% of those births were home births (Knox and Katherine 2006).

Midwifery in Ontario—and in several Canadian provinces—has a combination of structural characteristics that makes it unique. These include the following:

- A model of clinical care that emphasizes continuity of care, choice of birth place, and informed choice
- Public funding, which helps ensure that all women experiencing normal pregnancy and birth have access to their services regardless of income[8]
- An independent, direct-entry model of education at the baccalaureate level

In this next section, we look at each of these structural characteristics in turn, focusing on the ways in which they support midwifery as a birth model that works, that is, in terms of supporting a model of clinical care that is continuous, is personalized, and involves the wishes and shared responsibility of the birthing woman in her choice of birth setting. A birth model that works must also function for midwives as workers in a highly bureaucratic health care system.

Autonomous Professional Status and Scope of Practice

Midwives in Ontario are autonomous professionals. The scope of midwifery practice in Ontario is defined in accordance with the International Definition of a Midwife, which stipulates the particulars of training, licensure, and scope of practice. Specifically,

> The midwife is recognised as a responsible and accountable professional who works in partnership with women to give the necessary support, care and advice during pregnancy, labour and the postpartum period, to conduct births on the midwife's own responsibility and to provide care for the newborn and the infant. This care includes preventative measures, the promotion of normal birth, the detection of complications in mother and child, the accessing of medical care or other appropriate assistance and the carrying out of emergency measures. (ICM 2005)

Midwives in Ontario are primary care providers with hospital privileges, who follow women throughout their pregnancies, attend them in labor at home or in the hospital, and care for the mother and newborn for six weeks postpartum. Their work is not overseen by physicians, but they do consult family physicians and specialists when necessary as specified by a set of clinical guidelines. Most midwives work in practice groups made up of between two and eight midwives (often with a steady rotation of students).

The Ontario model of care stipulates two midwives at every birth in both home and hospital settings: the primary (for the mother) and the secondary (for the baby). This model differs from those of other provinces such as British Columbia, where there are two midwives at home births, but nurses provide the backup in the hospital. Solo practitioners in rural and remote areas of Ontario work with a provision for the use of second attendants who are not registered midwives. Second attendants may be nurses, but they may also be women in the community who have an interest in midwifery and have learned neonatal resuscitation. Full-time midwives attend forty births per year as the primary midwife, and forty as the secondary midwife.

Continuity of care is central to the midwifery model of practice, allowing a trusting relationship to build between midwife and client, and ensuring the presence of a known caregiver during labor and delivery. The model of continuity that worked well before legislation—one-to-one care—was ideal for the smaller caseloads midwives had then and the fewer bureaucratic requirements necessary for remuneration and legislation. Since regulation, however, continuity of care has been adapted by some midwifery practices into what is sometimes called *shared care*, whereby a client builds a relationship with two, three, or even four midwives, and is then assured of having two of these caregivers at her birth. Shared care is being employed as a practical way of balancing the principle of continuity with the reality of professional midwifery work (Bourgeault, Luce, and MacDonald, 2006). (We discuss shared care further in the section on challenges and opportunities facing midwifery in Ontario.)

Choice of birth place is another unique aspect of the Ontario midwifery model of care. Even though home birth is not uncommon around the world, what makes it special in Ontario is that midwives won the provision for home birth in a province where hospital birth had been the norm for more than half a century. More importantly, *all* Ontario midwives are required to maintain their clinical skills at both home and hospital by attending a minimum number of five births in each setting each year. This means that home birth is not just optional but central to Ontario midwifery— an aspect of the new profession that upholds the ideals of midwives working in the community prior to legislation. Offering choice of birth place to women also means that midwives must have access to hospitals.

In the months and years following legislation, hospitals across the province had to develop new policies and alter existing policies to accommodate these new professionals in their midst. Hospital departments in some cases had to be created or existing ones opened up to accommodate midwives; the use of hospital spaces—including work and personal space—had to be negotiated; lines of formal and informal communication between midwives and other clinicians and hospital staff had to be built; and perhaps most significantly, midwives had to be granted hospital admitting and discharging privileges. Midwifery without hospital access would restrict access to women who planned home births. Thus, a special provision was made for midwifery within the regulatory structure governing hospital admitting privileges.[9] Ontario midwives' admitting and discharging privileges are similar to those of physicians, in contrast to being salaried staff of hospitals as nurses and many midwives around the world are. Individual midwives must apply to individual hospitals just as physicians do, and the specific processes to gain and maintain privileges vary from hospital to hospital. Some midwives experienced delays in obtaining privileges for several months after their official integration in January 1994 as local hospitals worked out their policies.[10] Unfortunately, securing and maintaining hospital privileges has been an ongoing concern for midwives. Hospital integration was, and in some communities continues to be, a difficult transition both for midwives (some of whom had not attended births in hospitals before) and for hospitals. For that reason, we have described here how hospital integration ideally works and is working in many places in the province, and will discuss the issue further in the section on challenges still facing midwifery in Ontario.

It is also important to note that Ontario midwives function as part of a network of medical professionals, including obstetricians, family physicians and pediatricians, with whom, according to College of Midwives' protocols, midwives must consult for conditions of the mother or newborn that fall outside the midwifery scope of practice, such as hypertension during pregnancy. Other conditions, such as twins, require a complete, irreversible transfer of care. Sometimes when a transfer is required and the problem is later resolved, the care may be referred back to the midwife (as is also the case in the Netherlands—see Chapter 1). Consults and transfers may work the same way during labor, as in the case of a woman with an abnormal labor pattern who is transferred out of midwifery care. If the labor pattern is "normalized" by pharmaceutical augmentation, the attending physician can choose to transfer the care back to the midwife—depending on the particular physician and particular hospital where the care is being provided. Midwives can also refer clients to regulated health professionals who may be considered alternative or complementary, including chiropractors, naturopaths, homeopaths, nutritionists, physiotherapists, and massage therapists. Finally, emergency services for women giving birth with midwifery care in the hospital or at home are also available, just as they would be for a woman under a physician's care.[11] In these ways, midwives form part of a larger maternity care system that includes appropriate and timely access to medical specialists and emergency services when required.

Funding for midwifery services is provided by the Ontario Ministry of Health and Long-Term Care (MOHLTC) through its Community Health Branch to practice groups and solo practitioners in rural/remote locales.

At present, midwives are "dependent contractors" to the province, and midwifery is run as a specific program of the MOHLTC—the Ontario Midwifery Program (not to be confused with the Ontario Midwifery Education Programme). Midwives do not bill on a fee-for-service basis as do most physicians, but rather are remunerated based on fulfilling a requisite number of courses of care per year, with a full-time equivalent defined as attending forty births in a primary role and forty as backup. Full-time midwives earn approximately C$73,000–C$95,000 a year, depending on the number of years of experience the midwife has in Ontario and the number of clients seen each year. There are also provisions for part-time caseloads if midwives so choose. In the other provinces where midwives are integrated and publicly funded—such as in British Columbia and Quebec—similar course of care arrangements exist, but in the province of Manitoba, midwives are salaried employees of one of the province's regional health boards. Alberta is the one Canadian province that regulates the practice of midwifery without the provision of public funding, despite being one of the wealthiest provinces in the country (see James and Bourgeault 2004 for details).

Direct-Entry Education: The Midwifery Education Programme

Entrance to the Ontario Midwifery Education Programme (MEP) does not require a prior degree in nursing or health sciences. Despite recommendations from both the nursing and medical professions that prior nursing training should be a prerequisite for midwifery education, the AOM and provincially appointed policy makers disagreed. It was clear that midwives' educational credentials would have a major bearing on the legitimacy of midwives as practitioners, their ability to maintain a primary caregiver model, and their ability to offer choice of birth place. A direct-entry education model in a university setting was deemed preferable for two reasons: (1) a university degree would be necessary to ensure both the autonomy and the legitimacy of the profession in the mainstream health care system (Bourgeault 2006); and (2) hospitals would be unlikely to grant hospital admitting and discharging privileges to anyone with less than a baccalaureate-level degree.

The MEP was established in the fall of 1993 and currently operates at three sites—Ryerson Polytechnic University, which offers the program part-time; McMaster University, where it is part of an affiliated health sciences center; and Laurentian University, which offers the program in French as well as in English. The four-year program involves both a rigorous academic component and clinical placements with pregnant women, practicing midwives, and physicians, the intention being to combine standardized academic qualifications with a hands-on apprenticeship approach to learning.

Most faculty members are midwives with advanced degrees, who must also be in active practice in order to ensure that their clinical skills remain sharp and to prevent the emergence of different classes of midwives (i.e., those who teach and those who practice). Practicing midwives across the province act as clinical preceptors for students in the academic programs and receive remuneration for their mentoring work. Because the profession is relatively small, most practicing midwives in Ontario have a fairly constant rotation of students working with them. The cooperation of nonteaching midwives and midwifery clients is thus critically important in the education of midwifery students. Between September 1993 and the fall of 2002, 153 students completed the program (Kaufman and Soderstrom 2004). The number of graduates from the three campuses each year has increased from 18 to over 40 in 2004; the plan is to graduate at least 60 per year. New registrants join existing practices around the province and undergo six to twelve months of supervision with an established practice before they can set up on their own. Almost two-thirds of the registered midwives in the province have graduated within the last ten years—a fact that reminds us how new the profession really is.

A direct-entry university program is not the only way to become a midwife in Ontario. Access to the profession has grown through the introduction of the Prior Learning and Assessment (PLA) program. The PLA was set in place in 1996 by the College of Midwives after a period of intense criticism and lobbying against what was perceived and experienced as the "exclusionary practices" of the new profession. A group called the Committee for More Midwives (CMM) sprang up to fight against what its members saw as an unacceptable situation for midwives who were not considered experienced enough to be admitted to the preregistration program. Scholarly critiques tracing the experiences of foreign-trained midwives and immigrant women of color "excluded" by midwifery professionalization (Nestel 2004) also contributed to the push for another mechanism for registration. The first group of PLA midwives graduated in the fall of 1996 and became registered midwives. The PLA was later renamed the Prior Learning and Experience Assessment (PLEA) process. In 2001 the College of Midwives of Ontario won public funding to expand and enhance the PLEA process and house it at arm's length from the CMO in Ryerson University's Continuing Education Department; it then became known as the International Midwifery Pre-registration Program (IMPP). Headed by midwifery pioneer Holiday Tyson, the expansion of the IMPP includes an approximately nine-month "bridging program" that internationally educated midwives can undergo to prepare for registration with the college. The IMPP also prepares midwives for registration in other provinces. This mechanism for integrating foreign-trained midwives is another significant strength of Ontario midwifery, and it is critically important in a province where so many immigrants will continue to settle. Finally, midwives who have been registered in another province for a minimum of one year may apply to the CMO for reciprocal status in order to practice in Ontario.

The creation of these multiple routes to midwifery education and registration has been significant for a number of reasons in terms of expanding access to the midwifery profession in Ontario. Midwifery as a social movement was largely a white, middle-class phenomenon, a fact reflected in the makeup of the new profession and its clientele in the 1990s. Given the cultural and linguistic diversity of the province, especially in major cities such as Toronto and Kitchener-Waterloo, the need to diversify the profession was evident from the beginning. It is a critically important issue not just in midwifery care but in health care more generally. Together, these programs provide the opportunity to bring foreign-trained midwives with diverse cultural, linguistic, and religious backgrounds into the midwifery profession; they, in turn, encourage the use of midwifery services by a diversity of clients who may otherwise not have considered them.

Improving Access for Midwifery Clients

Midwifery is now legally and economically accessible to all Ontario women with normal, uncomplicated pregnancy and birth who live within current midwifery catchment areas. Approximately two-thirds of the sixty-four hospitals in the province that offer maternity care include midwifery services (Knox and Katherine 2006). This geographical inequity of access is a problem recognized by the MOHLTC.[12] Ensuring access to midwifery care for diverse cultural, linguistic, and religious communities—especially in the larger urban centers—has been another critical issue throughout the integration process. Neither of these issues has been fully addressed by public funding, but equity in access to midwifery as a profession and as a service has come a long way. As mentioned above, having multiple routes of entry to registration and practice helps increase diversity within midwifery as a profession, which in turn, helps facilitate access to care for various cultural communities. Women whose first language is not English or French are now more likely to find a midwifery practice with someone who shares their first language and cultural background. Indeed, midwifery practices across the province typically advertise the range of languages spoken. Further, midwifery practices are developing ways to outreach and then adapt their work to the particular needs of various groups in their communities: teenage mothers, incarcerated mothers, nonstatus immigrants, and low-income families. Midwifery practices that outreach to nonstatus immigrant women who lack public health insurance, for example, also work with hospital administrators and obstetricians to set nominal fees in case their clients need to transfer to hospital and into physician care.

Another feature of Ontario midwifery having to do with diversity is the fact that the Midwifery Act included an exemption for Aboriginal midwives serving Aboriginal women, thus leaving an opening for the development of a unique form of midwifery in the province created by and for Aboriginal Peoples. Quebec and the territory of Nunavut also have legal provisions and community-based Aboriginal midwifery training programs. In British Columbia, an exemption applies only to Aboriginal midwives who were practicing within Aboriginal communities prior to midwifery legislation. The College of Midwives of British Columbia is developing an Aboriginal category of registration, but it is not yet in place (CMRC 2007). The province of Manitoba has also established a unique Aboriginal Midwifery Educational Program particularly for those wanting to work in the northern regions (CMRC 2007).

Midwifery Outcome Data and Client Satisfaction

Because of the relative newness of midwifery in Ontario and across the country, there are very few studies that explore clinical outcomes, patient satisfaction, and cost effectiveness. The data that are available, however, do confirm midwifery in Ontario as a birth model that works. A review of midwifery undertaken by the Ontario Ministry of Health and Long-Term Care (MOHLTC) in 2003 found that midwifery was not only cost effective, but was cost saving for the provincial health care system (Association of Ontario Midwives 2007a). The savings derive from a number of factors: (1) normal births are not handled by specialists, whose services cost more; (2) home births do not require the use of hospital beds and services such as meals and housekeeping; (3) planned hospital birth clients typically leave the hospital sooner because midwives provide follow-up postpartum care at home—a feature of midwifery that also translates into lower hospital and emergency room re-admission rates; (4) midwifery is associated with less technology and medication use during labor as well as lower rates of interventions generally (Johnson and Daviss 2005). For example, when compared to family physicians with a comparable cohort of low-risk cases, midwives have lower rates of episiotomy (7.2% versus 16.6%), forceps/vacuum deliveries (5.4% versus 14.4%), and referrals to cesarean section (12.7% versus 20.6%). The Ministry report also found that midwifery had both very high client satisfaction rates (98.7%) and good clinical outcomes, with both maternal and infant mortality and morbidity rates being comparable to both national rates of all births and rates of family physicians following a comparable cohort of low-risk cases (Kaufman et al. 2001a and b; Association of Ontario Midwives 2007b).

A recent study in the province of British Columbia also demonstrates the safety of planned home births and documents the lower rates of intervention at midwife-attended births at home and in a hospital when compared to

Aboriginal Midwifery in Ontario

At the Six Nations Maternal and Child Health Centre in Ohsweken in southwestern Ontario, Aboriginal midwives have been providing maternity care services to Aboriginal women since 1996. The Centre's Aboriginal name, *Tsi Non:we Ionnakeratstha Ona:grahsta'*, combines the Mohawk words for "the place they will be born" and the Cayuga word for "birthing place." All Six Nations midwives are recognized and authorized to practice by the Band Council of the Six Nations reserve and are accountable to the community. Most have been trained at the center in a three-year training program that combines academic course work, clinical placements, and the teaching of traditional knowledge. The first class graduated in 2003. Funding for the Six Nations Maternal and Child Health Centre comes from the government of Ontario's Aboriginal Health and Wellness Strategy—a unique policy and funding body made up of representatives from four provincial ministries and sixteen Aboriginal groups from across the province.

There are currently four full-time midwives employed by the Maternal and Child Health Centre, who see approximately fifty women a year. Clients can give birth at home, at one of the center's three birthing rooms, or in nearby Brantford General Hospital, which cooperates with center midwives in cases of emergency and nonemergency transfers of care. Because the Six Nations midwives do not have hospital privileges, when a transfer of care occurs, they accompany the birthing woman to hospital in an advocacy and supportive care role only.

The scope of practice of the Aboriginal midwives at Six Nations is in accord with the College of Midwives of Ontario standards, but is ultimately determined by members of the center's advisory council, who have the power to adapt the standards to meet local needs and ideals. The supervisor of the center is Ruby Miller, a registered nurse and member of the Six Nations reserve. She oversees its clinical, educational, and community programs. She emphasizes that midwifery care at the center is not only about pregnancy and birth but also about "strengthening the family" through creating a welcoming environment and through the broader health and well-being programming offered.

Midwives are very involved in such activities as breastfeeding support for all women in the community (whether they are midwifery clients or not), educational workshops for young women, a child nutrition program, and a fetal alcohol syndrome education program (Miller, personal communication 2006). Midwives, in turn, are supported in their expanded role by the broader community. For example, a special group called the Grandparents—a group of elders—provides guidance and support on issues that intersect with midwifery care, including teaching parenting skills and traditional ethics, and conducting traditional ceremonies, such as welcoming ceremonies for babies. Center midwives have also enjoyed mutually supportive relations with non-Aboriginal registered midwives in nearby communities, getting together for clinical peer review, for example.

In the words of Katsi Cook, a practicing Aboriginal midwife with more than twenty years' experience, who worked at the center in the 1990s, the Maternity and Child Health Centre offers "the integration of traditional knowledge and the best of medical knowledge" (Aboriginal Health and Wellness Strategy 1996: 2). According to Ruby Miller, aboriginal women in the catchment area choose midwifery not only because they are looking for the type and quality of care midwives offer, but also because they want to have their babies "on their own territory" as part of "reclaiming birth" and rebuilding aboriginal families (personal communication, 2006).

physician care in a hospital (Janssen et al. 2002). Midwifery clients in Ontario had higher rates of breastfeeding uptake and continuation at six weeks postpartum (90.7%) compared with physician care (71.5%) (Association of Ontario Midwives 2007b). The outcome data, however, do identify some areas worthy of further research: rates of intervention that distinguish home from hospital cohorts and rates of transfers to the hospital that distinguish primiparous women from multiparous women are two examples (Kaufman et al. 2001a and b). The MOHLTC has recently introduced the Ontario Midwifery Clinical Data Base—a mandatory Web-based reporting and analysis program that will take over from the previous AOM system and continue to generate important midwifery clinical data (Knox and Katherine 2006).

FACING CHALLENGES, CREATING OPPORTUNITIES: SUSTAINING A MODEL THAT WORKS

In this chapter we have described the historic transition of midwifery in Ontario from a grassroots social movement to a full profession within the mainstream health care system. We have also shown the unique combination of elements that make midwifery in Ontario a birth model that works. Indeed, the province has acknowledged the success of midwifery and is showing its commitment to the profession with recently announced increases in provincial funding that will expand the availability of midwifery services to women across the province as the demand continues to grow (Ministry of Health and Long-Term Care 2005). Predictions are that by the year 2020, midwives will attend 20% of all births in the province. The sustainability of midwifery as a profession, however, is more complex than these apparently positive projections. A number of challenges still face this young midwifery profession.

In the years following integration in 1994, a relatively small number of new registered midwives were grappling with the huge demands of setting up a new profession and the new Midwifery Education Programme while continuing to care for clients within the new, regulated system and its institutions. At this time a number of issues were front and center, including getting used to working in hospitals, working the bugs out of the funding mechanism, dealing with fears that midwifery was becoming medicalized as a result of integration, and confronting the problem of access for women as clients and for midwives aspiring to enter the profession. Some of these problems are well on their way to being resolved (as discussed above), others are in still in progress, and others have been doggedly persistent. How can midwifery continue to "nurture normal birth" in the face of these challenges?[13] In this final section, we describe and reflect on three key challenges facing midwifery in Ontario (though not necessarily unique to this Canadian province), including hospital integration, medicalization of midwifery practice, and issues facing midwives as workers—including interprofessional relationships. We take the position that such challenges may be seen as opportunities for refining midwifery in Ontario as a model that works and is sustainable for midwives and the women they serve.

Hospital Integration

Prior to midwifery regulation, physicians, nurses, and hospitals were not always welcoming to midwives, and in some cases they were openly hostile. Having previously seen midwives and their clients only when there was a need to transfer care, most nurses and physicians knew only what they viewed as "midwifery disasters" and "botched home births." They did not recognize such transports as appropriate care and had little knowledge of all the midwife-attended home births that occurred without incident. The professional bodies of nursing and medicine had not objected outright to the implementation of midwifery per se, but they had expressed concerns about what kind of midwifery it would be, preferring exclusively hospital-based nurse-midwifery practice. Interestingly, even as physicians and nurses in Ontario recognized the midwives they knew as knowledgeable and competent, they often viewed midwifery—which they understood as "political"—with suspicion. These concerns did not disappear overnight (MacDonald 2007).

Although in some Ontario hospitals, nurses and physicians have welcomed midwives and the new approach to maternity care that midwifery brings, in general the transition has been marked by tension. Some physicians objected specifically to midwives' autonomy and rates of remuneration, and questioned their training and skills. They also objected quite rightly to the fact that a system for payment for consults was not initially in place when midwives were integrated. On this latter point, some of these physicians' anger was unfortunately directed toward midwives rather than toward their own College of Physicians and Surgeons or the Ontario Ministry of Health, which had failed to foresee this problem or address it in a timely manner. Nursing staff, for their part, were concerned about the implications of this new profession for their job security and turf in the hospital. They were and are frustrated in everyday ways, too, when midwives with little prior hospital experience cannot remember routines or paperwork or where to find supplies. Kornelsen and Carty similarly describe how midwifery integration in the case of British Columbia "has not gone smoothly" (2004: 112). Although the situation there is slowly improving, they describe it as characterized by tension and competition rather than collaboration.

As for midwives' feelings about working in a hospital, many—especially those who practiced prior to the formal integration of midwifery into the hospital system—were uncomfortable in a hospital with its institutional spaces, unfamiliar routines, and bureaucratic paperwork, or they were highly critical of the standardized approaches to childbirth taken by the nurses and doctors who worked there. They did not all take easily to the new routines, and many resented the new, bureaucratic demands, which they felt impinged upon their clinical authority and distanced them from their clients (Bourgeault 2006; MacDonald 2007). The scholarly literature on midwives' integration into hospitals generally points to how midwives are constrained within that setting from providing care within their full scope of practice (Annandale, 1988; Benoit, 1991; Harvey, Kaufman, and Rice, 1995; Rothman, 1983). Furthermore, many in the midwifery profession regard the move from domiciliary practice to hospital-based practice as limiting midwives' autonomy.[14]

To adjust positively to practicing in hospital, midwives often speak of "taking the home into the hospital" in simple but effective ways: closing the door to the hospital room to help ensure a woman's privacy and their own authority, changing the lighting, bringing in their own "tools of the trade" such as crock pots for hot compresses, and encouraging women to bring their own clothing and food to personalize the space (Bourgeault, Luce, and McDonald 2006; MacDonald 2007). Midwives accept that it is imperative to practice in the hospital so as to ensure women choice of birthplace and continuity of care in the case of a transfer from home. The experience

Midwifery in the Hospital

One midwifery practice covers three large rural counties, and the midwives who live and work in this area are committed to providing care to rural women—a labor of love that began long before regulation. As a consequence of the large catchment area, the midwives here have admitting and discharging privileges at three different hospitals. They describe the initial reception to midwifery integration at these hospitals as largely positive, praising the smaller rural hospital especially for having "rolled out the red carpet" for them. (In fact, it was the first hospital in the province to give midwives privileges.) Despite the warm welcome, one of the midwives at this practice who worked outside the system prior to midwifery regulation maintains, "It's always my first choice to be out in the community partly because I'm using my own equipment that I sterilised and I packed and I know where it is. . . . And you know in the hospital, it's just—it's just not a comforting environment for me because all my experience prior to legislation was in people's homes."

An obvious challenge for midwives in this practice is that they must learn about and follow slightly different sets of clinical protocols at each hospital. As one of them explains, "We have our College [of Midwives] list. We have mandatory consultations and transfers of care, but within each institution, there's also a subset of those that could be different. And so that has influenced the way we practice." She continues, "One of the things we are learning is how to step on the least toes, how to piss your consultants off the least and, you know, try to walk that fine line where we're are being true to our clients and the way we would like to practice midwifery in as holistic a way as possible."

of midwives in hospitals is affected to some degree by their training and prior experience. For example, midwifery students who trained partly in a hospital often have higher comfort levels there.

Overall, midwives' integration into hospitals as professionals was, and in some communities, continues to be a difficult transition, whereas in others this integration was handled with relative ease. In some places, it is still the case that physicians and midwives appear locked in bitter battles that are troubling to them as professionals and persons, and for the public.[15] Although the negative consequences of working in a hospital for midwifery seem clear, a review of three hospital-based midwifery projects in Canada (Harvey, Kaufman, and Rice 1995) points to some of the advantages of midwifery practice in hospitals. These advantages include (1) increasing the availability and visibility of midwifery; (2) providing medical and nursing students with an opportunity to observe practicing midwives, fostering positive and up-to-date images of midwifery practice; and (3) providing the opportunity for obstetric health care providers to learn about the ability of a midwifery model to change standard hospital practice.[16]

In February 2005 the AOM and the Ontario Medical Association (OMA) created *A Joint Statement of Professional Relations between Obstetricians and Registered Midwives in Ontario,* which states that "optimal patient care is achieved when obstetricians and midwives collaborate . . . [and] establish clear mechanisms for consultation and transfer of care, recognizing and understanding their respective roles in the provision of care" (AOM 2005: 1). The document goes on to affirm the professions' goal to "facilitate communication and collegial relationships between obstetricians and midwives" (AOM 2005: 1). Another recent joint statement concerns *Guidelines for Maternal/Neonate Transfers from Home to Hospital,* which is intended to help physicians and midwives establish clear lines of communication and protocols in their communities to make transfer situations go smoothly and reduce interprofessional tension. Though these joint statements clearly speak to past difficulties, they also speak to the commitment to refine and redress the trouble spots of midwifery integration.

Medicalization

One of the most commonly heard concerns of midwives and their clients in the years following professionalization was that midwifery would become medicalized. First of all, the ratio of home births to hospital births among midwifery clients in Ontario is slowly declining—from 50:50 in 1993 (Van Wagner 2005) to 25:75 in 2003 (MOHLTC 2005) and to 20:80 in 2006 (Knox and Katherine 2006). This is a concern because the scholarly literature on midwifery in hospitals in a variety of jurisdictions describes how the setting alters midwives' work as they experience more pressure to conform to standard obstetrical proscriptions, for example, for the length of various stages of labor (Foley and Faircloth 2003; Rothman 1983). "Midwives are more inclined to medicalize birth in a hospital," De Vries (2004: 267) concludes. Even though the clinical data from Ontario at this time, as discussed above, still find midwifery comparing favorably with physician care in terms of its lower intervention rates approach, a recent study that compared planned home births with planned hospital births in British Columbia seems to indicate that medicalization in the hospital is a concern. Janssen et al. report that "women who gave birth at home attended by a midwife had fewer procedures during labour compared with women who gave birth in hospital attended by a physician" (2002: 315), but that women who gave birth in hospital attended by midwife had more procedures compared to the home birth group.

The specter of medicalization, of course, had arisen long before in the debates leading up to the decision to pursue professionalization, and in the difficult process of defining the midwifery scope of practice. Yet one of the key reasons why midwives chose to pursue professionalization was to gain legitimate access to institutional settings, consultations with other health care providers, and the kind of diagnostic and therapeutic medicine that was not directly or uniformly available to community midwives and their clients outside the system. Midwives do use more medical technology now than they did prior to having professional status: they order diagnostic tests throughout pregnancy and manage births that may involve an array of technology (such as continuous fetal monitoring) and medication (such as narcotics for pain relief, and IV drips for prophylactic antibiotic drips or augmentation). Further, they are held to clinical standards that are often derived not from the most recent scientific evidence but from traditional obstetrical practice, including such things as specific allowances for length of stages of labor, the implications of which are potential interventions such as pharmaceutical augmentation for slow labor or cesarean for a long pushing stage. Such standards often impinge upon the noninterventionist character of midwifery care.

Exacerbating this situation is the concern around professional liability, particularly in the cases of consults and transfers of care. In theory, the principle of informed choice mitigates against the possibility of litigation in the event of an adverse outcome. In reality, however, as several recent inquests into infant deaths have shown, medical technology wielded by an authoritative expert trumps client choice in the eyes of the public (as represented by jurors), and in some cases retrospectively, in the eyes of clients themselves. In other words, the imperative to use technology weighs heavily on midwives' practicing in hospitals leading de facto to a degree of medicalization. Yet many midwives and clients would also argue that even as medical technology takes its place within a fully integrated midwifery, it does so in a new way. As MacDonald (2002, 2007) suggests, contemporary midwives and clients in Ontario seem to work to naturalize medical technology; that is, when trust characterizes the midwife-client relationship, and informed choice governs negotiations around medical interventions, midwifery care, even as it involves medical technology, may not be experienced as medicalized by clients.

Midwives as Workers

Creating and sustaining midwifery as a profession in Ontario has been a challenge these past thirteen years. That challenge is ongoing. The integrated model of midwifery work organization is notable for the manner with which it balances the needs of midwives as workers and the needs of midwifery clients as recipients of care. Specifically, the positive aspects of the organization of midwifery work for childbearing women include these:

- The assurance of continuity of care and caregiver (midwives are available twenty-four hours on call)
- Long pre- and postnatal visits; choice of birth place (all midwives practice both at home and in the hospital)
- Shared decision making expressed in a model of informed choice
- Public funding to help ensure access
- Clinical outcomes that indicate midwifery care and home birth are safe, even preferable

The aspects of midwifery work organization that make it manageable for midwives include these:

- A moderate birth caseload
- Remuneration to work in pairs (and many work in group practices)
- Provisions for part-time work and time off call

In these ways, midwifery in Ontario has been organized to minimize the "caring dilemma" that arises when workers' duty to care for others is promoted over their personal lives and unpaid work as partners and parents (Benoit and Heitlinger 1998). The true litmus test of midwives' caring dilemma, however, is the everyday experiences of practicing midwives. When we talked with twenty-six midwives practicing across Ontario, we found that many are inundated with work that does not directly involve caring for women: committee work to maintain hospital admitting privileges; preceptor work to mentor new midwives; and the paperwork involved in being financially accountable to the Provincial Ministry of Health for public funding. One midwife ruefully describes her work as "with chart" rather than "with woman" (MacDonald 2007). Several midwives also detail how their work, particularly being on call twenty-four hours a day, often results in personal and familial conflict (Bourgeault, Luce, and McDonald 2006). That is, midwives' caring dilemma seems to be salient not only in their roles as workers, but also in their roles as spouses and mothers. In response to this challenge posed by continuity of care as a central pillar of midwifery work, as noted above, some practices are introducing shared care models in which three or more midwives offer continuity of care to one client.

Shared care is an innovative response to an otherwise unsustainable ideal of continuity of care. It is also an excellent example of how Ontario midwifery is still in the process of adapting and perfecting its model in the first decade or so of its professional incarnation.

CONCLUSION

In this chapter we have described the creation of professional midwifery in Ontario as a birth model that works. We have touched on the key debates as midwifery moved toward professional status from its social movement roots and have highlighted the challenges of integrating it into a sometimes ambivalent health care system. We argue that midwifery in Ontario is a birth model that works because the unique place of midwives within the health care system facilitates the philosophical goals of midwifery everywhere with relative success: to offer continuous, personalized care that involves the wishes and shared responsibility of the birthing woman, and when necessary, a collaborating network of health experts and emergency services. Both client satisfaction and clinical outcomes confirm its success. Yet we have also shown that midwives must continue to engage in creative and adaptive ways to face the challenges they experience within the system, and in so doing, to refine their vision and their clinical work. Ontario midwives must also continue to respond to changing political and social trends that affect a highly institutional, bureaucratic, and publicly funded health care system, as well as to constantly emerging new clinical evidence. In keeping with their roots in a social movement, midwives *respond* rather than acquiesce to the formal health system of which they are now a part in order to maintain their commitment to the principles of midwifery and vigilance against their erosion. In agreement with other observers, clients, and midwives, we believe professionalization has strengthened Ontario midwifery, offering greater choice to more women as a regulated profession than it ever could as an underground practice focused exclusively on home birth. Ontario midwifery—an autonomous, publicly funded profession in the public sphere—is a birth model that works.

ACKNOWLEDGMENTS

The authors would like to acknowledge financial support from the Social Sciences and Humanities Research Council of Canada through a doctoral and postdoctoral fellowship (MacDonald) and through a doctoral and postdoctoral fellowship and standard research grant (Bourgeault). We would also like to thank the editors of this volume—Robbie Davis-Floyd, Lesley Barclay, Betty-Anne Daviss, and Jan Tritten for offering many insightful comments on earlier drafts of this chapter.

NOTES

1. Margaret MacDonald conducted fourteen months of intensive ethnographic fieldwork in Ontario from 1996 to 1997, which involved participant observation at midwifery clinics, births, and conferences as well as more than fifty formal interviews with midwives and their clients. Ivy Bourgeault collected over twenty years' worth of primary and secondary source documents on the integration of midwifery in Ontario as well as held over sixty interviews with key midwifery and policy informants. Both authors remain current with changes in midwifery since that time.

2. Midwifery was retained in some Mennonite, Hutterite, and First Nations communities as well as in remote and rural areas of Canada (Benoit 1991; Biggs 1983; Campanella, Korbin, and Acheson 1993). British-trained nurse-midwives were also recruited to staff nursing outposts in remote and northern regions until the 1960s (Kaufert and O'Neil 1993; Plummer 2000).

3. See Barrington (1985), James-Chetalet (1989), Mason (1988), and Shroff (1997) for examples of this tendency.

4. A forerunner of the El Paso clinic *Maternidad La Luz* was operated by midwife Shari Daniels, who, as a speaker during a local home birth conference in Toronto in the 1980s, had issued an open invitation to the Ontario midwifery community to come and train at her clinic, which served a largely migrant Mexican clientele. Sociologist Sheryl Nestel (1996/97:327) points out the irony in aspiring Ontario midwives traveling across borders to improve their skills on the bodies of "others" and thereby gain their qualifications, while immigrant women of color in Ontario possessing formal qualifications from their countries of origin did not dare practice outside the law.

5. The term *independent* or *lay midwife* was used in the United States in the 1970s and 1980s to distinguish these midwives from Certified Nurse-Midwives (CNMs). Lay midwifery was not a term used much in Canada because, as several midwives and commentators have pointed out, the term "lay midwives" is inaccurate and often is used as a pejorative. Midwife and scholar Betty-Anne Daviss notes that midwives in Ontario at this time often referred to themselves as "practicing midwives" to distinguish themselves from nurse-midwives trained in other countries who were working as obstetric nurses in hospital (personal communication 2006). It is also common now to hear midwives who are not nurses refer to themselves as direct-entry midwives, referring to their educational route to becoming a midwife.

6. For detailed accounts of these inquests see Fynes (1994) and Bourgeault (2006).

7. The group of largely foreign-trained midwives practicing a limited scope as obstetric nurses in a hospital.

8. There are, however, limitations depending on geography—outside of midwives' catchment areas.

9. At the time midwifery was being integrated in the early 1990s, only physicians, and in special circumstances dental surgeons, had hospital admitting privileges. Several other health professions, however, such as chiropractors and psychologists, had also sought hospital admitting privileges, and there was some resistance within the Ministry of Health to "open the floodgates."

10. Consequently, some midwives had to transfer care of their hospital clients during this time either to another midwife who did have privileges or to a family physician or obstetrician for these bureaucratic rather than clinical reasons.

11. To ensure access to emergency services, some midwifery practices limit the geographical radius of their home birth services. This means that women in northern settings, for example, who may live more than thirty minutes from a hospital providing full emergency services, including cesareans and newborn intubation, cannot choose home birth.

12. As mentioned above, only two-thirds of Ontario hospitals where births are conducted have midwives.

13. The title of the 2005 Association of Ontario Midwives Annual Conference.

14. For example, Benoit's (1991) research on midwives in Newfoundland and Labrador found that as more midwives moved from local midwifery clinics into the hospital setting, midwives' scope of practice and autonomy became severely restricted not only by supervising physicians but also by hospital administration.

15. For example, at the 2002 inquest into an infant death in the city of Guelph, Ontario, which involved an emergency transfer of care from a midwife to the on-call obstetrician, it was publicly stated by participants and reported in the media that the relationships between midwives and nurses, obstetricians and pediatricians at Guelph General Hospital were *terrible*—not simply a case of growing pains. Further, it was stated that part of the problem was the dysfunctional, institutional culture of the hospital—a situation not isolated to Guelph (Bruce 2001; Shuttleworth 2002).

16. Though this study involved nurse-midwifery in hospital, there are parallels relevant to newly integrated community midwifery.

REFERENCES

Aboriginal Health and Wellness Strategy. 1996. *Tsi Non:we Ionnatakeratstha Is Born*, vol. 1.3.

Annandale, Ellen C. 1988. "How Midwives Accomplish Natural Birth: Managing Risk and Balancing Expectations." *Social Problems* 35.2:95–110.

Association of Ontario Midwives (AOM). 2005. *A Joint Statement of Professional Relations Between Obstetricians and Registered Midwives in Ontario.* http://www.aom.on.ca/Communications/Position_Statements/Joint_Statements.aspx. Accessed November 25, 2008.

———. 2007a. "Benefits of Midwifery to the Health Care System." http://www.aom.on.ca/Communications/Government_Relations/Benefits_to_Women_Needing_Obstetrical_Care.aspx. Accessed April 15, 2007.

———. 2007b. "Benefits to Women Needing Obstetrical Care: A Case for Sustaining Midwifery." http://www.aom.on.ca/Communications/Government_Relations/Benefits_to_Women_Needing_Obstetrical_Care.aspx. Accessed April 15, 2007.

Barrington, Eleanor. 1985. *Midwifery Is Catching.* Toronto: NC Press.

Benoit, Cecilia. 1991. *Midwives in Passage.* St John's, NF: Institute of Social and Economic Research.

Benoit, Cecilia, and Alena Heitlinger. 1998. "Women's Health Care Work in Comparative Perspective: Canada, Sweden and Czechoslovakia/Czech Republic as Case Examples." *Social Science and Medicine* 47.8:1101–11.

Biggs, C. Lesley. 1983. "The Case of the Missing Midwives: A History of Midwifery in Ontario from 1795–1900." *Ontario History* 75:21–35.

———. 2004. "Fragments of the History of Midwifery". In *Reconceiving Midwifery*, edited by Ivy L. Bourgeault, Cecilia Benoit, and Robbie Davis-Floyd, 17–45. Montreal: McGill-Queen's University Press.

Bourgeault, Ivy L. 2006. *Push! The Struggle to Integrate Midwifery in Ontario*. Montreal: McGill-Queen's University Press.

Bourgeault, Ivy L., Jacquelyne Luce, and Margaret MacDonald. 2006. "The Caring Dilemma in Midwifery: Balancing the Needs of Midwives and Clients in a Continuity of Care Model of Practice." *Community, Work and Family* 9.4:398–406.

Bruce, Andrew. 2001. "Midwives, MDs Urged to Cooperate; Baby Death Inquest Calls for Change." *Toronto Star*, December 6, A04.

Campanella, Karla, Jill Korbin, and Louise Acheson. 1993. "Pregnancy and Childbirth among the Amish." *Social Science and Medicine* 36.3:333–42.

Canadian Midwifery Regulators Consortium [CMRC]. http://cmrc-ccosf.ca/node/19. Accessed November 25, 2008.

College of Midwives of Ontario. 1994. *The Midwifery Model of Practice in Ontario*. http://www.midwivesgreysimcoe.org/informed%20choice%20binder/H-MOP.pdf. Accessed September 8, 2008.

College of Physicians and Surgeons of Ontario (CPSO). 1982. *Statement on Home Birth*. Toronto: CPSO.

Davis-Floyd, Robbie. 2006. "ACNM and MANA: Divergent Histories and Convergent Trends." In *Mainstreaming Midwives: The Politics of Change*, edited by Robbie Davis-Floyd and Christina Johnson, 29–80. New York: Routledge.

Daviss, Betty-Anne. 1999. "From Social Movement to Professional Midwifery Project: Are We Throwing the Baby Out with the Bathwater?" M.A. thesis, Carleton University, Ottawa.

De Vries, Raymond. 2004. *A Pleasing Birth: Midwives and Maternity Care in the Netherlands*. Philadelphia, PA: Temple University Press.

Ehrenreich, Barbara, and Deirdre English. 1973. *Witches, Midwives, and Nurses: A History of Women Healers*. Old Westbury, NY: Feminist Press.

Foley, Lara, and Christopher A. Faircloth. 2003. "Medicine as Discursive Resource: Legitimation in the Work Narratives of Midwives." *Sociology of Health & Illness* 25.2:165–84.

Fynes, Mary. 1994. "The Legitimation of Midwifery in Ontario." Master's thesis, University of Toronto.

Harvey, Sheila, Karyn Kaufman, and Alison Rice. 1995. "Models for Midwifery: Canada." In *Issues in Midwifery*, vol. 1, edited by Tricia Murphy-Black. Edinburgh: Churchill Livingstone.

International Confederation of Midwives (ICM). 2005. *Definition of the Midwife*. The Hague: ICM. http://www.internationalmidwives.org/Portals/5/Documentation/ICM%20Definition%20of%20the%20Midwife%202005.pdf. Accessed December 2, 2008.

James, Susan, and Ivy L. Bourgeault. 2004. "To Fund or Not to Fund: The Alberta Decision." In *Reconceiving Midwifery*, edited by Ivy L. Bourgeault, Cecilia Benoit, and Robbie Davis-Floyd, 131–49. Montreal: McGill-Queens University Press.

James-Chetalet, Lois. 1989. "Reclaiming the Birth Experience: An Analysis of Midwifery in Canada from 1788 to 1987." Ph.D. thesis, Carleton University, Ottawa.

Janssen, Patricia, Shoo Lee, Elizabeth Ryan, Duncan Etches, Duncan Farquarson, Donlim Peacock, and Michael Klein. 2002. "Outcomes of Planned Home Births versus Planned Hospital Births after Regulation of Midwifery in British Columbia." *Canadian Medical Association Journal* 166.3:324–26.

Johnson, Kenneth C., and Betty-Anne Daviss. 2005. "Outcomes of Planned Home Births with Certified Professional Midwives: Large Prospective Study in North America." *British Medical Journal* 330:1416–23.

Kaufert, Patricia, and John O'Neill. 1993. "Analysis of a Dialogue on Risk in Childbirth: Clinicians, Epidemiologists, and Inuit Women." In *Knowledge, Power, and Practice: The Anthropology of Medicine and Everyday Life*, edited by Shirley Lindenbaum and Margaret Lock, 32–54. Berkeley: University of California Press.

Kaufman, Karyn, John C. Hogenbirk, Raymond Pong, and L. Martin. 2001a. "Midwifery Care in Ontario: Client Outcomes for 1998, Part 1; Maternal Outcomes." *Association of Ontario Midwives Journal* 7.2:56–64.

———. 2001b. "Midwifery Care in Ontario: Client Outcomes for 1998, Part II; Fetal and Newborn Outcomes." *Association of Ontario Midwives Journal* 7.4:147–53.

Kaufman, Karyn, and Bobby Soderstrom. 2004. "Midwifery Education in Ontario: Its Origins, Operation, and Impact on the Profession." In *Reconceiving Midwifery*, edited by Ivy L. Bourgeault, Cecilia Benoit, and Robbie Davis-Floyd, 187–203. Montreal: McGill-Queens University Press.

Knox, Sarah, and Wendy Katherine. 2006. *Ontario Midwifery Clinical Data Base.* http://www.apheo.ca/resources/events/06/confo6/Program.htm. Accessed November 25, 2008.

Kornelsen, Jude, and Elaine Carty. 2004. "Challenges to Midwifery Integration: Interprofessional Relationships in BC." In *Reconceiving Midwifery*, edited by Ivy L. Bourgeault, Cecilia Benoit, and Robbie Davis-Floyd, 111–31. Montreal: McGill-Queens University Press.

Laforce, Helene. 1990. "The Different Stages of the Elimination of Midwives in Quebec." In *Delivering Motherhood: Maternal Ideologies and Practices in the 19th and 20th Centuries*, edited by Katherine Arnup, Andrée Levesque, and Ruth Roach Pierson, 36–50. London: Routledge.

MacDonald, Margaret E. 2002. "Postmodern Negotiations with Medical Technology: The Role of Midwifery Clients in the New Midwifery in Canada." *Medical Anthropology* 20:1–36.

———. 2004. "Tradition as a Political Symbol in the New Midwifery in Canada." In *Reconceiving Midwifery*, edited by Ivy L. Bourgeault, Cecilia Benoit, and Robbie Davis-Floyd, 46–66. Montreal: McGill-Queens University Press.

———. 2007. *At Work in the Field of Birth: Midwifery Narratives of Nature, Tradition, and Home.* Nashville, TN: Vanderbilt University Press.

Mason, Jutta. 1990. *The Trouble with Licensing Midwives.* Ottawa: CRIAW/ICREF.

———. 1988. "Midwifery in Canada." In *The Midwife Challenge*, edited by Sheila Kitzinger, 99–133. London: Pandora.

Michaelson, Karen (ed.). 1988. *Childbirth in America: Anthropological Perspectives.* New York: Bergin and Garvey.

Ministry of Health and Long-Term Care (MOHLTC). 2005. *McGuinty Government Increases Access to Midwifery.* http://ogov.newswire.ca/ontario/GPOE/2004/08/13/c1159.html?lmatch= &lang=_e.html. Accessed April 15, 2007.

Mitchenson, Wendy. 1991. The Nature of their Bodies: Women and their Doctors in Victorian Canada. Toronto: University of Toronto Press.

———. 2002. *Giving Birth in Canada 1900–1950.* Toronto: University of Toronto Press.

Nestel, Sheryl. 1996/97. "A New Profession to the White Population in Canada: Ontario Midwifery and the Politics of Race." *Health and Canadian Society* 4.2: 315–41.

———. 2004. "The Boundaries of Professional Belonging: How Race Has Shaped the Re-emergence of Midwifery in Ontario." In *Reconceiving Midwifery,* edited by Ivy L. Bourgeault, Cecilia Benoit, and Robbie Davis-Floyd, 287–305. Montreal: McGill Queen's University Press.

Plummer, Kate. 2000. "From Nursing Outpost to Contemporary Midwifery in Canada." *Journal of Midwifery and Women's Health* 45.2:169–75.

Rothman, Barbara Katz. 1983. Midwives in Transition: The Structure of a Clinical Revolution. *Social Problems* 30.3:262–71.

Rushing, Beth. 1993. "Ideology and the Reemergence of North American Midwifery." *Work and Occupations* 20.1:46–67.

Shroff, Farah (ed.). 1997. *The New Midwifery: Reflections on Renaissance and Regulation.* Toronto: Women's Press.

Shuttleworth, Joanne. 2002. "Hospital Manager Says Disputes Being Ironed Out." *Guelph Daily Mercury,* June 13, A1.

Tyson, Holliday. 1991. Outcomes of 1,001 midwife attended home births in Toronto, 1983 to 1988. *Birth* 18.1:14–19.

Vadeboncoeur, Helene. 2004. "Delaying Legislation: The Quebec Experiment." In *Reconceiving Midwifery,* edited by Ivy L. Bourgeault, Cecilia Benoit, and Robbie Davis-Floyd, 91–110. Montreal: McGill-Queens University Press.

Van Wagner, Vicki. 1988. "Women Organizing for Midwifery in Ontario." *Resources for Feminist Research* 17.3:115–18.

———. 2005. "Who's Afraid of Midwives?" Oral presentation, New Brunswick Advisory Council on the Status of Women, February 18.

Chapter 4

Samoan Midwives' Stories

Joining Social and Professional Midwives in New Models of Birth

Lesley Barclay Utumuu

INTRODUCTION

This chapter challenges the assumptions, still held in many postcolonial countries, that the migration and replication of a Western model of birthing is necessarily a desirable goal. The system of maternity care left behind in the Pacific Rim as New Zealanders, Australians, French, or British colonialists moved out is at the very least disappointing. This chapter demonstrates how a group of leaders in one country, Samoa, have made considerable progress in both reconceptualizing and developing a "postcolonial" model of maternity care.

Samoa is a small Pacific island nation northeast of Australia and New Zealand and over 3,500 kilometers west of Hawaii. It consists of two main islands with a small population of 176,848, as recorded in the 2001 census (*Health Department Annual Report* 2002). Samoans mainly live on these large islands and on a few other tiny islands. The total of births recorded across a range of health service facilities in 2002 was 3,264 (Community Health Nursing Information System [CHNIS]).

Samoa's birth model integrates social systems and practitioners with professional nurse-midwives in a model of health services delivery that appears to be unique. I describe in this chapter a new, non-Western birthing model that seems to work, and contrast this with my own experience as a midwife, midwife teacher, and maternity services consultant in Papua New Guinea and India over a decade ago and more recently in Jordan. In these countries, the Western professional culture dominates health care and birth rituals. These are imposed on normal birth, irrespective of local cultural values, evidence, cost effectiveness, and their capacity to increase risk. As data we have collected from traditional and professional midwives show, the experience in Samoa paints a much more positive picture and demonstrates a convincing and successful transformation from colonized birthing models. I would describe Samoa as developing a "postmodern midwifery" (Davis-Floyd 2004) and indeed a postmodern system of maternity care. Although this model is still evolving, it is more advanced in integrating social systems and practitioners with the advantages of professional health care than many others.

"Informed relativism"—a key characteristic of postmodern midwifery (Davis-Floyd 2004; Introduction, this volume)—is played out in Samoa to the full in their rapidly evolving system of birth. The philosophy that underpins nursing and midwifery is Samoan and has repositioned cultural values and competence alongside professional competence (Barclay et al. 1998). This repositioning is unique and has significantly influenced professional development and behavior. The chapter explores these issues. I draw on research data and published work with Samoan colleagues with whom I have been working for fifteen years. I believe the Samoan model of birth illustrates a postcolonial birth system that is developing in ways that not only are economical and pragmatic but that also go beyond attention to physical outcomes to meet women's individual needs for good spiritual, emotional, and social outcomes of birth as well—needs that are poorly recognized in Western systems of birth.

BACKGROUND

In the late 1980s, I worked on sabbatical for some months in India studying village-based systems of health care. During the visit, I spent a short time observing in a labor ward in one of the best hospitals in the country. I was interested to see how care was provided for those village women who chose or could afford to bypass the local, traditional midwives, who had been trained by the health system to provide village birth, a well-functioning and impressive service that I had also observed. The hospital had been established by a Christian church, was well supported, and was internationally connected: many members of its medical staff had studied in the United Kingdom, North America, or Australia. The hospital was a respected educational center for undergraduate and postgraduate medical, nursing, and midwifery students. Despite the international linkages and educational status of the hospital, I saw women "being delivered" without any social or family support—lying flat on their backs, undergoing routine episiotomy, being shaved of their pubic hair, and having their bowels emptied with enemas. That is, women were still receiving as "routine" the kind of non-evidence-based care that was unnecessarily distressing and did not improve outcomes (Barclay 1998).

A few years later, I was visiting the highlands of Papua New Guinea (PNG) as preparation for providing technical advice for the World Health Organization (WHO) and the PNG government on nursing and midwifery education. The professional nurse-midwife proudly described how she would undertake an elective episiotomy on every woman and then suture it later. I had serious concerns about her overuse of this procedure that I did not share with her at the time. My concerns were not only related to the unnecessary nature of this procedure and the pain and costs attached, but also to unnecessary blood loss and risk of infection in PNG women, who were frequently anemic and often poorly nourished, at least by Western standards. In addition, there were few scissors available for use, and sterilizing practices were deficient. The women were laboring on their backs in a large room, without privacy and virtually naked, and without company or support from female relatives (Barclay 1998).

I was new to working outside my own country and had hoped that respect for local culture and common sense might have ameliorated some of these excesses of Western pseudoscientific practice. These were battles that I was fighting every day in my practice and research in Australia, where at least we had ready access to facts that could/should be used to guide maternity care, even if we also were too slow in implementing this evidence.

These unnecessary birth practices, in postcolonial as well as Western countries, were redolent with potent professional symbolism and antithetical to my understanding of women and their needs. My experiences overseas confronted me with the strangeness of the common assumption that Western-style maternity systems are appropriate in non-Western countries where resources, human and monetary, are so scarce. This assumption becomes even more curious when we consider that Western systems themselves are under criticism for lack of implementing evidence (World Health Organization 1996; National Health and Medical Research Council [NHMRC] 1996), overuse of technology (Roberts, Tracy, and Peat 2000), increasing risks, and ever-escalating costs (Tracy and Tracy 2003). Furthermore, Western systems still too often devalue women's own needs for social and emotional support despite evidence that attention to these needs improves outcomes (for examples, see Department of Health Expert Maternity Group 1993; Hodnett et al. 2007).

DEVELOPING HEALTH SYSTEMS AND BIRTH WORKERS

Samoa has been independent and responsible for the development and maintenance of its own health and education systems for over forty years (Barclay et al. 1998). Colonization left nurses and nurse-midwives with Western understandings of health services and resentment of the experience of colonization that strongly influenced professional developments in nursing (Barclay et al. 1998). Other legacies, also shared with other countries establishing independent governments and health systems, included inadequate health worker education systems and non-Western budgets. Traditional cultural systems of birth were often hidden and denigrated as a result of many years of Western influence.

When I started work in Samoa, it had a highly regarded and safe social system of birth run by respected women who are often called traditional birth attendants (TBAs) in development discourse, but whom we also respectfully refer to in this volume as traditional midwives. This system worked in parallel, but often covertly, with successive German- and New Zealand–led health services. Our research and the earlier work of Aiavao (1993) showed that social rather than professionally managed birthing, paradoxically, was stimulated by "TBA trainings" introduced in the late 1970s (Barclay et al. 2005). These training programs were designed to improve the practice of existing traditional midwives, but they actually became responsible for more women undertaking this calling.

International policy recognizes that TBAs fulfill an important social and emotional support role in delivery, but it has less often acknowledged that they may have lessons to teach the dominant health system (Kruske and Barclay 2004). Nevertheless, in some places a pragmatic inclusion of traditional practitioners in health systems is occurring. For example, WHO (World Health Organization 1998: 1) exhorted health services "to establish or strengthen linkages between TBAs and the formal maternal health care system . . . and ensure that health centres and hospitals will accept referrals from TBAs." Yet achieving this strengthening of linkages has not been as easy or straightforward as it sounds: many researchers (for example, see Rozario 1998) challenge the "generalism" inherent in these policies.

When I began working in Samoa, it appeared to me as an outsider that the social system of birth in Samoa was either largely ignored by most of my medical, nursing, and midwifery colleagues or perceived as problematic. (Exception to this view were those working in TBA training programs, led most often by my friend and colleague Kaisarina.) Even though Pelenatete Stowers, the senior nurse in Samoa, and I challenged the categorization of traditional home birth as a problem because we found little evidence to support it (Barclay et al. 2005), senior health services personnel persisted with the colonial notion that birth must be hospital centered and professionally managed. Despite this persistent notion, the work of traditional midwives was and remains a significant part of the total number of births in this small country. For example, in 2004 there were only thirty-one professional nurse-midwives in practice in Samoa, but at least eighty-nine active TBAs (Barclay et al. 2005). There are very few doctors qualified to work in obstetrics, with only one fully qualified obstetrician in practice in the government service (*Health Department Annual Report* 2002). Traditional midwives are now regarded as an important part of the Samoan birthing system, as attitudes have changed and the social system of birth is becoming a respected and integrated part of the national system that brings together social and professional models of birth.

ANALYZING CHANGE IN SAMOA

Together with a group of Samoan colleagues, including Pelenatete Stowers, Fulisia Aiavao, and Kaisarina Tooloa Papua, over the last fifteen years I have explored a clash of birthing cultures common in countries introducing Western health care into traditional systems of birth. Pelenatete is an experienced midwife as well as the country's director of nursing, who has led major reform in the way maternity care is provided in Samoa. Her understanding and subsequent leadership of birth models changed, beginning in 1986, when she audited six out of seven maternal deaths that had occurred within one year. She found that six of these deaths had occurred with licensed health workers present, and that the mistakes made by traditional midwives were the same kinds of mistakes made by professional medical and nurse-midwife staff. Her report was unpopular with some of her senior health service colleagues because it made clear that it was no longer possible to blame the TBAs for mistakes also made by those in the professional system (Barclay et al. 2005). She found that although professionals were focusing on what was bad about social/traditional systems of birth, they had lost sight of the fact that they also needed to examine their own practices and refocus on the safety of the mother.

Fulisia is not only the dean of nursing at the National University but is one of two nurse-midwives who have conducted research into midwifery in Samoa. Fulisia has led the shift in nursing education from hospital certificate through diploma to university degree over a decade of professional contribution. She also led the introduction of the graduate diploma of midwifery into the university, undertaken by registered nurses, which was coordinated by Tauaitala Lees, the other Samoan researcher on midwifery. The third person most influential in this work is Kaisarina, who passed away in 2005. She was the most respected clinical midwife leader nationally, taught students, contributed to policy and data collections around maternity care, and led the training programs provided for traditional midwives. She lived in a village with her extended family, including her mother-in-law, one of the most venerable and respected traditional midwives in the country, who also passed away in 2005. Our past discussions have been informed more recently by research with both the traditional and professional nurse-midwives in Samoa, who contributed to our joint published work (Barclay et al. 2005).

My work in Australia as a midwife researcher leading maternity care reform and the introduction of new birth models locally, such as government-authorized home birth, has overlapped with this period of international work. For example, in Australia, there is still considerable prejudice against home delivery, although this is lessening, and small, government-run home birth services are now operating in four of eight states. Hospital services remain slow in taking up policy directives from national and state governments to introduce midwife-led care and create family-friendly and flexible services (National Health and Medical Research Council [NHMRC] 1996). This reluctance to implement women-friendly, evidence-based home birth services has been less evident in the United Kingdom, where policies have encouraged a return to planned home birth (Department of Health Expert Maternity Group 1993). In New Zealand, at least at the level of government policy and rhetoric, home birth with midwives or general practitioners in attendance at home is being promoted as a viable option to birthing in under-resourced and often undermaintained hospital facilities, and home births are increasing (Hendry 2003; Chapter 2, this volume).

My Samoan colleagues and I have grown together in our thinking and learning over a range of projects that have brought me to Samoa many times over the last fifteen years. A major impetus that enabled us to move beyond discussion and into focused research activity, including the collection of the experiences of midwives, was a Safe Motherhood project sponsored by WHO from 1999 to 2002. I was a short-term consultant on this project with other colleagues from Australia. The information we produced from this project and from two additional research projects resulted in further action that guided national policy and service development in Samoa. One of the issues that stimulated and intrigued me in Samoa was how my Samoan colleagues were able to reconcile the paradoxes they had lived out daily over many years. They were part of two worlds of midwifery.

For example, Kaisarina, while working as the leading professional nurse-midwife in the country during a time when home birth was frowned upon, and leading hospital practice herself, simultaneously assisted her mother-in-law with traditional midwifery at home when situations became difficult. She would listen when her mother-in-law went out at night to a birth and then wait for her return. If she did not come back, then Kaisarina would go to find her. During our work together, Kaisarina told me how when she started assisting her mother-in-law, she was not very confident doing deliveries at home, but became so over time. She also described how she continued to learn from her mother-in-law, who transmitted her knowledge the "old" way by "washing off her hands"—a phrase used to describe how the traditional midwives learned from another, more experienced woman. Kaisarina said, "When I watch her closely, it appears similar to abdominal palpation for detecting abnormalities. She [also] massages women with infertility problems. . . . The idea of the massage is to straighten the uterus. Some are retroverted, and some are posterior. My mother-in-law is 'washing her hands' to me; she has given me about a quarter of her knowledge of this special massage treatment but not all. For me, this learning takes time. I am a busy mother, not only at work but at home" (modified from Kaisarina's Story, Barclay et al. 2005: 141).

Vipula Maiava is a professional midwife and nurse educator in the undergraduate nursing program in Samoa. When Vipula was young, her mother, a traditional midwife, delivered many babies in the village, and Vipula went with her. She was told to sit outside while her mother and the other women helped at the birth. When Vipula became a nurse, although she never went to any births with her mother, she knew that people in the village relied on and trusted her. Vipula's first experience giving birth herself was in New Zealand. She was very lonely, left in the room by herself. When she became pregnant a second time, she was in Samoa and attended the hospital antenatal clinic during her pregnancy. At the last minute, she decided to stay home for the birth with her mother attending her, and she had a traditional birth. She was much happier with this birth and her subsequent births at home. Vipula had much shorter labors at home than in the hospital in New Zealand, and did not feel the pain as much because her husband kept rubbing her back all the time. Her father was also around outside. Her mother did not use medicines or herbs, just encouragement (Barclay et al. 2005).

My discussions with Samoan colleagues over the years of work together as well as our research showed that the notion of superiority of "safety" promulgated within the Western health system was not convincing to professional midwives who were related to traditional midwives. For example, Mesepe Mulitalo, one of the senior professional nurse-midwives on the large island of Savai'i, also had her mother, a traditional midwife, support her birth at home. Importantly, Mesepe, a professional, also saw herself carrying on the tradition of her mother and aunt, who were traditional midwives.

Despite these personal decisions and perceptions of the traditional midwives, the professional nurse-midwives themselves had become agents for biomedically oriented change in the 1970s and 1980s. They heightened the "colonization" of their own birthing traditions and taught the traditional midwives Western techniques, while at the same time trying to provide professional midwives for all women. The paradox was that they often chose a traditional midwife for their own births and supported, or at least condoned, the practices of the traditional midwives close to them. When I inquired how this was possible, it appeared that each individual saw the traditional midwife they knew, worked with or whom they chose to birth them, as *exceptions*. Somehow they were "different" from the traditional midwives criticized by other professional colleagues. These "others" were the midwives who were unsafe and who, they believed at that time, would eventually be replaced by professional midwives.

Our research highlights clashes that occur in many countries as Western medical hegemony attempts to introduce a "safer" system of childbirth. This system defines safety within biological parameters only and in a peculiarly idiosyncratic, Western cultural form. This narrow definition denies the social, emotional, and cultural safety so valued by women across a range of societies, and often ignores that even the most expensive private obstetric care may decrease physical safety and increase morbidity (Roberts, Tracy, and Peat 2000).

WHY DID POSITIVE CHANGE OCCUR IN SAMOA?

Cultural Patterns

The traditional midwives of Samoa have historically been of high status and were often chosen by the community for this role because of their leadership—a practice that has continued in well-educated families, including those of health professionals, as well as at the village level. This situation differs from other cultures in which traditional midwives may fill a very different role, as for example with the low-caste women who manage the pollution aspects of birth in India or Bangladesh (e.g., Rozario 1998). The utility of cross-cultural generalizations about traditional birth attendants and midwives is very limited. In their edited collection *Maternities and Modernities: Colonial and Post-Colonial Experiences In Asia and the Pacific* (1998), Ram and Jolly demonstrate the futility of defining TBAs as one and the same despite country or culture, as well as of trying to find generalizable solutions to the risks of birth—physical, social, or emotional (Rozario 1998). They also make clear the difficulty in unraveling local reconfigurations of maternity services from colonial or Christian impositions.

A Samoan example of this lack of cross-cultural generalizabilty stems from research conducted in the 1980s by Patricia Kinloch (1985), who found that one-third of the women labeled TBAs by the Department of Health (and for whom that department had provided a training program) became TBAs only *after* the very brief training program they attended. Research conducted by Fulisia Aiavao (1993) that I supervised confirmed this finding, though she also managed to find a few midwives who had learned their skills on their own or from mothers or other experienced women. In her studies of TBAs in Nepal, Stacy Leigh Pigg (1997) also found that many TBAs were created not by tradition but by government-funded programs.

Pelenatete Stowers, the director of nursing in Samoa, finds that as a Samoan woman, she is uncertain about what constitutes the contemporary Samoan cultural pattern of birth. Her uncertainty stems not only from the fact that this cultural pattern is always changing, but also she believes, because professionals always define TBAs through the eyes of the professional. Professional midwives have assumed that because traditional midwives work at home, are not regulated, and may have little or no formal training, they are not qualified to safely attend birth (Barclay et al. 2005). Yet as the result of her change in perception, Pelenatete now encourages her staff to go and learn from the TBAs, noting that she would have liked to have been given an opportunity to follow and work with a TBA when she had been a practicing midwife. She believes that learning from traditional midwives can also help the nurse-midwives understand why their own services are sometimes rejected in favor of those of the TBA.

To recap, our work and that of others shows that in Samoa, as in other countries, there exist traditional midwives who learned through the "washing off hands" as well as TBAs who began their work only after attending professionally led training courses. One of the women whom we interviewed for our research, Kaisarina's mother-in-law, Soonalote Siutavae, received her training prior to World War II in yet another way—from a doctor and nurse at the hospital in her village in an apprenticeship model. She claims to have never lost a mother or an infant in nearly fifty years of midwifery.

Spiritual Reasons

Samoa has incorporated and integrated Christianity within an emphasis on the spiritual dimensions of life that existed long before Christianity arrived in the 1800s. The power of God was very real and tangible to the women who contributed to our research. In the stories we collected, professional and other midwives alike put their trust and faith in God. God guides, gives confidence, and supports them as women birthing or supporting birth. For example, Mere, a health professional herself, preferred to birth alone with only God's support. During an interview, she described how she delivered her own baby in her bedroom. Locking the door to keep others out, she prayed to God to support her. She felt his presence, which gave her confidence to birth alone.

My colleague Fulisia recorded and transcribed data from a traditional midwife, Iao, who described how God influenced her in her own life as well as her "calling" to be a midwife.

> Mother Sooleupu was doing this work in my village and I observed her. She was instrumental in inspiring me to do this job of assisting women

[to] deliver their babies. I considered very seriously the idea of practicing midwifery and prayed to God to help me with what I intended to do. . . . At that time I had a very small family, there was only my husband and me. . . . I was convinced in my heart and mind that God would help me with [my] pregnancy. . . . So when the pains started I didn't tell him [my husband] or anyone. He was at work. When it was time for the baby to be delivered, according to God's will, I quickly sat on the floor and had one foot against one of the posts of my house and the other foot against the other post. I gave one big push and the baby came out. I sat up, reached for the towel and dried my baby, then I wrapped the baby and put her aside. I then turned on my side, and gave another push and my placenta came out. I then stood up and tidied the things that I used for the delivery. I had my shower and then collected the things for bathing my baby. When my husband arrived I was preparing our food. He was surprised that I had delivered and expressed his concern of what had happened. I said to him, "*Loto tele*, have courage, the best thing that has happened to us is that you have arrived and I am alive and have delivered due to the love of God." (Modified from Iao's Story, Barclay et al. 2005: 43)

Pragmatic Reasons

For many families in Samoa, the absence of a cash economy remains an important consideration in where and how they will birth. Although the health service does not charge at cost recovery rates for services, some families have little or no money to contribute toward birthing at all. They do have, however, the capacity to provide food, cloth, or mats and therefore "gift" rather than pay for the service they receive. The nature of the "contract" that exists between a birthing woman and her attendant at birth differs between traditional and professional midwives, including how their work is reimbursed or reciprocated. Our research showed that in Samoa the traditional midwives worked out of a sense of obligation, duty, and social contribution and were not paid with money for their services (Barclay et al. 2005). They were and still are reimbursed with gifts of food or fine mats, while the nurse-midwives are salaried members of the staff of the Ministry of Health.

There are relatively few medical practitioners in Samoa and no competition for births. There are also too few professional midwives and overstretched hospitals. Distances around the island are relatively short, and transport is usually available. It is helpful that women can remain outside the health system and have a safe birth, and it is important that those attending them can summon an ambulance for transport (at no personal cost), work closely with professionals in an atmosphere of mutual respect, and achieve a successful referral.

The Importance of Education

Samoa has made rapid progress in the improvement of its education systems, with a bachelor's degree preparation at the university the requirement for entry to nursing practice. A one-year postgraduate diploma midwifery program, taught in partnership between the National University and the health service, is also available. These courses are based on a Samoan philosophy developed in association with Samoan cultural studies experts in 1991 (Barclay et al. 1998). This philosophy has continued to guide course design and content development. Numbers of staff have continued their own education formally and informally despite many difficulties and considerable sacrifice. The two master's-research-prepared educators who have studied midwifery and who are experienced midwives are Fulisia Aiavao (Aiavao 1993) and the person responsible for the midwifery course, Tauaitala Lees (Lees 2004).

Tauaitala and other experienced midwives, such as Kaisarina, worked with me to develop a new Samoan midwifery curriculum in 1998. This new curriculum was designed to prepare a specialist midwife with a high level of professional skill *and* a high level of cultural preparedness and skill in negotiating partnerships between professional and social systems of birth. This curriculum appears to be quite unique in its capacity to prepare midwife practitioners who are far more suited to their own cultural and resource context than those prepared from Western-based curricula introduced under colonial governments. Although some elements are the same, much is different and is designed specifically to meet Samoan priorities. For example, Tauaitala described her rationale for change and the importance of students learning new ways to work with and learn from traditional midwives. It was her suggestion that students should be placed with selected traditional midwives during their clinical placement to learn about and develop confidence in home birth (Barclay et al. 2005: 180).

Stable, High-Quality Leadership

During the early 1980s, Pelenatete Stowers undertook training in midwifery in New Zealand that she describes as consolidating her Western conceptions of nursing and midwifery. This training taught her that it was essential for women to birth in hospital with professionals. (Much has changed in New Zealand since that time; see Chapter 2). She also was originally against the idea of the Health Department, through WHO, developing training and support for TBAs. Pelenatete has by now been the leader of nurses and midwives for more than two decades, and during this time she has changed, learned, and guided colleagues from her own field as well as those in medicine into these new ways of thinking (Barclay et al. 1998).

> During that decade [the 1980s] the responsibility shifted to the midwives themselves, to us. We were required to work with and train the traditional birth attendants. . . . Most of the time [this relationship worked well and collaboration improved]. Our midwives identified the kinds of mothers that could be managed [locally] and those that should be referred to the professional midwife. The midwives who were most successful and skilled at working in their communities . . . allowed the TBAs to [assess women] and . . . bring . . . them in to the district hospital. If it was a normal delivery, the TBA undertook the delivery in there under supervision or with the midwife as an observer. (Barclay et al. 2005: 193)

Pelenatete powerfully described how the nurses and midwives had started to take their own culture into account, actively resisting the Western medical model of health and birth care. She also realized that long-term strategies were needed to assist her to reform the services and help her build new models of birth beginning with the education system for midwives:

> While we said we have a health focus and are culturally appropriate . . . when we looked at our actual curriculum there were no links. . . . So that's when we decided to ask Lesley to review our . . . midwifery program and work out how we could actualise what we put in our philosophy. The process that we went through forced us to rethink, to re-conceptualise what we had and it was not very easy . . . all of us needed to rethink and relearn before we got this curriculum done. We needed to look at the curriculum from . . . what a normal Samoan mother thought, what she expected from us and start from there rather than from what we thought obstetrics and science believed the mother needed. (Barclay et al 2005: 195)

One of Pelenatete's plans is to work toward contracting those professional nurse-midwives who are interested in independent practice at home to be paid by the Ministry so that the mothers will not be charged large fees to have a professional midwife attend them. She is clear also that if women do choose to use traditional midwives, these TBAs will also be working closely with the local, salaried nurse-midwives. She believes these partnerships help the professional nurse-midwives develop understanding of the social and cultural benefits a mother can receive from the care provided by TBAs. Additionally, if the mothers chose to use traditional midwives, they would be assured of safety in terms of having ready access to the technical support and emergency measures available from the health services.

In my experience in a number of countries, Samoa appears to be unique in that the health leadership now acknowledges that the *mother* is the determinant of the best form of care. She can decide whom to see and where to go to give birth, and it is the Ministry of Health's responsibility to ensure that wherever she goes, she comes out better supported than she has in the past.

There are risks attached to this model of leadership, and it is not always safe or comfortable. Pelenatete took the ultimate risk in the 1980s when, as director of nursing, she went on strike against the Health Department, along with the whole nursing service. This strike was to address long-standing problems facing nurses in their employment that were not being addressed by the leaders of the health service, as well as the focus and quality of the education programs that were available to nurses. Pelenatete was stood down for nearly a year until a formal inquiry vindicated her stand and reinstated her (Barclay et al. 1988). Her leadership has always been fearless, and subsequent to this court case, she was supported by stable medical leadership at the top level of the health service. Her leadership is also forward looking, strategic, and in contemporary bureaucratic parlance, "manages risk." She is aware of nuances and power more acutely than most. For example, she describes how the Health Department executive must understand that getting the TBA to work with nurse-midwives does not mean that the professional tells the traditional midwife how to work; rather, that they create a partnership. She recognizes this as a challenge that might cause resistance over time. A major concern she has not resolved is how to include a traditional midwife as part of a review team in the event of a maternal death (Barclay et al. 2005).

There were only two director generals (now called the chief executive officer) of the health service in the decade before we published our research. Both were medically qualified. These men were supportive of innovation from the nursing and midwifery leadership group. It appears to me, as the outsider who has also been privileged to work with them as a consultant, that these medical leaders have wisely capitalized on their nursing and midwifery colleagues' achievements.

SAMOAN BIRTHING: WHAT HAS BEEN ACHIEVED?

In Samoa, I found that the recommendations for inclusion of traditional midwives within health systems were being taken further than in other countries in which I had worked—and frequently within a spirit of partnership and mutual respect. This was a long process, predominantly locally led, although my input and curiosity as an informed outsider probably assisted. More than any other individual, Pelenatete has been responsible for driving positive change. Very slowly to start with, Pelenatete; Fulisia, who led educational developments; Kaisarina, who was a conduit for the health service interaction with the social system of birth; and I, who concentrated on policy and research, worked on reforms. These involved policy, health services structure, education, and information systems, and used research to inform changes.

In a number of the interviews I undertook for one of our research projects, traditional midwives told me how they were encouraged by professional nurse-midwives, including Kaisarina and others, to bring the women they were caring for to the health center and use the facilities without interference from the nurse-midwife unless it was requested or necessary. This process started slowly, and was led by midwives already comfortable with the quality and leadership provided by the traditional midwife in the villages in which they worked. Gradually, this practice spread, in spite of resistance from some nurse-midwives. Professional midwives like Mesepe also described learning from traditional midwives how to be quiet and gentle at birth and how to use massage. Other midwives told about the benefits the professionals perceived that went along with the practice of working more closely with the TBAs. However, interviewees also intrigued me as they described the tensions and struggles those accommodating changes had to make to their own Westernized beliefs and previous practices. Those who were accommodating changes invariably said, when asked, that they were prepared to make these changes because they knew it would be better for the women so they would no longer bypass the health system altogether. Even if they still gave birth at home, the traditional midwife could ask for help if necessary, and women who did need professional care would be transferred promptly and respectfully from one system to another. Although it is not common for the traditional midwife to go with women to the main hospital and stay there during the labor and birth, by the time we completed our research, traditional midwives were quite frequently in attendance in small hospital clinics at the village level.

As part of our Safe Motherhood work, we conducted a second study, a national audit of all maternity services in the country (Barclay, Homer, and Davis 2001). This study was published in a research thesis prepared by Tauaitala Lees (2004), who led the team that conducted this audit under the supervision of myself and Caroline Homer, another Australian midwife working on the WHO project. The National Steering Committee that guided us through the Safe Motherhood work developed and articulated a National Safe Motherhood Policy, describing in part the role of the traditional midwife in Samoan birthing as "a strong cultural system of assistance in childbirth . . . retained alongside modern medicine" (Barclay, Homer, and Davis 2001).

All settings managed by the Ministry of Health where women give birth now use evidence-based guidelines for management of antenatal, birth, and postnatal care. Dr. Caroline Homer led the development and testing of these guidelines (Barclay et al. 2005). A national information system lacked sufficient detail about birth statistics, and birth register data kept on each birth in the hospital did not collect information on episiotomy and induction of labor rates. These have been added to the birth register in the main hospital, and can now be assessed and easily monitored without having to undertake a record audit. Audit work conducted by Lees under the auspices of the Safe Motherhood committee measured the progress in introducing evidence-based care. Her findings showed that episiotomy rates that had been unacceptably high previously had fallen to 20% (Barclay et al. 2005).

An international consultant and local leaders reviewed the Health Act in 2004, and we were able to feed information into this process. Our research led to recommendations to ensure that professional midwifery in the home was included in the revised Act. This was part of a strategy, along with reclaiming the title "midwife," to encourage confident, local leadership of birth by midwives, who like midwives in Australia, had been confident to practice only in institutional settings.

Extensive investigation led by Lees found over eighty known, active TBAs working in Samoa, who were then linked to the health system through partnerships with local nurses and midwives. Pelenatete describes what happened to build this relationship over time:

> We were required to work with and train the traditional birth atten-
> dants. . . . Most of the time this relationship worked well and collaboration
> improved. Our midwives identified the kinds of mothers that could be
> managed by traditional midwives and those that should be referred to the
> professional midwife. The midwives who were most successful and skilled at
> working in their communities . . . allowed the TBAs to [assess women] and . . .
> bring . . . them in to the district hospital. If it was a normal delivery the TBA
> undertook the delivery in there under supervision or with the midwife as an
> observer. This worked better in some places than in others and I guess what
> made the difference was attitude, staff attitude. (Modified from Pelenatete's
> Story, Barclay et al. 2005: 193)

My experience talking with both traditional and professional Samoan midwives confirms the importance of attitude and attitude change, and points to the friendships and respect that develop over time when persons have an opportunity to get to know each other, as well as to the opposite results. For example, some years ago, we talked with one traditional midwife on Savai'i who had little contact with the professional midwife who worked in the district hospital close by. When this traditional midwife recommended that mothers go to the hospital for stitches if they tore at birth, she faced resistance from women who refused hospital treatment, fearing the nurse-midwife would scold them. I believe that this is now the exception rather than a common experience (Barclay et al. 2005).

A directory of TBAs has been established so these women are formally recognized as part of the system. Each completes a record in her own register, described as a "Birth Book." The book was designed by Kaisarina and myself to fill some gaps in the deficient health information on births by recording details of the birth and outcomes of the mother and infant. Another important goal was to provide a way of linking the professional and traditional midwives. Both have a responsibility for these important statistics: The nurse-midwives who work nearby collect information from the villages and feed the data into the national system. During data collection, the traditional and professional midwives undertake a case review of all the births recorded in the Birth Book by the particular traditional midwife. Analysis of this Birth Book data is demonstrating excellent results in over 330 births attended by traditional midwives over two years, with no evidence of complications indicating unsafe or ill-informed practice—for example intrauterine infections, tears requiring suturing, or injured babies. There was one woman with a postpartum hemorrhage who was safely transferred (Barclay et al. 2005). Although these numbers are small, the total numbers of births in Samoa is fewer than 4,000 annually, and these low numbers, along with the quality, location, and availability of other data, make detailed comparison difficult. In our opinion, these results are as good as or better than the birth data of most hospitals.

Sustainability of Change

There are strong indications that the transformation of the service as reflected in the new model and in the understandings, skills, and motivations of the next generation of midwives will be sustained. Sustainability was exemplified in a project undertaken by a small group of young midwives and nurses as part of Quality Awards, introduced in a capacity-building project by the Ministry of Health in 2004. Participants were locally educated professionals who had completed the new, Samoan-designed educational programs. Their project focused on improving maternity care on Savai'i by establishing partnerships with traditional healers and midwives in their local communities. The group surveyed the traditional healers and midwives across eight villages, confirming findings of our own earlier research (Aiavao 1993; Barclay et al. 2005): even though 90% of women received antenatal care from professionals, only 40% of these sought professional birth care in a hospital. Reasons included the costs of professional care and transport to get to the health service and return. Acting on their study results, the group planned and undertook action around the importance of making an early referral if things are going wrong, ensuring that the traditional midwives had Birth Books and were linked to professional nurse-midwife partners, and offering them an update of skills and knowledge (Barclay et al. 2005).

These young staff members did not know about our research, the Safe Motherhood project, or the policy work at the "top" of the health system to reform maternity care and improve education. On their own, the nurses and midwives in the group were able to collect and analyze data in their communities to inform them about aspects of care that women preferred from traditional midwives, such as privacy, no-cost services, and massage. They then worked locally to change the style and therefore the acceptability of services. This new generation of potential leaders impressed us because they had insights and concerns that had taken us many years to gather and know how to address (Barclay et al. 2005).

CONCLUSION

The introduction of Western health care and birthing systems has not only ignored what was there before, but also denigrated and defined social midwives as "unskilled" (World Health Organization 1998; Kruske and Barclay 2004). This denigration reflects a medical hegemony no longer defensible in contemporary health care or health systems, and certainly unjustified by our experience and by the evidence of Samoa. However, it remains the way that many postcolonial health systems are managed today (Barclay 1998). The Samoan nurses and professional midwives I have worked with over the last fifteen years no longer believe that women have to fit into a postcolonial, hospital-preferred model to be safe. They know and have reinforced for them time and again that Samoan women will move outside the health system rather than be cared for in ways they do not like or cannot afford. This generation of nurses and midwives, led by people like Pelenatete and Fulisia, accepts multiple values and realities. These locally prepared health professionals have been educated within a uniquely Samoan philosophy that underpins the courses that have been taught in the national nursing and midwifery programs since 1991 (Barclay 1998), and have the skills and motivation to provide women- and community-focused care.

I believe we have been part of a transformation rather than a simple reform of the system. It is not perfect or complete, and we have evidence at times that some hostility remains between the traditional midwife and the professional, but it is on its way.

My colleagues have created, with some assistance from others, including myself, an overt alignment of traditional systems of birth with a modern health service developing in Samoa. The persistence of a village-focused economy, small numbers of medical practitioners, and the status and quality of traditional practitioners have combined to resist absorption or takeover of birth by a biomedical or Western health system. Traditional midwives in Samoa are not only high status and valued in traditional Samoan culture, but also in this new Samoan health system. The new model of birth has taken time and tremendous effort to put in place, but it has been with wise and proud Samoan nurse-midwives leading the transformation.

ACKNOWLEDGMENTS

I want to acknowledge WHO and AusAID, which agreed to fund most of the work that produced our findings. I also want to thank my Samoan colleagues mentioned in this chapter: they have provided me with the opportunity of a lifetime to learn and contribute. This chapter originally appeared in L. Barclay, F. Aiavao, J. Fenwick, and K. Tooloa Papau, *Midwives' Tales: Stories of Tradition and Professional Birthing in Samoa*.

NOTE

Utumuu: A chiefly title bestowed on Lesley Barclay by Samoan colleagues in recognition of her contribution to their nursing and midwifery services.

REFERENCES

Aiavao, F. 1993. "The Role of the Traditional Birth Attendant in Western Samoa through the Perceptions of Three Groups: Traditional Birth Attendants Themselves, Professional Midwives and the Mothers." M.S. thesis, Flinders University, South Australia.

Barclay, L. 1998. "Midwifery in Australia and Surrounding Regions: Dilemmas, Debates and Developments." *Reproductive Health Matters* 6.11:149–56.

Barclay, L., F. Aiavao, J. Fenwick, and K. Tooloa Papua. 2005. *Midwives' Tales: Stories of Traditional and Professional Birthing in Samoa*. Nashville, TN: Vanderbilt University Press.

Barclay, L., J. Fenwick, F. Nielson, B. Poston-Anderson, P. Stowers, and J. Wilkinson. 1998. *Samoan Nursing: The Story of Women Developing a Profession*. Sydney: Allen & Unwin.

Barclay, L., C. Homer, and G. Davis. 2001. "Safe Motherhood Final Report: Safe Motherhood Steering Committee Policy Statement." Manila: Department of Health Samoa and WPRO WHO.

Callaghan, H. 2003. "Birth Dirt: Relations of Power in Childbirth." Ph.D. thesis, University of Technology, Sydney.

Community Health Nursing Information System [CHNIS]. Nursing Division Department of Health Samoa (an informal collection of data held within the Nursing Department of the Ministry of Health).

Davis-Floyd, R. 2004. "Daughter of Time: The Postmodern Midwife." Unpublished.

Department of Health Expert Maternity Group. 1993. *Changing Childbirth*. London: Department of Health HMSO.

Health Department Annual Report. 2002. Pago Pago: Government of American Samoa.

Hendry, C. 2003. "Midwifery in New Zealand 1990–2003: The Complexities of Service Provision." Doctoral thesis, Faculty of Nursing, Midwifery & Health, University of Technology, Sydney.

Hodnett, E. D., S. Gates, G. J. Hofmeyr, and C. Sakala. "Continuous Support for Women during Childbirth." *Cochrane Database of Systematic Reviews* 2007, Issue 3. Art. No.: CD003766. DOI: 10.1002/14651858.CD003766.pub2.

Kinloch, P. 1985. "Midwives and Midwifery in Western Samoa." In *Healing Practices in the South Pacific,* edited by C. D. Parsons, 199–212. Provo, UT: Institute of Polynesian Studies, Brigham Young University.

Kruske, S., and L. Barclay. 2004. "The Effect of Shifting Policy on Traditional Birth Attendant Training." *Journal of Midwifery and Women's Health* 49.4:306–11.

Lees, T. 2004. "Safe Motherhood in Samoa: A Needs Assessment." M.S.N. thesis, University of Technology, Sydney.

National Health and Medical Research Council [NHMRC]. 1996. "Options for Effective Care in Childbirth." Canberra: Australian Government Printing Service.

Pigg, S. L. 1997. "Authority in Translation: Finding, Knowing, Naming and Training 'Traditional Birth Attendants' in Nepal." In *Childbirth and Authoritative Knowledge Cross-Cultural Perspectives,* edited by R. Davis-Floyd and C.F. Sargent, 233–62. Berkeley: University of California Press.

Ram, K., and M. Jolly (eds.). 1998. *Maternities and Modernities: Colonial and Postcolonial Experiences in Asia and the Pacific.* Cambridge: Cambridge University Press.

Roberts, C., S. Tracy, and B. Peat. 2000. "Rates of Obstetric Intervention among Private and Public Patients in Australia: A Population Based Descriptive Study." *British Medical Journal* 321:728–38.

Rooks, J., N. Weatherby, E. Ernst, S. Stapleton, D. Rosen, and A. Rosenfield. 1989. "Outcomes of Care in Birth Centers: The National Birth Center Study," *New England Journal of Medicine* 321.26:1804–11.

Rozario, S. 1998. "The Dai and the Doctor: Discourses on Women's Reproductive Health in Rural Bangladesh." In *Maternities and Modernities: Colonial and Postcolonial Experiences in Asia and the Pacific,* edited by K. Ram and M. Jolly, 144–76. Cambridge: Cambridge University Press.

Tracy, S., and M. Tracy. 2003. "Costing the Cascade: Estimating the Cost of Increased Obstetric Intervention in Childbirth Using Population Data." *BJOG: An International Journal of Obstetrics and Gynaecology* 110:717–24.

World Health Organization. 1996. *Care in Normal Birth: A Practical Guide.* Geneva: Maternal and Newborn Health/Safe Motherhood Unit, Family and Reproductive Health, WHO.

———. 1998. *What's New?* Geneva: Maternal and Newborn Health/Safe Motherhood Unit, Family and Reproductive Health, WHO.

PART TWO

Local Models in Developed Nations

Hospitals and Birth Centers

Chapter 5

The Albany Midwifery Practice

Becky Reed and Cathy Walton

INTRODUCTION

Following the U.K. government report *Changing Childbirth* in 1993, a group of midwives working together and desperate for change won the setup money for a groundbreaking midwifery practice. The South East London Midwifery Group Practice (SELMGP) was inaugurated in April 1994 in Deptford, South East London. After three years of excellent outcomes and growing popularity, the group, renamed the Albany Midwifery Practice (AMP), successfully negotiated the first ever subcontract with a healthcare trust in the United Kingdom, becoming the first group of National Health Service (NHS) midwives working as a self-employed, self-managed practice, based in the community and offering continuity of care within an individual caseload model.

Our challenge was to prove that this model was effective and improved outcomes for women and babies in order for it to become accepted within mainstream midwifery practice. Since 1994 data have been collected on all the women who have given birth with the AMP. We now have data on over 1,500 births, and when compared with both local and national statistics, these show increased rates of normal birth, including an unusually high home birth rate, a low cesarean section rate, and high breastfeeding rates, all in a multicultural, inner-city population with recognized high levels of deprivation. An evaluation of the practice was undertaken in 2001 (Sandall, Davies, and Warwick 2001), which showed a positive response from the women receiving our care.

This chapter tells the story of the Albany Midwifery Practice. As two of the original midwives involved, we explain how we work and what the practice has achieved since 1997, and discuss our thoughts on why working in this way produces such excellent outcomes for women.

HISTORY OF THE PRACTICE

In the early 1990s, the midwives who would go on to form the SELMGP were working as independent midwives in South East London. Independent midwives are fully qualified midwives who choose to work outside the NHS and therefore are paid directly by the women. Working independently gives midwives increased autonomy and enables them to work on a one-to-one basis with women rather than in the fragmented system common in the United Kingdom. Although we all enjoyed working in this way, we felt passionately that the associated degree of continuity of carer could and should be available to women free of charge within the NHS. We believed that a midwifery model based on continuity of carer would not only improve outcomes for women and babies, but would also increase satisfaction for midwives. We came together in order to find a way to provide a model of midwifery care that would offer women choice, control, and continuity of care (Department of Health 1993).

The SELMGP evolved over a two-year period. Six of us, working in three pairs, were drawn together by a common philosophy and the practical need to provide support and cover for each other. We were all working within a closely defined geographical area, providing a service that offered continuity of carer and choice of place of birth. Believing fundamentally in the principles of the NHS that care should be free at the point of delivery and accessible to all, we felt strongly that all women should have access to this type of care. In order to accommodate these beliefs, we had been making our services available to local women on a sliding scale, with wealthier clients subsidizing those who were on benefits. We saw this as an interim measure while we worked toward secure funding to become an NHS project.

One of our intentions was to see whether the excellent statistics associated with independent midwifery in the United Kingdom (Weig 1993) could be maintained when the same model of care addressed the issues of inner-city deprivation and inequalities in health. Outcomes for the years in which we had been working independently were encouraging, showing a high rate of normal births and breastfeeding, and low rates of medical intervention.

Since the 1970s, maternity services in the United Kingdom have been organized around an increasingly medicalized, institutional model with a consequent erosion of the traditional, more autonomous role of the midwife. By 1980 the home birth rate had reached an all-time low, with less than 1% of women giving birth at home. This wholesale move to the hospital had led to fragmentation of care during pregnancy, birth, and the postnatal period, and a "production line" experience for the majority of women as they were herded into hospitals. Increasing dissatisfaction led to more and more support for consumer groups, whose members provided a voice for those women who, as described by Nicky Leap (one of the original SELMGP midwives), "were not prepared to tolerate a system that left many feeling powerless" (1996). The campaigning done by the Association for Improvements in Maternity Services (AIMS), the National Childbirth Trust (NCT) and the Active Birth Movement, together with that of the Association of Radical Midwives (ARM), paved the way for the groundbreaking Health Committee Report on Maternity Services (House of Commons Health Committee 1992).

The early 1990s were a time of change in maternity care in the United Kingdom. The 1992 Health Committee Report recommended that a medical model of care was not appropriate for all women, and that maternity services should be based around the needs of women and their families. The government response to this report was to set up an Expert Maternity Group, under the chairmanship of Baroness Cumberlege, to review NHS maternity care, including the role of professionals, to ensure that the service offered women choice, control, and continuity of care. The group took evidence from a variety of maternity service providers, including the independent midwives who were to become the South East London Midwifery Group Practice (SELMGP). The SELMGP model of midwifery care was recommended in the ensuing government report, *Changing Childbirth, Part 1:* "The (Expert Maternity) Group also heard and discussed evidence about midwifery group practices which aim to provide a high degree of support and continuity. . . . These appear to demonstrate high quality practice and the most complete continuity of carer. . . . The Group would like to see some experimental schemes being introduced within the NHS in the next five years" (Department of Health 1993).

Following the publication of *Changing Childbirth,* the SELMGP was successful in a bid to become one of three midwifery group practice pilot sites chosen by South East Thames Regional Health Authority (SETRHA). These pilot projects were launched in January 1994, and the (initially) two-year SELMGP project began in April of that year.

SETRHA awarded us £30,000 in setup money, but we still needed to fund the ongoing project. We embarked on a lengthy and complicated negotiation process with the local health authority, and by the end of the first year, we had managed to secure funding for the care of 150 women. We made a decision to become a partnership, employing a practice manager. We would be self-employed, having direct contract with the local health authority, the first midwifery practice in the United Kingdom to be set up in this way. We held a firm commitment to providing a midwifery

The SELMGP

- Was a community-based project offering a self-managed midwifery service ensuring continuity of care and carer to women living in a deprived inner-city area

- Targeted women who were most vulnerable in terms of socioeconomic need; worked with women choosing either hospital or home birth, including those with known medical or obstetric complications

- Operated from storefront premises in a busy community center, offering free pregnancy testing, antenatal and postnatal groups, walk-in advice and information, and midwifery care that was free at the point of service

- Eventually undertook the total midwifery care of 200 women per year: each woman was allocated two midwives who looked after her throughout her pregnancy, labor, and the first month of her baby's life

- Performed a national and international function as a resource for all those interested in this type of innovative midwifery practice

service within the NHS that would serve as a replicable model for implementation nationwide.

From the start, we have collected our data in order to perform an ongoing audit of the midwives' practice. We set up an advisory group, of which half were users of the service and half were professionals with relevant expertise, including heads of midwifery and consultant obstetricians from the local hospitals. During the following three years, funding proved to be an ongoing problem, necessitating continuing negotiations with a succession of different representatives from the health authority. The SELMGP model of care, however, quickly proved to be very popular with the women, and our work soon became both nationally and internationally acclaimed as groundbreaking.

Toward the end of 1996, despite its success, SELMGP was under serious threat. The health authority, although clear in its desire to see the project continue, had massively overspent its budget, and it became apparent that funds would no longer be available to support SELMGP after the end of the financial year. We began to explore ideas for moving forward with the project; with satisfied customers and excellent clinical outcomes, we decided it was unthinkable to give up at this point. It was obvious that a different route for funding would be necessary. In the light of SELMGP's excellent outcomes, predicted cost-effectiveness, and health gain within the local population, both the midwives and the health authority were hopeful about making the SELMGP model of care more mainstream. We approached Cathy Warwick, the director of midwifery of a neighboring healthcare trust, who had been a very supportive member of the advisory group for the SELMGP. She agreed to work with us and the health authority to negotiate a subcontract with Kings Healthcare Trust, and although this would mean relocating and losing the innovative storefront premises, it was an opportunity for secure funding and thus the survival of the model.

We signed our first contract on April 1, 1997, and the SELMGP was renamed the Albany Midwifery Practice, after the Albany Community Centre, where we had first set up as the SELMGP three years previously. In this unique contract, we were able to maintain our self-employed and self-managed status, which we saw as fundamental to the principle of an autonomous midwifery model. We were very interested in continuing to audit practice outcomes and believed the caseload should be either geographically based or generated by local general practitioners (GPs), thereby ensuring equity of access to the service. This would address any criticism that self-selection might affect outcomes. The group, now consisting of six whole-caseload-equivalent midwives, would take on the care of 216 women per year. It was agreed that the caseload would be generated by three GP practices located on a housing estate in Peckham, an area of South East London recognized as having high levels of social deprivation. A budget was agreed on, to be paid directly to the practice in quarterly installments. This funding came directly from the hospital trust, which planned to use available finances from midwifery vacancies, with the health authority making an initial contribution in recognition of the value of this arrangement. The trust agreed to indemnify the midwives in accordance with clinical protocols and trust policies, and Cathy Warwick agreed to manage the contract.

Initially, the practice was based in a condemned building that housed the GPs. However, we felt strongly that working from a community base in a nonmedical environment was crucial to our model of care, and the following year, we moved to a newly built local health and leisure center, the Peckham Pulse, with an office and access to other rooms for antenatal visits and ante- and postnatal groups. The center has swimming pools, a gym, a children's play area, meeting rooms, and a café, as well as a health suite for complementary practitioners, and is well used by local women and their families.

Philosophy of the Practice

- Pregnancy and birth are seen as a normal part of a woman's life.
- Midwifery care is a trusting, mutually respectful partnership between the woman and her carers.
- Each woman is entitled to get to know the midwives caring for her throughout her pregnancy and childbirth regardless of recognized risk factors, complications, or place of birth.
- Women should be able to give birth to their babies in a safe and satisfying way in the place of their choice.
- The midwife "follows the woman," thereby enabling care either at home or in the hospital, as appropriate to the woman's needs and choices.
- Women have the right to be given evidence-based information in order to make informed choices throughout pregnancy, birth, and the postnatal period.

THE MODEL

The Albany Practice provides woman-centered care as recommended by the *Changing Childbirth* report (Department of Health 1993). In the early years of the SELMGP, we developed a philosophy that continues to be the cornerstone of the current practice.

We offer continuity of midwifery care with two known midwives for each woman. These midwives provide antenatal and intrapartum care, and postnatal care for up to twenty-eight days. The caseload continues to be generated by local GP practices, with occasional self-referrals, and some referrals from consultant obstetricians at the hospital. We look after all the women referred to us, regardless of their perceived obstetric, medical, or social risk. Each whole-caseload midwife looks after thirty-six women per year as a primary midwife and a further thirty-six women as a second midwife; each of the two half-caseload midwives looks after eighteen "primaries" and eighteen "seconds." We are on call for our own caseload at all times unless we are on vacation; we have twelve weeks of vacation time a year, organized well in advance in order to facilitate the allocation of bookings. The women know that they can contact their midwives at any time if they need to, but are asked not to call with nonurgent messages after 8 P.M. or at weekends. We arrange time off between ourselves and liaise with each other to cover special, unmissable social or family events. Fundamental to the model are the two support workers, who between them ensure the smooth, day-to-day running of the practice and its continued place in the wider midwifery world. The practice administrator handles referrals and does general secretarial work for the midwives, while the manager deals with media requests, organizes workshops, and serves as the contact point for national and international interest in the practice.

The practice administrator, who coordinates the bookings according to the midwives' holidays as the referrals arrive, allocates each woman booked with the practice a primary and a second midwife. The primary midwife is responsible for the woman's midwifery care and provides an overview of her individual situation. This midwife meets the woman at home for a first visit, during which she takes all the booking details and discusses a pattern of care appropriate to the individual woman, including relevant referrals and screening tests. Further antenatal visits are usually at the practice at a time that is convenient for both the woman and her midwife. The second midwife also builds up a relationship with the woman, sharing her antenatal care and attending the Birth Talk visit at around thirty-six weeks in the woman's home. The primary midwife arranges any necessary consultations with other professionals and always accompanies a woman on an obstetric visit to act as her advocate. We have a link consultant obstetrician with whom we work very closely, meeting regularly over lunch to review ongoing practices and discuss different aspects of care.

Choice of place of birth is discussed at the booking visit, and women with healthy normal pregnancies are encouraged to keep their options open until labor is established. Home birth is always presented positively, since we know that for most women, this option will optimize their likelihood of having a normal birth and provide an empowering start to their lives as mothers. Throughout the pregnancy, the midwives continue to discuss the safety and benefits of home birth, illustrating these with stories and photographs from previously attended births.

Both of the woman's named midwives plan to attend the birth, the primary midwife calling the second when the birth is near or at any time she feels in need of support. The midwives carry their equipment with them at all times, and plan to visit all women at home in labor, giving them the opportunity to make a final choice about place of birth at this time. In a long labor, the two midwives share the care, and try to ensure that the woman's primary midwife is with her when her baby is born. The primary midwife provides the majority of the postnatal care, with the second midwife usually doing one visit. We are on call for the women up to twenty-eight days postnatally, and arrange to visit them at home when appropriate during this time, encouraging them to start attending the postnatal group at AMP when they feel ready.

This model ensures a very high level of continuity of carer: our statistics from the last five years show that 84% of women were attended by the primary midwife during labor, and a further 10% were attended by the second midwife if the primary midwife was unable to be there (for example if she was with another woman in labor, or if the woman was having her baby unexpectedly early or late). Two percent of women were cared for in labor by another Albany midwife who was not one of their original named midwives; 2% of women gave birth before their midwife arrived, usually at home with a very rapid birth; and 2% either gave birth at another hospital or were attended by a hospital midwife (giving birth very quickly after arriving and perhaps before the Albany midwife arrived).

Farida, who had a vaginal birth at home following a previous cesarean section, made some comments that illustrate the importance to women of this model of care: "Seeing the same person . . . you're not afraid. . . . It's nice to see the same friendly face. You can also express your feelings more about any problems you may have. Just to know that you know who to contact, and you know who you're contacting at the same time."

We each work with different midwives in the group, which enables us to develop and maintain a shared philosophy and approach. We enjoy the opportunity to be together at births, in order to learn from each other and to be able to debrief together. Each midwife organizes her own working week depending on births and domestic commitments. Every week we all attend our two AMP meetings, and we each have a weekly session at the practice where we see the women in our caseload for their antenatal visits. A midwife with a full caseload will attend on average eight births a month; some births will obviously be more difficult or more time-consuming than others, but the total workload eventually evens out.

In this model, each midwife is on call only for the women in her own caseload, ensuring that the women know their midwives and the midwives know the women who will be calling them. In the "team" model of care, a group of midwives jointly share the care of a large number of women. Women in the team system do not identify with a particular midwife, and often see midwives they haven't met before. The team model doesn't provide a high level of continuity of carer, and is associated with high levels of burnout for midwives (Sandall 1997). With an individual caseload model, a trusting, respectful relationship is built up between the midwives and the women. This ensures that women rarely call unnecessarily at any time of day or night, making it much easier for their midwives to be on call all the time. Farida added: "But you know the main thing is trust, that's the main thing. If you meet someone on a regular basis you build this trust within each other, 'cos to give birth you

The Albany Midwifery Practice

- Is a self-employed and self-managed midwifery group practice
- Is subcontracted to King's College Hospital NHS Trust
- Employs seven midwives in partnership, with two practice support workers
- Serves a nonclinical community base
- Provides antenatal, intrapartum, and postnatal care to women with two named midwives
- Keeps individual caseloads for midwives
- Provides care to 216 women per year
- Serves women referred by local GPs
- Is based in an inner-city part of South East London, with recognized high levels of deprivation
- Provides antenatal and postnatal groups free to local women
- Follows shared philosophy
- Commits to normal birth, home birth where appropriate, and breastfeeding
- Believes in women's ability to give birth with minimal assistance
- Believes in women's ability to work with pain in labor
- Provides the thirty-six week Birth Talk
- Visits women at home in labor and keeps decision about place of birth open

need to trust the person. Your life is in the midwife's hands in a way. If I didn't trust [my midwife] I wouldn't have listened to her, and I wouldn't have felt safe to give birth at home, 'specially after the CS and the way that whole thing went."

We have always held regular meetings with each other and the practice manager for support, peer review, skill sharing, and discussion of organizational matters. At the start of each week, all the midwives and the practice manager meet to discuss any practice business and organizational issues. During this meeting, we also have a "how are we?" session where we all share what has been happening and how we are feeling; this is very important because we are working so closely together. The midwives also meet over lunch later in each week to share knowledge and discuss any interesting clinical issues.

The Birth Talk

The Birth Talk takes place at the woman's home at around thirty-six weeks, attended by the two midwives, the woman, and her chosen birth partner(s). This is our opportunity to bring together all the information we have been giving the woman throughout her pregnancy, and to begin to focus on, and look forward to, her birth. At this visit, we discuss such important issues as the onset of labor, with particular emphasis on pre-labor; how and when to call the midwife (and when not to call); how labor may progress; and the role of the birth supporters. We use visual aids such as Birth Atlas diagrams and a doll and pelvis to explain clearly the process of labor. We show photos of births given to us by other mothers: through these we aim to instill in women and their families a confidence in the birth process and the idea that birth can and should be a joyful event. Photos are also useful to illustrate, for example, positions in labor and birth, perineal stretching, and the physiological third stage. Seeing a photo of a woman smiling as she pushes her baby out, or seeing an empowering image of a new mother kneeling and picking up her baby as her placenta drops into a bedpan beneath her can make a real difference to a woman's belief in her own possibilities for her forthcoming birth. As Farida said, "And the belief that she gave me . . . my belief was on a thin piece of thread and she gave me the strength to believe in myself. Not just me but my husband as well . . . we didn't have belief and she gave us hope, which no one else gave us."

At the Birth Talk we discuss the pain of labor, explaining about natural endorphin production and emphasizing that a woman is more likely to labor well if she feels safe and comfortable, and trusts those around her. We explain the difference between the normal pain of a normal labor, which we believe all women are equipped to cope with, and the abnormal pain of a dystocic labor, where pharmacological pain relief may be appropriate. Perhaps most importantly, we emphasize that we visit all women at home in labor, giving them the freedom to make a final decision at this time about where to give birth.

Debbie, a student midwife on placement with the practice, made the following observation about the Birth Talk: "During my time with the Practice, I came to realise that although the Birth Talk is a fundamental and unique aspect of the care given by the Albany, it is just building on all the work that has gone before. From the very start of the care, the women are encouraged, supported and given real informed choice. All aspects of care build and complement one another, giving women the confidence and knowledge to birth their babies in the most normal and natural way possible."

Antenatal and Postnatal Groups

And you've got loads of talks, antenatal talks which are happening . . . and I'm sure that's why lots of people come and tell their birth stories, because of the personal contact and they want to express how the level of service has helped them. And they want to encourage other people by giving the same belief that they got from the midwives at the Albany Centre to other women in general.

FARIDA

We run antenatal and postnatal groups on a weekly basis. There are two antenatal groups each week and one postnatal; one of the antenatal groups is for women only; the other is held in the evening, and partners are welcome. The groups are free and open to all local women regardless of whether they are booked with the practice. The groups are women-led, facilitated by a midwife but with no planned program. Women can attend at any time and as often as they wish during their pregnancy. Learning takes place through the sharing of concerns and experiences, and particularly through birth stories, as each new mother returns to the group with her baby to tell her own individual story. We have achieved national and international recognition for our innovative work in developing these client-led groups.

EVALUATION OF THE ALBANY MIDWIFERY PRACTICE

An evaluation of the Albany Midwifery Practice was undertaken by King's College, London, in 1999–2001 (Sandall, Davies, and Warwick 2001). It was commissioned by King's College Hospital as "an independent review of the operation and outcomes of the Albany Practice." The aims and objectives of the evaluation were these:

- Investigate processes of interprofessional work since integrating into King's NHS Trust
- Examine the implications of self-employment for the midwives and the trust
- Describe the processes of care
- Examine the outcomes of care

The evaluation included a questionnaire sent to 447 women who gave birth in King's Health Care Trust in 1999, including 106 women cared for by the AMP. This enabled comparison with women receiving care from other midwifery group practices that do not provide such a high rate of continuity of carer, and where the midwives are not self-employed, and with women receiving care in the conventional hospital system.

There were a number of important differences in the findings for women cared for by the AMP. Women booked with the AMP reported being given more choice over where to have their babies, including a choice of home birth. Among AMP women, 97% stated that they felt fully involved in the decision about where to have their babies, compared to 83% of other women. Women cared for by AMP were less likely to describe their midwives as "rushed" and more likely to describe them as "kind" and "warm." They were also less likely to describe their midwives as "unhelpful," "offhand," "condescending," "bossy," "inconsiderate," or "insensitive." Of AMP women, 95% reported they were given an opportunity to discuss their wishes about labor and birth, compared to 80% of other women. More AMP women also reported being given more information about pain relief, monitoring of the baby, and emergency backup during home birth than other women.

When asked about continuity of carer, 73% of AMP women said that it mattered that they had met their midwives before. Of AMP women, 97% had met their midwives before, and AMP women were almost twice as likely as other women to have done so. In fact, during the evaluation period, 98% of AMP women had their primary midwife or another Albany midwife with them in labor, and 93% of AMP women had the same midwife throughout labor. Significantly more AMP women said it was very important to receive care from someone they knew (58% compared to 35% in the other mid-wifery group practices).

Reflecting on the care they received during labor, more AMP women reported that their midwives explained what was happening, told them enough about necessary interventions, took enough notice of their views, and were kind and understanding. It is notable that during the evaluation period, 69% of AMP women did not use pharmacological pain analgesia, compared with 18% of women cared for by the other midwifery group practices. This figure is in line with the rate of nonpharmacological analge-sia use reported later in this chapter. Importantly, significantly more AMP women said that "no pain relief was required" than other women (49% versus 24%), suggesting that AMP women may have been either better prepared for labor or better supported to cope with pain in labor.

Albany midwives were more likely to arrange to visit women postnatally at a specific time than other midwives: 89% of AMP women saw only one or two midwives postnatally, compared to 44% of women with the other prac-tices. AMP women were also much more likely to have met these midwives before and to say that this mattered to them (78% versus 43% of other women). And 90% of AMP women reported being given enough informa-tion about feeding their babies, compared to 76% of other women.

The evaluation comments that "throughout the women's responses, there is a clear pattern of woman centred care being offered and of partnership with women, which may contribute to the positive evaluations of antenatal care and good clinical outcomes" (Sandall, Davies, and Warwick 2001: 57). The evaluation concludes that the aims and objectives of the AMP are being met, and that the practice is providing a form of maternity care that women feel positive about, as well as producing good clinical outcomes.

OUR FEEDBACK

We collect feedback on the service we provide and continue to evaluate our own practices. The practice manager sends out anonymous client evaluation questionnaires at intervals, which she then collates. Below are some characteristic responses taken from evaluation questionnaires:

Q: *Why was it important to know your midwife?*

A: Vital to strengthen the relationship, give continuity, birth confidence.

Because these people are the ones who are going to handle (sic) in labor and delivering the baby.

It helped to build up a personal bonding before the birth.

Getting to know the women who would bring my baby into the world was very important to me; it made me feel confident and relaxed about labor and birth.

Q: *What did you find helpful about the antenatal groups?*

A: My fears and anxiety were calmed down. They made me feel strong and confident to face any matters that might arise during the course of the pregnancy and birth.

How to endure pains when in labor. Also it helped me to know what to take to the hospital and what is good for my new born baby.

Information to cope with the pregnancy pains/to reduce the pregnancy pain myself.

Q: *Other comments made on care received by the practice?*

A: Despite an eventual emergency caesarean instead of my planned home/water birth, my birth experience was really positive. My midwives gave me such special support before, during, and after my baby's birth that I really miss seeing them!

I have had 2 babies with Albany and 2 under Kings and the difference is amazing. Being with the Albany gave me confidence and a feeling of being in control during such an important time. I felt cared for and listened to. I felt that my partner and other children were listened to and thought about. I always felt I could discuss any issue with my midwives. It was empowering yet still very supportive.

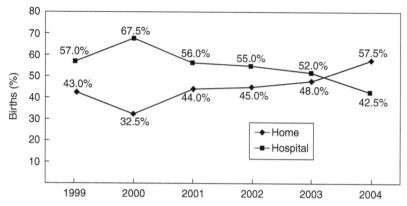

Figure 5.1. Trends in place of birth.

STATISTICAL OUTCOMES, 1999–2007

One of the criticisms of new ways of working or new models of midwifery is that they are expensive and do not make much difference to outcomes for mothers and babies. Between 1999 and 2007, we provided midwifery care to 2,064 women. Our data for this period show a home birth rate of 44%, a spontaneous vaginal birth rate of 80%, a cesarean section rate of 16%, and a forceps/ventouse rate of 3%. The cesarean section rate for England in 2007 was 23.5%, and the instrumental delivery rate (forceps and ventouse) was 11.1% (Birthchoiceuk 2008).

Ethnic Origin

The practice caseload has a higher proportion of Black African women than King's College Hospital as a whole, but otherwise it is representative of the general population served by the hospital. The data reflect the demographic mix of the geographical area of the practice, demonstrating that the practice provides care to a nonselective group of local women. Women who describe themselves as Black (African, British, Caribbean, or other) make up more than 50% of our caseload, with a further 14% of women from ethnic groups other than White.

Place of Birth

Figure 5.1 shows trends in the place of birth since 1999. The home birth rate has steadily increased since 2001 and overtook the number of hospital births in 2004. This increase reflects how the practice over time has had an

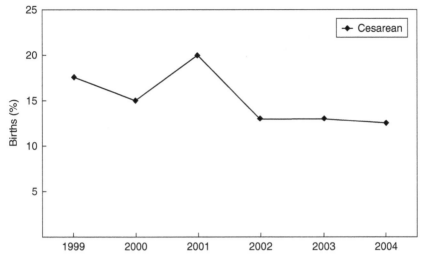

Figure 5.2. Cesarean section rate.

influence on local birthing culture. Going to women's homes during early labor and helping them keep their options regarding place of birth open until labor is established undoubtedly contributes to this high home birth rate, which was 57.5% in 2004.

Normal Birth

In the United Kingdom there has been much discussion over the amount of intervention now occurring even in vaginal births. Birthchoiceuk published a normal birth rate for England of 46.6% for 2004. This definition includes women who had a spontaneous onset of labor, no anesthesia during labor, and a spontaneous vaginal birth without an episiotomy. Using this definition, 72% of all AMP women giving birth spontaneously had a normal birth.

Our induction rate has remained consistently low, ranging between 4% and 9%, 6% overall. The rate of induction for England in 2007 was 20.2% (Birthchoiceuk 2008).

Cesarean Section

The AMP cesarean section rate for the years 1999–2007 was 16.4%. This includes 12.3% emergency cesarean sections (9.6% in labor) and 4% elective cesarean sections. Figure 5.2 shows that, contrary to national trends, cesarean section rates are declining in our practice.

Pain Relief in Labor

Fourteen point five percent of women used Entonox in labor, and 11% had an epidural. Seventy percent of women did not use any type of pharmacological analgesia in labor. This includes 22% who labored in water. This unusually large percentage is at odds with the prevailing philosophy of the "menu" approach to pain relief promoted by many centers in the United Kingdom, where women are routinely offered a range of pharmacological techniques (Leap and Anderson 2004).The high rates of satisfaction with our care suggest that women are not feeling deprived of pain relief.

Breastfeeding

The midwives actively promote an expectation of breastfeeding and work hard to maintain high rates of exclusive breastfeeding. Ninety-two percent of women breastfed their babies at birth; 74.5% were exclusively breastfeeding at twenty-eight days, and a further 17% were mixed feeding. The breastfeeding initiation rate for the United Kingdom was 76% in 2005 (Information Centre Part of the Government Statistical Service 2006).

Perinatal Mortality

The perinatal mortality rate (PNMR) for the practice was 4.9/1000 for this period. This compares with a PNMR for England and Wales in 2006 of 7.9/1000 (CEMACH 2008) and 11.4/1000 for Southwark (the Borough of London where the practice is based).

HOW DO WE ACHIEVE THESE RESULTS?

We summarize below the factors we believe have contributed to these excellent results:

- Shared philosophy
- Individual caseloads
- Commitment to normal birth, home birth where appropriate, and breastfeeding
- Antenatal and postnatal groups
- Belief in women's ability to give birth with minimal assistance
- Belief in women's ability to work with pain in labor
- The thirty-six-week Birth Talk
- Visits to women at home in labor, and keeping decision about place of birth open

All the midwives in the AMP have a fundamental belief in its philosophy and are committed to achieving the best possible outcomes for the women, the babies, and their families. It is worth reviewing the aspects of the model that we believe contribute to our remarkable statistics.

We work with individual caseloads, not a shared team caseload. We are able to build a relationship with each woman for whom we provide care, enabling the development of mutual trust and respect. We share a commitment to helping women have as normal a birth as possible. Knowing the woman's family, history, and social context helps us support her in her choices throughout her pregnancy, birth, and postnatal period. The woman benefits from having two midwives who not only know her but are on call for her 24/7, and who are also committed to being there for her in labor. Looking after individual women enables us to work with them throughout pregnancy, helping them to prepare for their individual labor and birth. We believe that as a result, women feel more confident as they approach their labors, thus increasing the likelihood of starting labor normally, and using their own resources (and those of their chosen birth supporters) to cope with labor positively.

Women tell us that the antenatal groups have a powerful influence on the way they feel about the birth. Listening to real women telling their birth stories helps them and their partners think about their options in many different situations. We believe that our high home birth rate is partly due to women learning from each other in these groups: women are discovering what is possible for them and making it happen. Starting with the first visit in the woman's home, we are able to offer her an ongoing level of support that is impossible in any other system of care. It is difficult to measure the effect this has on a woman's confidence in her ability to give birth, but the following example illustrates this well. One of the authors was booking a Vietnamese woman, pregnant with her third baby. She had had two "normal" births in two different hospitals, and in both labors had had an epidural. When told that the midwife this time would be with her in labor, her immediate response was, "I won't need an epidural then, will I?" After further discussion, she decided that she would like to give birth at home, and eventually had a beautiful water birth, so very different from her previous experiences.

Not every woman will discover quite so quickly and easily what is right for her. But with the same two midwives participating in antenatal care and discussing choices in a positive way, each woman has the opportunity to make truly informed decisions about what is best for her and her baby. We have discovered that by altering the usual pattern in the United Kingdom and actively promoting home birth, many women are choosing to have their babies in their own homes, where they feel both comfortable and safe. We have shown that the Albany model of midwifery care works for both women and midwives, achieving remarkable outcomes and reversing trends in the increasing medicalization of childbirth.

REFERENCES

BirthChoiceUK. 2008. www.birthchoiceuk.com. Accessed November 2008.

CEMACH 2008. *Confidential Enquiry into Maternal and Child Health (CEMACH) Perinatal Mortality 2006: England, Wales and Northern Ireland.* CEMACH: London 2008

Department of Health. 1993. *Changing Childbirth, Part 1 (Report of the Expert Maternity Group).* London: Her Majesty's Stationery Office (HMSO).

House of Commons Health Committee. 1992. *Second Report: Maternity Services.* London: Her Majesty's Stationery Office (HMSO).

Information Centre Part of the Government Statistical Service. 2006. *Infant Feeding Survey 2005: Early Results.* www.ic.nhs.uk. Accessed November 13, 2006.

Leap, N. 1996. "Woman-led Midwifery: The Development of a New Midwifery Philosophy in Britain." In *Baby Friendly Mother Friendly*, edited by S. Murray, 135–147. London: Mosby.

Leap, N., and T. Anderson. 2004. "The Role of Pain in Normal Birth and the Empowerment of Women." In *Normal Childbirth Evidence and Debate*, edited by S. Downe, 25–39. London: Churchill Livingstone.

Policy Studies Institute. 1997. *A Leading Role for Midwives?* London: Policy Studies Institute.

Sandall, J. 1997. "Midwives' Burnout and Continuity of Care." *British Journal of Midwifery* 5.3:106–11.

Sandall, J., J. Davies, and C. Warwick. 2001. *Evaluation of the Albany Midwifery Practice.* London: Kings College.

Weig, M. 1993. *Audit of Independent Midwifery, 1980–1991.* London: Royal College of Midwives.

Chapter 6

Small Really Is Beautiful

Tales from a Freestanding Birth Center in England

Denis Walsh

INTRODUCTION

Birth centers have evolved in many developed countries as an important alternative model to hospital-based, obstetric-led care (Rooks et al. 1989; Saunders et al. 2000; David et al. 1999). Though they are an alternative on the margins, representing just 2%–4% of births in the United Kingdom, their profile is high in the childbirth literature. Increasingly, both quantitative and qualitative research is being undertaken in these settings, and I have been part of these investigations (Walsh and Downe 2004; Walsh 2006). Birth centers contrast to large hospital maternity services in a number of ways: midwife led, small in scale, and premised on a social model of care (Kirkham 2003).

This chapter summarizes the findings from an ethnographic study I conducted of the Lichfield Maternity Unit, a freestanding birth center (FSBC) in the United Kingdom. I used ethnography because this technique specifically engages with the culture of an environment (Hammersley and Atkinson 1995) and reveals the inner workings of the birth center, from how it is organized and run to the relationships and care offered by the staff. This approach allowed me to reflect on and engage with the values, underlying structures, and nuances of this model of birth.

I chose this qualitative approach to augment what is already known about the clinical outcomes of birth centers to see whether it would shed light on the noninterventionist childbirth care typical of these settings. Some earlier qualitative research revealed birth centers as complex environments of both empowerment and conflict, and of both clear and ambiguous values driving childbirth provision (Esposito 1999; Annandale 1988). Esposito's study of a New York birth center showed how most women who had previous negative experience with hospital birth internalized the active birth values of the birth center and went on to have empowering birth experiences there. Annandale's study, also from the United States, revealed conflicts between the birth center and the host hospital, with the latter imposing strict criteria for referral, which the birth center midwives tried to subvert. The remainder of this chapter outlines the methods and findings from my study of the Lichfield Maternity Unit.

SETTING AND METHOD

The Lichfield Maternity Unit is situated in Lichfield, a large market town in the midlands of England. At the time of my study (January 2002– May 2003), it catered to the births of around 300 women per year. It was sited next to a small district hospital, which stood on the town periphery, surrounded on one side by open fields and on the other by a new housing estate. The birth center was a single-story building with its own car park and was situated at one end of the district hospital. The nearest obstetric maternity hospital was fifteen miles away. The center was staffed by midwives and Maternity Care Assistants (MCAs), who provided twenty-four-hour service. MCAs are assistant nurses who have undertaken a basic nursing training over one year in a maternity hospital. There were two birth rooms, each with attached wash and toilet facilities and a birthing pool room. There was capacity for five postnatal women, fours beds in one room and a single. Since then, the center has moved to a new building.

My aim in the Lichfield study was to explore the culture, beliefs, values, customs, and practices around the birth process as experienced by both midwives and women. After gaining ethics approval for the study, I undertook participant observations over a nine-month period that included all hours of the day and all days of the week. Although I am a midwife, my role in this study was as an observer. In addition, I interviewed an opportunistic sample of thirty women approximately three months after they had given birth at the center. A purposive sample of ten midwives and five MCAs, representing a breadth of clinical experience, was also interviewed. The interviews were participant led and very unstructured.

I transcribed all interviews and field notes, undertaking analysis concurrently with data collection. This dialectical interaction between data collection and analysis required me to carefully consider both activities simultaneously while maintaining an open orientation to what was going on and what this meant theoretically. I found that tension is often created between emerging theory and fresh data that may endorse, refine, challenge, or contradict the theory. The findings that emerged represent my own interpretation of the data and are structured under nine key themes:

- Staff empowerment through a struggle to prevent the closing of the birth center
- Postmodern leadership styles
- Altered temporality
- Rejection of Fordism (assembly-line birth)
- Nonbureaucratic, noninstitutional ways of working
- Focus on the birthing environment conceptualized as "nesting" behavior
- Matrescent or "becoming mother" care by birth center staff
- Communitarian ethos conceptualized as an expression of social capital
- Labor and birth beyond the biomedical model

I will address these key themes in turn. In what follows, all client names have been changed, but those of the staff have not.

EMPOWERMENT THROUGH COLLECTIVE ACTION

When I began data collection at the birth center, it had just been reprieved from the local health authority's plans to close it. Their rationale was based on cost—they believed that centralizing provision at the closest maternity hospital would be cheaper. Many of the details of the two-year campaign to keep it open were recounted to me during the staff interviews and my observational visits.

The staff had written hundreds of letters to past patients, the patients' families, and local businesses asking for support in keeping the center open. They undertook substantial fund-raising to support their campaign. They got themselves represented at all the consultation meetings and sought private meetings with the health authority representatives overseeing the decision. One of the women who had given birth at the center was skilled at desktop publishing; she designed orange protest postcards inscribed with "We want our Unit saved." These were given out in the city center shopping mall at lunchtimes. Staff members discovered the name and address of the chief executive who was to make the decision and "flooded him with postcards." They had little orange ribbons made to attach to clothing and distributed them at every opportunity. A local member of parliament (MP) was approached, and he became central to the public profile of the campaign, commenting in the local paper on a weekly basis.

This group of activists, both women who had birthed at the center and the staff, made two trips to London, the first when their MP presented questions to the House of Commons regarding the plans for closure, and the second to participate in the all-parliamentary group consulting on the new National Service Framework for Women and Children (Department of Health 2002).

As time moved on, these staff members and women formed a representative steering group to orchestrate the campaign. The steering group consisted of some of the staff, the manager, a supportive general practitioner (GP), a National Childbirth Trust (lobby group) member and a user representative. Attendance and representation at all meetings was planned in advance. Particular individuals handled the media side, and others managed the fighting fund. In fact, every member of the staff contributed to the campaign in some way.

The campaign culminated in a Saturday rally in the city center, and a march and a meeting at a city park. The rally idea had come from one of the birth center women. Advertisements for the rally were disseminated as widely as possible through the local area. The staff still did not really know how many would turn up. Shirley, a midwife at the birth center, continues:

> A most emotional day. You couldn't believe it. It was overwhelming. I was at the front with the banner and all the staff that led it were up the front and we were walking and all my family came. My mum was there, my daughter and my sister, my husband, everybody. We were walking down the road and I remember getting to Abbey Park, and the thing with Abbey Park is you can look up the main street and see the whole of the city, and I just turned round and the whole of the road was full of people. There must have been 2,000 people there. And I was like, "God!" Everybody was blowing whistles and it was really amazing! (Transcript 38: 17)

Most of the crowd were women who had had babies at the center and their families. The rally was a sea of orange balloons. The local media turned up in force, and the story was on the regional television as well as in the regional papers. After the rally, hundreds of women wrote personal letters to the health authority praising the center for the care they received and protesting against the closure plans. In addition, the staff started a petition that was 10,000 strong by the end of the campaign.

The struggle around the birth center's viability has many of the classic tenets of David-versus-Goliath contests. On one side was an alliance of local midwives, consumers, and representatives of community groups, who are predominantly female, and on the other side, the patriarchal structures of health care institutions, their bureaucracies, and the medical professions (obstetrics, pediatrics, anesthetics). Because of the mismatch of power between these two, stories of successful resistance were inspiring.

The center supporters' story is characterized by the politicization of the campaigners, their dogged persistence in the face of powerful antagonists, their skillfulness in marshaling public opinion, their astute management of the media, and their willingness to commit time away from paid employment to the cause (Walsh 2004). For the birth center staff, there was much more than job security and job satisfaction at stake. As detailed later in this chapter, they had built up considerable social capital at the birth center over the years and were driven by solidarity and resolve.

After two years, the health authority and the local primary care trust that owned the hospital building relented, and the birth center's future was secured. This success was a powerful demonstration of personal and collective agency, and of resistance to hegemonic discourse and development planning. The effects on personal empowerment are demonstrated by Shirley's comments: "I really wouldn't mind having a go at anything. That's not how I was a few years ago! But now it's another dimension! We've really grown here. I feel much more responsible. I don't want to sound arrogant, but I am important, I am doing things, I am making a difference. I go home and I'm thinking about what we can do, where we can go" (Transcript 38: 13).

This sense of confidence was obvious to visitors to the birth center and is typified by an entry in their photo album and scrapbook, proudly displayed on the corridor table near the entrance. The first page has a letter sent to the wife of the then prime minister, inviting her to have her baby at the birth center. She had politely declined, but clearly the birth center staff wanted to let everyone know about their service. The birth center's legacy is about empowerment but also inspiration: a "bottom-up" campaign of "little people" defeating a large and powerful bureaucracy, making possible what seemed improbable. Since securing the future of the center, the number of births has steadily increased from 340 in 2002 to a projected 390 in 2008.

POSTMODERN LEADERSHIP

Leadership was critical to coordinate and lead the campaign to prevent closure. Anita created a new approach to leadership when she was appointed the lead midwife at the beginning of the 1990s. She came with a clear vision of an ideal midwifery service, predicated on a personal value system that stressed the centrality of women's care. Reflecting on Anita's vision, Helen, then deputy and now current lead midwife, noted: "She always knew this type of midwifery was right, even in the height of the seventies when the technology was coming. She has had battles every day of her working life. She wouldn't worry about stepping on anybody's toes really. If she thought it was for the patients' benefit, she was really, really motivated. You know the patient should come first and not the system.

And she put into words what I always thought was right. Hers was a courageous leadership" (Transcript 45: 18).

This durability and courage were not born of an aggressive, dominating manner, and several of the staff commented on Anita's gentleness. Her vision unfolded over five years, during which time an explicit philosophy of active birth was cultivated. Prior to her coming, the staff structure was very hierarchical, and relationships with the women and each other were formal and deferential. Anita, it was reported to me, addressed staff by their first names, expanded the role of the MCAs to include maternal support in labor, introduced informal visits for women considering booking at the center, and instigated the use of birth plans. She relaxed the institutional feel of the center by deregulating visiting times and abandoning maternal postnatal observations and morning routines like bed making. She brought in midwifery-led care by negotiating the withdrawal of GPs from intrapartum care and the setting up of an antenatal clinic at the unit, run by the midwives. She continued the refurbishment of the unit and deregulated staff work patterns.

In all these initiatives, she used a variety of methods in bringing about change. She worked with a supportive GP who mediated the changes in GP practice. For clinical changes, she used a combination of explaining her rationale and leading by example. Other staff were especially interested in upgrading the décor, and she gave them the freedom to lead this initiative. She built a team ethos by organizing regular social outings and shared, fund-raising activities. She eschewed role demarcations by encouraging all staff to be involved in the upkeep and cleanliness of the facility. I was struck by the legacy of this leadership when I started observations. One of my field note entry records the following: "Helen (current clinical manager) is vacuuming the carpet after a woman vacated her bed. This house-keeping idea, house-cleaning idea is something that anyone who is here feels a responsibility to do. It is not really delegated to the cleaner or the MCAs—the midwives do it as well" (Observation 7: 3).

Helen's willingness to do the mundane tasks endeared her to the staff. Nancy, an MCA, said, "She would never say to us, could you make them a cup of tea? She would clean the kitchen out just like the rest of us" (Transcript 42: 11). Over time, older members of staff who did not like the changes Anita instituted left to be replaced with new ones, who were inducted into the new philosophy.

There are a number of interesting aspects to Anita and Helen's approach to leadership that confront modernist leadership tenets and resonate with emerging postmodern leadership ideas. McCambridge (2002: 1) makes the following observations regarding some differences of emphasis between modernist and postmodern organizations:

Modern	*Postmodern*
One best way to organize, plan, and perform work	More flexible
Requires management oversight, planning, and standardization for integration	More integrated, more team based
About uniformity	About diversity
Aim to control	Aim to empower
Stability as value	Change as constant
Things (tasks, materials)	People and relationships

One can see the resonance between the changes Anita introduced and postmodern organizations. A deconstruction process has occurred here, where the assumptions behind the order and efficiency of hierarchical and authoritarian models of birth are not only challenged but also usurped by a different paradigm that values flexibility over regulation, client needs over system needs, and relationship over task. Similarly, the old leadership paradigm was top-down, authoritarian, coercive, and reliant on surveillance. Anita's leadership was through service, resisting autocratic and transactional approaches (Cross 1996). Her way had more in common with "transformational leadership" styles. Ritscher (1986) wrote of the inner or spiritual qualities of this kind of leader, noting that they are not techniques, but attributes—ways of *being*, not doing. Inspiration, courage, and enablement are central to a transformational leader's methods.

This transformational leadership requires nurturing and training if what was achieved at this birth center is to be replicated elsewhere. Roberts has written of the "leadership of compromise" (2000: 74) common within oppressed groups like nursing and midwifery, where the aspirations of person-centered care are often sublimated to the organization's priorities. To forsake the hierarchical and authoritarian model requires courage and vision. These qualities first need recognition in potential leaders and then encouragement to flourish.

Anita's influence was felt in many of the other changes in the birth center over that time—none more so than the fundamental reframing of the labor and birth events away from time-determined processes.

REJECTION OF ASSEMBLY-LINE BIRTH

I'm having a mini-crisis here. I've had four cups of coffee and been offered more and it is not even lunch time. There are no women in labour and just three postnatals. Either this place is over resourced or under-used or something else but I don't know what that is yet.

Reflective Diary, Day 1

This was my first diary entry on my first day of observation, and it identified a theme that would keep recurring during the data-collection phase of my research in the birth center. Coming from a practice background of a busy consultant maternity unit, I was steeped in a busyness culture and had to confront on day one of data collection something entirely different. At the end of day one, a new perspective was struggling to emerge as a further diary entry recorded: "I know about 'process mentality' in maternity hospitals (moving labouring women through a large busy hospital based on an assembly-line model) and I am very critical of it, so why does it feel so strange to be in a place where processing is not in the vocabulary? I can see already that the quality of the interactions among the staff, and between the staff and the women, is different" (Reflective Diary, Day 1).

The absence of a process mentality within the birth center has important resonance with the temporality of labor and birth. These events are by their very nature unpredictable. Huge variations exist between the lengths of women's labors, from hours to days. The need to measure progress in labor, which has been a major factor in labor care since Friedman's (1954) studies, was predicated on clinical concerns related to long labors. There is a surprising lack of attention in the literature to an additional reason for a focus on labor length, which is the requirement of large hospitals to keep women moving through the system. In my experience, midwives and women frequently complain about "conveyor-belt" labor care (see also Davis-Floyd 2004). Rarely, though, has the organizational model of care been explored as a regulator of labor length, where the objective is organizational efficiency, not clinical efficacy. By default or design, placing restrictions on labor length has had the fortuitous spinoff of enabling bigger and bigger hospitals to cater to more and more women. Shorter labors enable more births to be managed in the one space.

REJECTION OF FORDISM

A preoccupation with labor progress and length reached its zenith with the development of the active management of labor protocol, which guarantees women a maximum labor length of no greater than ten hours (O'Driscoll and Meager 1986). The National Maternity Hospital in Dublin, Ireland, where this model is most prevalent, regularly accommodates in excess of 8,000 births per year and has clear commonalities with the industrial model of Fordism (Giddens 2001). Both arrange activity around disassembled stages and with clear demarcations for employees' roles. As a car is "birthed" following linear and discrete processes on an assembly line, so laboring women are processed through "stages" using a mechanistic model. Both have a timescale for completion of the product, and both have a highly sophisticated regulatory framework. Women interviewed in this study echoed this kind of language. Commenting on her perception of birth in a nearby consultant unit, Agnes said, "At the consultant unit, you felt almost like you were on a conveyor belt and all the nurses were a bit robotic towards you" (Transcript 1). Jo, one of the midwives, used the same metaphor in her interview when she said, "Consultant units are like baby factories" (Transcript 33).

Procrastination and delay cannot be accommodated, because of a cascade effect for other stages. In their study of a large delivery suite, Hunt and Symonds (1995) observed that the labor procrastinators ("nigglers," or women in early labor) did not constitute real work in the eyes of midwives in their study, and that this activity needs sifting out if the system is to work efficiently. Delays after a process is started are dealt with by acceleratory interventions such as artificial rupture of membranes.

The following stories illustrate how staff members perceive labor progress in the birth center. The stories also have important implications for trust, both for the woman in accurately reading her body's signals, and between the woman and the birth center staff. Denise said:

> It was the week before Christmas and I had one lady who was five centimetres when she came in. Actually she was really more six but she was desperate to get her Christmas shopping done—you know she had this little window of time to do it and now this! So because the labour wasn't that strong, we decided she could go shopping and come back afterwards. She came back and delivered a couple of hours later. . . . I was still here when she came back and she got her shopping done and then she went home that night after the baby was born. You have got to be flexible here. That's one of the nice things here, you can use common sense. (Transcript 31)

Jenny, who was expecting her first baby, came in at midday. Her husband was with her, but she was in very early labor so they decided to return home. They came back in the early evening, but again her cervix was just two to three centimeters dilated. Jenny was contracting but comfortable. Her husband had a commitment as a DJ for a local rugby club that evening, and they decided he should go and do it. Jenny stayed behind until about 9:00 P.M. but was becoming bored and "fed-up." My field note entry continues: "She says 'I think I would just rather go and be with him,' so she went and sat with him at the rugby club do. He's doing the DJ-ing and she is at the back, sitting down, and while all that's going on she is obviously quietly labouring because when she comes back at 12:30 A.M., she delivers" (Transcript 3: 2).

These variations from the labor norms are not perceived as deviant if the lens of process is removed; rather, they serve to illustrate the obvious: Different women have different labors. Each labor is unique. Just as is it impossible to pinpoint when labor will start, so it is impossible to predict its exact course or when it will end. Recent understanding of the role of birth hormones and their sensitivity to environmental and relational effects reinforce this idea of the diversity of labor experience (Odent 2001). Therefore, situating birth within a Fordist, industrial model is bound to be problematic. The context and person-specific nature of birth physiology will not fit easily within a systemized, production-line model. Labor at the birth center suggests the possibility of a temporality different from labor in other settings. But the deconstruction of assembly-line birth at Lichfield could not have happened had not another model—bureaucracy, also borrowed from industry—been similarly dismantled.

RESISTING BUREAUCRACY

Anita's advent as the new clinical leader in the 1990s brought a dramatic change away from bureaucratic and institutional processes. My early data collection capturing the history of the center revealed the different ethos that was now operating. One of the most remarkable aspects was the complete makeover of the interior of the building over a fifteen-year period. What the staff achieved here was typical of their approach to running this small-scale institution. Helen, the current clinical leader, told the following story about the conversion of one of the center's rooms: "I just thought, well, why don't we have a Complementary Therapies room then? This room is not really used for anything because it is so horrible you wouldn't want to deliver in here, so it just became a bit of a storeroom, and then before we knew it, as it always happens here, somebody comes up with an idea and six hours later we have got a master plan and three days later it was painted and done" (Transcript 45: 16).

Some of the detail was filled in by Shirley, the midwife mentioned before, who told me her version of the story. "Helen—I call her 'wants it done yesterday.' She wants to paint the room now so I got the money from petty cash. I went out and did the shopping. We just put up the paper and painted it. We did it there and then and the therapy room was born, decorated that in a day!" (Transcript 38: 12).

Such flexibility and spontaneity are very different from the procedural detail that has to be followed in hospitals before upgrades in décor can occur. Who is paying, and where is the money coming from? Spending needs approval, fund-raising has to be organized and approved, and capital improvements have to be sanctioned by budget holders. There is a process to purchase of materials. Government health services usually have approved suppliers, and procurement of materials takes time. The work itself has to be done by in-house contractors, but they have to schedule it in among other competing demands.

Contrast this with what happened here: a day to consult with staff and decide the plan; ongoing fund-raising, so there was enough money to purchase what was needed—an amount is always held in the safe as petty cash; paint and wallpaper bought in town shops as soon as convenient for a staff member to do so; necessary tools (paint brushes, wallpaper paste, and table) kept in the store room within the unit; staff do the work either on their own time or, if the unit is quiet, at the earliest available opportunity. In the hospital example, a number of bureaucratic mechanisms have to be negotiated, mostly to do with external approval and regulation; at the birth center, the process more closely resembles home decorating, just as the process of giving birth there more closely resembles home than hospital birth.

Helen told me that their smallness and isolation helped them because they were not under constant surveillance. Their employer, the host consultant unit, did not own the buildings, so it showed little interest; the local primary care trust assumed, because someone else employed the birth center staff, that the staff were not really their responsibility. The reality that escaping surveillance may facilitate nonbureaucratic ways of achieving goals reinforces Foucault's (1973) concept of panopticism and its constraining effects, in this case as a demonstration of resistance to institutional surveillance. By being outside the "gaze," the staff experienced a freedom and autonomy that seemed to drive a creative zeal.

Resisting bureaucratic processes opened up possibilities for upgrading the buildings, so the entire space was redecorated over a relatively short period. During this time, the staff raised many thousands of pounds and undertook much of the decorating themselves. Their pragmatic and "can do" philosophy freed them to realize their ideas. The impact on the women of these changes was particularly interesting. This next section explores the significance of the changed birth environment.

A RETURN TO NESTING

The centrality of the environment and setting for women's decision to book at the birth center was apparent from the first interviews. I asked all the women I interviewed why they had chosen this option. For some, their own childbirth history influenced their decisions. Seven had already had babies in the unit before and wanted to return there. The majority, though, had not used the unit previously. Thirteen women were pregnant for the first time, and eleven had had babies elsewhere. Their reasons had to do with recommendations from family and friends; the birth center's proximity to their homes; and the relaxed, informal, and friendly atmosphere there.

Impact of the First Visit

Further clues came from the women's reactions to their first visits to the birth center. These visits generally occurred in the second trimester, between eighteen and twenty-eight weeks. One woman said, "We went to have a look, and as soon as we walked in we thought—yep! This is the sort of place. I think it was so small and it's not like a hospital. We thought it would be a nice, relaxing place to go." Another woman said, "The birth space is somewhere you could relax." Carmel noted the homelike effect: "The psychological effects of being there, it was like being at home really in terms of environment, it was very, very comfortable and calming, relaxing. It was the room itself, the way it's made up. It's got homey things in it. Most of the instruments are hidden away. They're not on display" (Transcript 10: 4).

These environmental features were repeated often as women spoke of the different pace, lack of frenetic activity, and the smaller, more intimate surrounds. Some contrasted this with their previous experience of births in hospital where they felt they were "processed." Sarah thought she would find this atmosphere of busyness when she visited the center. "You feel a bit like you are imposing on them because you get a general impression that hospitals are very busy, but they had all the time in the world to answer questions. You kind of get a sense that they want to help you rather than just a sense of you are just another person coming in the door and you have got to get in and out as quickly as possible" (Transcript 8: 6).

In addition to environmental features, women commented on the friendliness and welcome they received from the birth center staff. Many did not expect to be offered cups of tea and toast. Some turned up without appointments and were made welcome. One woman commented on the fact that she was greeted at the door by a staff member holding a baby—she concluded that this was a baby-friendly environment. Another woman was impressed by how promptly and efficiently the staff sorted out an antenatal scan for her. She had moved during the pregnancy, and her maternity care records had been lost in the post. Several days of anxiety were cleared up in an afternoon, and she promptly booked to have her baby at the center.

"Nesting" Responses

These interviews emphasize the importance of environmental, organizational, and emotional ambience to women as they consider an appropriate space for birth. In explaining these emphases, I would like to examine a possible link to an old-fashioned midwifery concept: nesting. Nesting was mentioned in midwifery textbooks up to the mid 1980s, where it was used to explain maternal behaviors during pregnancy (Myles 1981). During the first twelve weeks of gestation, nesting was said to cause tiredness and lethargy that slowed women's activity during the critical embryonic phase of fetal development. Nesting behaviors returned in the weeks preceding the birth and were marked by a drive to prepare the baby's immediate environment. Decorating the nursery, purchasing the layette, cleaning, and tidying the home were said to be manifestations of nesting. For reasons that are not immediately apparent, references to nesting disappeared from midwifery textbooks around this time and only rarely appear in midwifery books today (England and Horowitz 1996). They survive in populist magazines on new motherhood (*Parents* 2005) and in the self-help literature around childbirth (Robertson 1997).

Nesting links humans to the large mammalian species in which these behaviors are usually understood to be grounded in instinct—a much more problematic notion for humans because of the layers of socialization and learned behaviors that suffuse human learning and development. Some authors (Davis-Floyd and Arvidson 1997) recast grounded and primordial behaviors as intuition, which can then encompass emotional and thinking components, enabling the exploration of instinct-related phenomena without the charge of essentialism. Using the characteristics of an intuitive response as identified by Bastick (1982), I want to explore some of the women's data that may relate to nesting, from this perspective. Bastick named these characteristics of intuition:

- Sudden immediacy of awareness
- Association of affect with insight
- Nonanalytical, nonrational, nonlogical, gestalt nature of experience
- Empathic, preverbal
- Sense of certainty of the truth of insights

The women's comments are suggestive of some or all of these features:

> "As soon as we walked in we thought—yep! This is the sort of place."
> "I got stuck on it."
> "I could picture myself there."
> "It's really something you can't definitely put your finger on, which makes it so difficult when you're talking about it because it's so much in a woman's own mind. It's a feeling rather than an empirical value system. A woman knows immediately when it's the right atmosphere." (Transcript 9: 10)

The sense of immediacy and certainty about the birth center being an appropriate site for birth comes through here. The final comments articulate clearly the difficulty of explaining exactly why that certainty is felt, and the visualization confirms the involvement of the nonrational, emotionally mediated brain functions.

Vicarious Nesting

A remarkable feature of activity at the birth center, already mentioned, was the single-minded staff focus on upgrading and maintaining the center's physical environment. They had turned a traditional maternity unit into a modern birth center. Clues as to why it was so important came in phrases the staff used from time to time. The midwives spoke of "creating an oasis of calm," of the place "mimicking home," of providing "a nurturing environment," "a quieter more relaxed ambience." Sue, an MCA, said "a calming space and not like a hospital" (Transcript 35: 3).

There is a resonance between these ideas, women's reactions on visiting the center, and women's reasons for booking there. It appears to lead back to nesting, now manifesting vicariously through staff activity around honing the birth environment. In a sense, staff members themselves spend their working lives "preparing for a baby." At any moment, women may come through the door in labor, and the staff's raison d'être is providing for that eventuality. Their preparing is not an idle pastime but a sustained, continuous activity as they are constantly adapting, making over, and maintaining the birth space. It is environmental nurture.

The Implications of Nesting

Nesting may have been sidelined by the "irresistible metaphor" of biomedical birth (Machin and Scamell 1997: 78), by the institutionalization of labor care (Kirkham 2003), and by evidence-based medicine's discrediting of intuition (Wickham 1999). Some would argue that society at large has embraced a discourse of risk that weds us to technological solutions for problems including pain and travail (Beck 1992). Little wonder, then, that nesting has disappeared from the vocabulary and writing of maternity care professionals. Yet as latent (or dormant) as the notion of nesting may have become, it continues to emerge as a reality in the ongoing interest in place of birth, style of care, and ambience of the birth setting.

Reexamining nesting as central to decision making around the place of birth and to the preparations of maternity care staff for receiving a baby throws up distinctive challenges to current service provision. Though one might argue that women in this study are atypical, it is likely that their nesting behaviors would resonate with other women's behaviors on some levels. Four issues are worth considering for further research and practice: How do women construct the notions of protection and safety in relation to the birth space? How would women structure environmental ambience to counterbalance their internal stress over the physicality of the experience of labor? What qualities would women choose to characterize human relatedness within the birth environment? What would women's ideal mix and number of birth attendants be?

MATRESCENCE

I now want to explore the possibility that nesting and nurturing skills can be conceptualized as *matrescence*—a term whose meaning I want to expand to "the nurturing of the becoming mother." The following story is suggestive of a particular kind of nurture. It is taken from an interview with one of the midwives:

> A teenage girl [Rachel] came in with her mother and sister. The girl became extremely distressed in the middle of the labour. She was thrashing around on the bed so we took the bed out. Julie [the midwife] wondered whether her distress was due to the awesome responsibility of parenthood that she felt she wasn't ready for, so Julie asked her Mum and her sister to leave the room. Then she just sat with her for two hours on the floor and this girl was just sobbing into her lap, just sobbing, and then after two hours—almost as if it was out of her system—she was completely more focused and she went on and had a really good birth (Transcript 7: 9).

Rachel had been in the latent phase of labor (early stage) a long time and was becoming very distressed. It appeared that through a cathartic experience of emotional release, when the midwife held her in an embrace lasting two hours as she wept, Rachel reached a place of accepting her labor and the imminent birth of her baby. In this situation, the midwife could be said to have intuited an appropriate response to the girl's distress that would not be found in textbooks or within the paradigm of the technocratic model (Davis-Floyd 2004). Leap and Anderson (2004) have written that a common response of midwives to the distress of labor is treating it with a variety of pharmacological pain-relieving agents. These authors argue for an alternative approach, which they call "working with pain" (2004: 25). This recognizes that labor pain has a physiological purpose, but that it can also indicate emotional distress. The midwifery skill is in discerning these differences. For Rachel, the "becoming mother" journey had been a traumatic one, and the midwife's empathic care for her in labor had smoothed her path.

Another episode of care illustrated a similar dynamic. An hour after giving birth, Sarah called the midwife, complaining of abdominal pain. It was so severe she felt cold, clammy, and faint. Judith, the midwife, examined her but did not think there was any serious clinical reason for her pain. The field note continues, "Judith managed it by just sort of cradling the woman in her arms, resting her head on her lap and holding it gently and massaging her hair and scalp in a very sort of motherly, maternal way. And she did that for a long time, 20–30 minutes. Just sort of held her safe I suppose." During the postnatal interview, I asked Sarah about her experience of care at this point. She answered, "She [midwife] was great afterwards because it was like having my Mum there. I remember having my head on her lap and she was just stroking the back of my head saying you will be all right. Just kind of nursing you which was invaluable. It was like you were her daughter." (Transcript 8: 7) Comfort and protection emanate from this incident. For Sarah, it was as a mother would care for her child.

Sketching Matrescence

In both of these stories, the midwives manifest intuitive-like responses: nonverbal, empathic actions that spring from spontaneous insight and awareness. There is no obvious logical or rational analysis guiding them to embrace the women in the ways they did. Their actions may have been preceded by a biophysical assessment that eliminated pathology in their minds, but then the midwives appear to tap into a protective, nurturing reservoir that could be understood as "matrescent" or "of matrescence" (Thomas 2001)—becoming mother. The term matrescence was first coined by Dana Raphael (1973: 23) to mean "the process of becoming a mother," emphasizing the fact that pregnancy and birth create a new mother as well as a new baby—an idea that has been echoed since by Wickham (2002) and Thomas (2001). Thomas writes of matrescence as spiritual formation, drawing analogies with the Judeo-Christian tradition. Using neglected Old Testament imagery of the fecundity of God in giving birth to creation, of nurturing the people of Israel as a mother suckles her child at the breast, and of protecting the nation from harm as a hen protects its chickens, she argues for a new, spiritual examination of birth as a rite of passage experience. These images of nurture and protection certainly apply to the caring by the birth attendants here. Sarah alludes to it in her extract—"it was like having my Mum there"—and Judith offers protection and nurture in place of the mother of the teenage girl described above. In another interview a woman said of labor, "You just want your Mum."

Thomas (2001) explores another, more clearly ethical dimension to matrescence in her reflections on the physicality of pregnancy (two in one), and of childbirth (one becoming two). Commenting on this ethical dimension, Cosslett (1994) notes that the concept can radically challenge the idea of the autonomous, individual subject. This connection between mother and child, though severed physically by the cutting of the cord, remains intact as the child grows, drawing selflessness and agape (the Christian notion of disinterested love as opposed to erotic love) from her. It is a kind of unconditional love that finds meaning in giving. Matrescent care, understood in this way, incorporates an ethical disposition. If authentic, it would manifest more broadly than in just relationships with the birth center women: one would expect to witness its effect among staff.

Mandy, an MCA who worked permanent nights, told me that "the girls here have been marvellous to me I have to say. Problems that I have had at home with elderly relatives dying of cancer. . . . I've had a load of hassle and they have been really good. I've come in on nights and been knackered, not had any sleep and they have tucked me up in bed for a couple of hours." Such behavior borders on the subversive—when I mentioned it to other midwives, some commented that sleeping on duty was a "sackable" offense (in other words, one could be fired). But here, it is an extension of the empathy shown to women and a poignant example of compassion to fellow colleagues. Little wonder that Mandy concluded her tale with "I love this place. It has been really good to me" (Transcript 38: 5). Such actions can be seen as matrescent in the sense of mothering, nurturing, and protecting work colleagues, demonstrating Cosslett's idea of connection to others, overriding the needs of the autonomous self.

Matrescence seems to tread a delicate path between listening, talking, showing, observing, and leaving alone. Alice alluded to this when she commented in relation to her labor, "They let me get on and find my own rhythm." Others, reflecting on their postnatal care, said "There was no fussing over you" (Transcript 19: 6). Previously, I have written of the difference between a "being" disposition and a "doing" disposition in the staff's approach to care, with the former being less time bound (Walsh, forthcoming) and making space for relational and emotional work. Matrescent care requires a level of nuance reading that is suggestive of an acute emotional intelligence (Goleman 1996) and is sometimes recognized more easily by the absence of unhelpful behaviors (paternalism, being patronizing) and attitudes (indifference, fear of intimacy).

These findings lead me to believe that midwives should seek ways to rehabilitate "nurture" and "love," derivative of matrescence, as familiar childbirth language and as mainstream caring activities in childbirth. These have been sidelined by the industrial model of birth, which reifies management rhetoric in labor care (Walsh 2003), and by a professional paradigm that locates midwives and women in different planes of being (Wilkins 2000). Matrescence as an attribute and attitude of care may also help professional birth attendants to reconnect with their empathic and intuitive selves (Fahy 1998).

The themes discussed so far hint at another dynamic at work within the birth center to do with community.

SOCIAL CAPITAL

All staff members were asked this question at the beginning of their interviews: What's it like working here? The response of my first interviewee, midwife Denise, set the tone for subsequent ones: "Working here is like having your favourite chocolate bar. You really want it, you get to have it and you still want some more. It's lovely." Denise's sentiments were to be repeated with slightly different emphases many times as the interviews continued. "I thank God everyday that I can work here," said Helen, a midwife. "I waited for ten years for this—it's my dream job," commented Jackie, one of the MCAs. Another midwife likened working there to "practising perfect midwifery," while another offered, "I just love working here; it's like a breath of fresh air" (Transcript 39: 1).

In searching for an explanation for the obvious fulfillment that the staff had in their work, one feature of their employment stood out. Twenty out of twenty-two permanent staff were on part-time contracts. There was only one full-time midwife and one full-time MCA. Only a few of the staff spoke unprompted about the advantages of part-time hours in their interviews. For many of them, it seemed self-evident that this should be an option. Only when questioned in more detail did they articulate the benefits: "There is more of an advantage because you have got more people to call upon if you need somebody to come in at short notice" (Jo, Transcript 44: 14). Helen, the clinical manager, expressed strong views about the value of the part-time option: "Most midwives are women who are married with children and so they can't work full-time because they don't function that well because they are feeling so guilty about what they have left at home. If they come part-time, they have got less guilt about their home life and can feel on top of it. They may actually overcompensate by doing both things at a higher level than if they were just doing one or the other" (Transcript 45: 18). Helen clearly engages with the whole reality of the staff's lives, at work and at home. Her comments open up for examination the interface between these two, which have been traditionally seen as opposites.

Deconstructing the Work/Life Split

The dualism of the work/life dichotomy has become well entrenched in Western industrial work practices (Hodgson 2004). Helen begins to deconstruct the division by talk of balancing the two. Other observations at the birth center provided evidence of a more fundamental subversion. My field notes recorded the following episode regarding a midwife who was working a weekend. "Jo had a phone call from home and twenty minutes later her husband and two daughters turned up at the birth centre. He couldn't manage to do their hair before taking them out horse riding so Jo said she would. The two daughters sat in the office, made themselves at home while she French-plaited their hair" (Observation 9: 2).

There were at least three other occasions when family members came in for a chat or on an errand while I was there. It was clearly quite a normal event in the activity of the birth center. These activities transgress organizational norms around work and nonwork. The Weberian response could be to sanction them as inappropriate in the workplace, judging them in the best light as inefficient use of time and in the worst as dishonest and deceitful, an abuse of trust. Yet there was a sense in which these events were related to me by other staff as an endearing feature of the organization and, when I observed them, as a poignant symbol of relational care. They simply fitted with the ethos of the birth center as a caring environment for new families and fit within all the other activities that served this purpose. In fact, to see them applied within the staff's own families suggested a congruence of values and an authenticity around their expression. Jackie, one of the MCAs, sums up the blurring of work/home borders in this paradoxical statement: "When you're here, it becomes your life. When I started, I felt like I was coming home. When I come to work, it is not like going to work, it's like going home." (Transcript 35: 2)

Supporting Each Other

If retention of staff is strengthened by a supportive work environment, then a number of features of birth center activity contribute to this end. There was a remarkable degree of flexibility in the day-to-day staffing of the center. I witnessed this countless times during the observation period. The informal, day-to-day accommodating of staff members requesting to come in later or go off earlier because of a variety of family/school/external commitments was surprising to me at first. I questioned interviewees about it later, and nobody complained, accepting it as "the swings and roundabouts" of flexible working. Everyone could recall a time they had been helped out, and so they were very willing to reciprocate. Though the comment was made that "the place runs on good will," it was said without resentment. Over the period of nine months that I was associated with the center, I did not hear one negative comment about having to attend meetings or training events in one's own time.

This level of flexibility extended to babysitting networks among staff and mutual childcare arrangements during the weeks of school holidays. "For the first two weeks of this summer holiday myself, Shirley and Jo have just shared each other's children. And it has worked brilliantly. I think we just sat down and thought Oh! This is a good idea. And the kids all get together so it's like a little network, you know the husbands, the kids, it's great" (Julie, Transcript 44: 6).

Staff interviews revealed a regular pattern of social outings throughout the year. These occurred at about monthly intervals, and all of the staff would attend at least some during that period. It was part of the culture of the place and served an important purpose: "If we feel that we need a lift or need a bit of support, we'll go out—have a girlie night out. It's really good" (Sue, Transcript 37: 10). Such outings also served to help staff get to know colleagues away from the work environment and contributed to a collective memory of their life together. Photos of special outings were in photo albums in the staff room, and stories would be retold about incidents and experiences they had shared. There was longevity to this tradition of social outings as retired staff continued to participate years after ceasing employment. I was not surprised when the analogy of "family" began to be spoken of as that concept seemed to capture what the staff was saying about working at the birth center. "We are family here," said Sue, an MCA. "It's like a family," "It's a family sort of thing," or "like a second family" were other comments (Transcript 35: 3).

Social Capital in the Life of the Birth Center

A strong communitarian ideal appeared to be at work in the birth center, and the theory of social capital seems to explain it best. A phrase with a diffuse meaning, most experts agree that *social capital* consists of "the networks, norms, relationships, values and informal sanctions that shape the quantity and co-operative quality of a society's social interactions" (Aldridge, Halpern, and Fitzpatrick 2002: 5). Three elements can be gleaned from this definition: social networks, social norms, and sanctions. Social networks have been further described at two levels: horizontal networks between family members or groups sharing similar demographic characteristics are referred to as *bonding* social capital; *bridging* or *linking* social capital refers to ties that cut across different individuals and communities (vertical networks). Both forms can operate on a micro level of local, or within small groupings, and at a macro level of larger geographical areas or larger populations of people (Baum and Ziersch 2003). Social norms are the values, understandings, and rules that govern behavior within the networks and provide an ethical framework for social activity. Though these may vary enormously according to cultural encoding, they tend to reflect values of cooperation, trust, altruism, and reciprocity (Edmondson 2003). Finally, sanctions encompass the processes that help ensure that network members comply with the social norms. These are often informal and vary from the withdrawal of certain privileges to complete ostracism.

There are a number of common threads between the theory of social capital and the internal and external dynamics of the birth center in this study. The first is to do with the idea of community. Community is central to social capital. In fact, some authors see social capital as simply repackaged older ideas about communitarian values, empowerment, and social support (Lynch et al. 2000). At the heart of community is the sense of belonging and commitment to each other. These often cluster around a shared identity. Edmondson (2003) cites examples of how social capital built up in communities exposed to threat. Parallels are clear with recent birth center history. As described above, in the late 1990s, an alignment of staff and consumers resisted health authority efforts to close it down. The solidarity of struggle was identity shaping for staff at the center, and it reinforced an existing sense of belonging cultivated by the lead midwife appointed in 1993. The attributes of identity and belonging lead to both reciprocal and nonreciprocal giving. This reciprocity is apparent in the working lives of staff at the birth center, where flexibility with work patterns is endemic. Nonreciprocal giving is manifest in the amount of birth center activity that takes place on the staff's own time, such as fund-raising, meetings, support for individuals in crisis through phone calls/visiting, and staff making themselves available to observe new forms of care like water birth.

Staff willingness to volunteer for activities and participate in the life of the birth center stands out as a further indicator of social capital. Though levels of participation varied, nobody, it seemed, was outside of the loop. Everybody went to at least some of the monthly social outings, everybody contributed in some way to maintaining and improving the upkeep of the center and to its fund-raising events. The level of staff involvement may reflect the operation of sanction, one of three key elements in social capital. Sanctions in social capital are more tacit and less formal than their legal expression in the judiciary and the law, but they are nonetheless powerful. Occasionally, toward the end of the observation period, I saw manifestations of sanction in disputes about holiday flexibility or reluctance to do night duty, when individual members of staff rescinded what were perceived as their unreasonable requests because of pressure from the majority.

Finally, trust is considered a cornerstone of social capital. It operates at an individual level between group members, at a social level between members and outsiders, and at a hierarchical level in relation to the governance of formal institutions. The birth center exudes trust at an individual level, in part facilitated not just by work relationships but by friend relationships among the staff. Compassionate responses to personal problems were one manifestation. Longevity of employment seemed to play a part in cultivating mutual understanding and tolerance for the mix of personalities. Trust exhibited by the women entering the birth center was also high, as demonstrated by the accommodation of women's choices for their labor and postnatal care (Walsh 2005, submitted). Trust in the institution was also evident but has evolved in a surprising way. By deconstructing staff and staff/patient hierarchies and the institutional trappings of how the birth center operated, trust became aligned to a community rather than to an institution. It, therefore, flowed out of flat structures and a shared identity and purpose, not as a consequence of benevolent, paternalistic, top-down management.

It is clear that the ethos of the birth center is enacted in contrasting ways with that of many maternity hospitals. Therefore, it is not surprising that the technocratic model, so dominant in childbirth services, is radically challenged in this setting.

LABOR AND BIRTH BEYOND THE TECHNOCRATIC MODEL

The viewpoints of the women who booked at the birth center indicated positive attitudes toward alternatives to the biomedical discourse. None of the women interviewed raised concerns about risk and safety at the birth center. They did not comment on an absence of doctors, epidural provision, electronic fetal monitoring, facility for obstetric procedures like ventouse or cesarean deliveries, or an ambulance journey of at least thirty minutes if complications arose. Instead, women focused on the social (family and friends' recommendations from their own experiences, proximity for visiting), the environmental (calm, homey, small scale, available parking, absence of busyness), and the personal (welcome, friendliness, helpfulness). In fact, their response to the technocratic model was negative if they had had previous experiences of birth at larger consultant units.

It was clear that, for many with whom I talked, the first visit to the birth center was very influential in their decisions to book there. In particular, the visit seemed to precipitate an immediate decision regarding the right place of birth for them. For many, this appeared an intuitive process that either simply felt right ("Yep—this is the sort of place") or could be visualized as the only appropriate place. As Rita, one woman, said, "I could picture myself at the Vic" (Transcript 13: 4). (The district hospital next to the birth center is called the Victoria, so for some decades now, local women have referred to the hospital and birth center as "the Vic.") This response portrays the affective component of decision making that is nonrational and nonscientific. It is immediate and right, rather than considered and weighed as probability-related decisions are. It serves to illustrate the complexity behind decision making. In the context of childbirth, scientific evidence about mortality and morbidity has been assumed to be pivotal to women's considerations around where to have a baby (MIDIRS 2002). In contrast, the decision-making process at the birth center seems to undermine the notion that evidence is the dominant factor of influence.

The focus on the safety and potential complications of childbirth reflects the technocratic model of childbirth, principally described by Davis-Floyd (2004). Her work was empirically rooted in anthropological studies of birth in the United States and built on seminal studies by Jordan (1993) of birth in four contrasting cultures. The following sections highlight some of the contrasts between the technocratic model's typical response to the embodied experiences of labor and the model of birth within the birth center, which is much more in line with what Davis-Floyd (2001, 2003) describes as the humanistic and holistic models of birth (see Conclusion, Appendix C3).

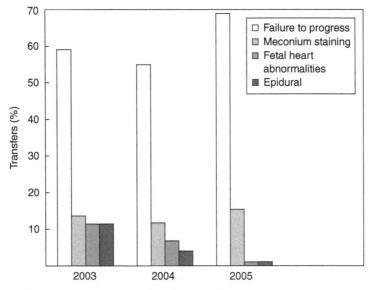

Figure 6.1. Reasons for hospital transfer.

Agnes's birth narrative is a powerfully illustration of the paradoxes of labor when not reduced to construction only through a biomedical lens. This was her first labor, and she primarily chose the birth center because she had been born there, and many of her friends had recommended it. Note the language she uses to describe her experience:

> I was shocked about how painful it was . . . right at the end when I was pushing, I just wanted them to cut me open. I'd just had enough. The pain was unbeliev-able, I really did not think it was going to hurt like that . . . like a knife being pushed up your backside. . . . But the moment he come out it was just the most unbelievable experience. And you just keep reliving it for days. The pain was like forgotten then. Brilliant, an amazing experience, nothing touches it . . . all of a sudden you just come alive. It's really bizarre. I think it's the adrenaline or something. As soon as he came out, because I think the pain as well, your body just tries to numb the pain for you and blocks it out. (Transcript 1: 6)

Agnes speaks here of a central ambiguity at the heart of the labor experi-ence, poetically described by Klassen (2000) as "sliding around between pain and pleasure" (45).

Transfer indications support this different attitude toward pain. Request for an epidural is an extremely uncommon reason for intrapartum transfer. Failure to progress in labor was by far the most common reason, followed by meconium staining of liquor, abnormalities of the fetal heart, and then epidural (see Figure 6.1).

Another story highlights the ambiguity inherent in the clinical assessment of labor when complications might be developing. After her water birth, Sarah asked the midwife to come and see her. The field note continues:

> She got really acute contraction like pain but about a couple of hours after the birth. They were so bad that they made her go cold, clammy and faint and sick feeling when they came. Judith [midwife] massages a bit of blood out of her uterus, not much, but it was pretty well contracted after that, but she really felt poorly when she got these contractions. I really did not know what they were. I thought, I wonder if she is bleeding internally or something, or God forbid, and ruptured uterus or something like that. Her vital signs weren't too bad. Her pulse was a little bit fast but blood pressure okay. Judith managed it by just sort of cradling the woman in her arms . . . for a long time, 20–30 minutes. (Observation 14: 4)

The woman settled and slept for the rest of the night. I was challenged by the midwife's nonclinical approach to the situation. She had made an assessment and had decided no clinical intervention was needed, so she just held the woman. I had the opportunity to ask the woman about this incident when I interviewed her three months after the birth.

Sarah told me that she had felt very faint in the days following the birth and had passed a large clot vaginally during this period. I asked if her hemoglobin level was taken and she replied that it was 7.1. Clearly, she had sustained significant intrauterine bleeding in the early postnatal period. Most maternity units would probably advise a blood transfusion for this, particularly if the woman was symptomatic. The staff gave her a choice of transferring to the host consultant unit for a transfusion or staying at the birth center, where treatment would consist of oral iron supplementation and an iron-rich diet. Despite her symptoms, she opted to stay at the birth center. Over the course of the next week, she regained her strength and was eventually discharged home ten days after the birth.

Sarah's care demonstrates that the midwife looking after her on that first night had a high threshold for judging whether pathology was developing in the situation. In other words, she was not "expecting trouble," a phrase used by Strong (2000) in his stinging critique of interventionist prenatal care in the United States. When I subsequently asked the lead midwife, Helen, about this episode, she explained the birth center midwives' normative mindset this way: "I think you have to look at the numbers of problems that have occurred postnatally through the unit and you keep the likelihood of it being something serious at the back your mind. And that's where it is, at the back of your mind and not the forefront" (Transcript 45: 18).

A midwife with more of a technocratic model mindset (and I recognized this in myself), may well have initiated medical intervention rather than

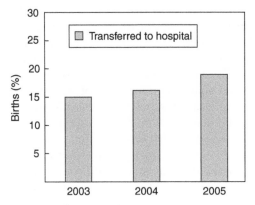

Figure 6.2. Transfer rates.

supportive midwifery care. Sarah's evaluation of the staff response to these events was unequivocally positive. "I was so glad that they did not transfer me. I absolutely wanted to stay at the Vic and I wanted to correct the anae-mia myself, by dietary means primarily" (Transcript 8: 10) was her conclu-sion. This clinical scenario occupies the gray area between physiology and pathology.

It is interesting to note that since I completed my research, the trans-fer rate has gone up steadily over a three year period (from 15% to 18%), though it is still commensurate with similar facilities elsewhere (see Figure 6.2).

Finally, it is worth noting that at the extreme end of the spectrum of what could go wrong (mortality rates), there have been no maternal deaths at the birth center and since 1995, and there have been only three perina-tal deaths out of 3,000 live births. These stories suggest that childbirth in this setting has moved beyond reflecting the influences of the technocratic model to an embracing of a nonmechanistic, more holistic understanding of birth physiology.

CONCLUSION

The findings from this birth center ethnography reveal a number of signifi-cant differences in the model of birth from mainstream maternity services in many developed countries. Here, in an unassuming building, care is delivered by ordinary staff to a tiny fraction of the women requiring mater-nity care in the United Kingdom. Yet, something quite countercultural and alternative, and quite efficacious, is occurring.

Many of the nine themes discussed here are linked to, and arise from, the accrued benefits of small-scale provision. The small scale impacted on chronological time and labor because there was no need to process women through a large institutional system, on the eschewing of a bureaucratic and institutional culture and the embracing of a homey/family feel, and on the communitarian ethos because relationships had the time and space to grow and mature. Even the birth center's struggle to resist closure was helped by the solidarity and shared commitment of the small team. There were probably follow-on effects of the postmodern leadership style demonstrated here, which could be realized more readily in a setting of this scale.

All of these features contributed to the realization of a different ethos of care, where nurture, matrescence, nesting, and intuition were expressed and valued at least as highly, and sometimes more highly, than the more ubiquitous, technocratic values of monitoring, regulation, and surveillance.

Though I know that qualitative research, especially the single-site ethnography, is vulnerable to the charge of being particular to that situation and therefore of limited generalizability, it would be shortsighted to dismiss the results out of hand. Their very peculiarity and detail reveal their power. I learned through this research of a real example of triumph over the odds, of doing childbirth beyond the technocratic model, and of experiencing genuine community at work. This is no fictionalized account or allegory of what could happen—it is the lived experience of birth center staff and the women they cared for. As such, its role is to inspire and model a different way of doing and being. There will be elements in these themes that lend themselves to adaptation to other settings. All those in maternity services who are critical of current large-scale models of service and the various discourses that accompany them can take heart and learn from the findings of this ethnography. There is a different way to do childbirth that is effective and sustainable and caring, all at once.

REFERENCES

Aldridge, S., D. Halpern, and S. Fitzpatrick. 2002. *Social Capital: A Discussion Paper*. London: Performance and Innovation Unit.

Annandale, E. 1988. "How Midwives Accomplish Natural Birth: Managing Risk and Balancing Expectations." *Social Problems* 35:95–110.

Bastick, T. 1982. *Intuition: How We Think and Act*. New York: John Wiley & Sons.

Baum, F., and A. Ziersch. 2003. "Social Capital." *Journal of Epidemiology and Community Health* 57:320–23.

Beck, U. 1992. *The Risk Society: Towards a New Modernity*. London, Sage.

Cosslett, T. 1994. *Women Writing Childbirth: Modern Discourses on Motherhood*. Manchester: Manchester University Press.

Cross, R., 1996. *Midwives and Management: A Handbook*. Cheshire, UK: Books for Midwives Press.

David, M., H. K. von Schwarzenfeld, J. A. Dimer, and H. Kentenich. 1999."Perinatal Outcome in Hospital and Birth Centre Obstetric Care." *International Journal of Gynaecology and Obstetrics* 65.22:149–56.

Davis-Floyd, R. 2001. "The Technocratic, Humanistic, and Holistic Models of Birth." *International Journal of Gynecology & Obstetrics* 75, Suppl. no. 1:S5–S23.

———. 2003. "The Technocratic, Humanistic, and Holistic Paradigms of Child-birth. *MIDIRS Midwifery Digest* 12.4:500–5.

———. 2004. *Birth as an American Rite of Passage*, 2nd ed. London: University of California Press. Originally published 1992.

Davis-Floyd, R., and P. Arvidson. 1997. *Intuition: The Inside Story; Interdisciplinary Perspectives.* New York: Routledge.

Edmondson, R. 2003. "Social Capital: A Strategy for Enhancing Health." *Social Science & Medicine* 57:1723–33.

England, P., and R. Horowitz. 1996. *Birthing from Within.* Albuquerque: Partera Press.

Esposito, N. W. 1999. "Marginalised Women's Comparisons of Their Hospital and Free-Standing Birth Centre Experience: A Contract of Inner City Birthing Centres." *Health Care for Women International* 20.2:111–26.

Fahy, K. 1998. "Being a Midwife or Doing Midwifery." *Australian Midwives College Journal* 11.2:11–16.

Foucault, M. 1973. *The Birth of the Clinic: An Archaeology of Medical Perception.* London: Tavistock.

Friedman, E. 1954. "The Graphic Analysis of Labour." *American Journal of Obstetrics & Gynaecology* 68:1568–75.

Giddens, A. 2001. *Sociology*, 4th ed. Cambridge: Polity.

Goleman, D. 1996. *Emotional Intelligence.* London: Bloomsbury.

Hammersley, M., and P. Atkinson. 1995. *Ethnography: Principles in Practice.* London: Routledge.

Hodgson, D. 2004. "Project Work: The Legacy of Bureaucratic Control in the Post-Bureaucratic Organisation." *Organisation* 11.1:81–100.

Hunt, S., and A. Symonds. 1995. *The Social Meaning of Midwifery.* Basingstoke, UK: MacMillan.

Jordan, B. 1993. *Birth in Four Cultures: A Cross-Cultural Investigation of Childbirth in Yucatan, Holland, Sweden and the United States.* Prospect Heights, IL: Waveland Press.

Kirkham, M. 2003. "Birth Centre as an Enabling Culture." In *Birth Centres: A Social Model for Maternity Care*, edited by M. Kirkham, 249–63. London: Books for Midwives.

Klassen, P. 2000. "Sliding between Pain and Pleasure: Home Birth and Visionary Pain." *Scottish Journal of Religious Studies* 19.1:45–67.

Leap, N., and T. Anderson. 2004. "The Role of Pain in Normal Birth and the Empowerment of Women." In *Normal Childbirth: Evidence and Debate*, edited by S. Downe and C. McCourt, 25–40. London: Churchill Livingstone.

Lynch, J., P. Due, C. Muntaner, and G. Smith. 2000. "Social Capital: Is It a Good Investment Strategy for Public Health?" *Journal of Epidemiological Community Health* 54:404–8.

Machin, D., and M. Scamell. 1997. "The Experience of Labour: Using Ethnography to Explore the Irresistible Nature of the Bio-Medical Metaphor During Labour." *Midwifery* 13:78–84.

McCambridge, J. 2002. *The Context of Leadership.* http://www.biz.colostate.edu/faculty/jimm/BG620/Session%201%20Ldsp,%20teams,%20ethics%20intro.ppt. Accessed 2005.

MIDIRS. 2002. *Place of Birth: Informed Choice Leaflet No. 1.* Bristol, UK: MIDIRS.

Myles, M. 1981. *Myles Textbook for Midwives.* Edinburgh: Churchill Livingstone.

Odent, M. 2001. "New Reasons and New Ways to Study Birth Physiology." *International Journal of Gynaecology & Obstetrics* 75:S39–S45.

O'Driscoll, K., and D. Meager. 1986. *Active Management of Labour.* London: W. B. Saunders.

Parents. 2005. http://www.parents.com.

Raphael, D. 1973. *The Tender Gift: Breastfeeding.* New York: Schocken Books.

Ritscher, J., 1986. "Spiritual Leadership." In *Transforming Leadership*, edited by J. A. Adams, 61–80. Alexandria, VA: Miles River Press.

Roberts, S. 2000. "Development of a Positive Professional Identity: Liberating Oneself from the Oppressor Within." *Advances in Nursing Science* 22.4:71–82.

Robertson, A. 1997. *The Midwife Companion.* Sydney: Ace Graphics.

Rooks, J. P., N. L. Weatherby, E. K. Ernst, S. Stapleton, D. Rosen, and A. Rosenfield. 1989. "Outcomes of Care in Birth Centres: The National Birth Centre Study." *New England Journal of Medicine* 321.26:1804–11.

Saunders, D., M. Boulton, J. Chapple, J. Ratcliffe, and J. Levitan. 2000. *Evaluation of the Edgware Birth Centre.* Middlesex: North Thames Perinatal Public Health.

Strong, T. 2000. *Expecting Trouble: The Myth of Prenatal Care in America.* New York: New York University Press.

Thomas, T. 2001. "Becoming a Mother: Matrescence as Spiritual Formation." *Religious Education* 96.1:88–105.

Walsh, D. 2003. "Feminism and Intrapartum Care: A Quest for Holistic Birth." In *Pregnancy, Birth and Maternity Care: Feminist Perspectives*, edited by M. Stewart, 73–84. London: BfM.

———. 2004. "'Becoming Mother': An Ethnography of a Free-Standing Birth Centre." Ph.D. thesis, University of Central Lancashire, Preston.

———. 2006. "Birth Centres, Community and Social Capital." *MIDIRS Midwifery Digest* 16.1:7–15.

Walsh, D., and S. Downe. 2004. "Outcomes of Free-Standing, Midwifery-Led Birth Centres: A Structured Review of the Evidence." *Birth* 31.3:222–29.

Wickham, S. 1999. "Evidence-Informed Midwifery 1." *Midwifery Today* 51:42–3.

———. 2002. *Reclaiming Spirituality in Birth.* http://www.withwoman.co.uk/contents/info/spiritualbirth.html. Accessed 2003.

Wilkins, R. 2000. "Poor Relations: The Paucity of the Professional Paradigm." In *The Midwife-Mother Relationship*, edited by M. Kirkham, 28–54. London: MacMillan Press.

Chapter 7

Transforming the Culture of a Maternity Service

St George Hospital, Sydney, Australia

Pat Brodie and Caroline Homer

INTRODUCTION

In this chapter we describe the process of transforming a maternity service at St George Hospital in Sydney from a traditional, medically dominated culture to one that is flexible, woman-centered, and embracing of innovative models of continuity of midwifery care. Both of us were employed to be part of this change, Pat as the clinical midwifery consultant and Caroline as a researcher whose PhD project addressed the research attached to the implementation of the first models we describe here. This process of organizational change and leadership has taken us and others who have worked with us the better part of ten years and continues today with ongoing new challenges.

The process of transforming the maternity service came after a number of government reports had been published that clearly showed women wanted more control and choice over their care during childbirth, and this included access to midwifery continuity of care in the community. These reports and the policy push for transformation are described later in the chapter.

Pat was recruited from another hospital in Sydney, where she had implemented one of the first team midwifery models of care. She was committed to developing midwifery continuity of care for women, and at the time was finishing her master's research on the experiences of the team midwives. Caroline had been away from midwifery for a couple of years and came back committed to continuity of care as a model. She had been working with people with HIV-infection in a model that highlighted the value and importance of known caregivers. Pat and Caroline met for the first time at St George Hospital in late 1996.

The principles that underpinned our work were based on a cultural change in this organization that included a shift to a woman-centered ideology—that is, to a midwifery model of care using midwives as the primary care providers for the majority of births, basing antenatal care in the community, and providing improved continuity of care for women. We have developed and evaluated a number of models of continuity of midwifery care over the past ten years. These include a team midwifery model, the St George Outreach Maternity Program (known as STOMP), and a caseload group practice model, Towards a New Group Practice Option (or TANGO).

The chapter begins by describing the models of care that we were involved in developing. We then describe the system and culture of the urban Australian maternity service that prevailed before the changes were introduced so that you can see the context in which the models were developed—a traditional, hierarchical, and medically dominated structure, with obstetricians being responsible for most women's care. The chapter then describes the events that combined to ensure that changes could occur. We expand on our experiences and describe how the models of care were developed, highlighting the key factors necessary for success. We discuss the "positive" influences—education, leadership, collaboration, shared philosophy and commitment, changing government policy directions, local knowledge, and evidence from other countries—that influenced and facilitated change. We also describe some of the "negative" influences (e.g., resistance to change by some stakeholders and staff, distrust of midwifery care, and preference for the status quo). Finally, we outline our vision for the future, which includes strategies to promote and support organizational change and practice development that enable the provision of high-quality maternity service that meets the needs of women, midwives, and the larger organization.

Some of this story and the positive clinical outcomes that ensued from our work have been published elsewhere (Homer, Davis, and Brodie 2000; Homer, Davis, et al. 2001; Homer, Matha, et al. 2001; Passant, Homer, and Wills 2003; Homer 2005). The purpose of this chapter is to provide our personal views on what worked and what did not work in our particular setting. We will also provide some ideas for future strategies to bring about cultural change in maternity service provision.

THE MODELS OF CARE: WHAT DID WE DO?

The STOMP Model

STOMP (St George Outreach Maternity Program) was the first model we established with others as part of our goal to change a culture of maternity care. There are two STOMP teams, one located in each of two separate areas in the southern suburbs of metropolitan Sydney: Hurstville and Rockdale. Each team consists of seven full-time midwives, giving a working roster of six midwives per team. The additional midwife is required to cover the annual leave entitlements within the team. The Rockdale team was established first in early 1997. The Hurstville team followed about six months later. Both remain viable and well supported over a decade later, and both have evidenced excellent outcomes.

The goal of each STOMP team is to book 35 women per month to provide a full range of care for thirty births per month or approximately 360 women annually. From our experience with this population of women, we have determined that thirty births per month is a feasible caseload for a team of seven midwives working in a team midwifery model. This equates to five births per midwife per month, given that, on average, there is usually one midwife on annual leave most of the time. Regardless of risk factors, all women are able to be booked with STOMP since it is a collaborative team with obstetric involvement in each team.

In the Australian system, most women receive care through a hospital-based system and give birth in a hospital. Women usually choose the STOMP model because it is convenient for them to attend as the antenatal clinics are based in the community. In the early days of this program, women were allocated to have care from the STOMP teams because the model was developed experimentally as part of a randomized controlled trial we and others initiated as a culture change strategy. Now, women who live in the areas close to the community centers are offered the STOMP model routinely, and most women take up this offer. Women who do not live in the areas served by the community centers are offered hospital-based care although they can still request the STOMP model. Most non-STOMP women do not receive continuity of caregivers through pregnancy, labor, and birth, or into the postnatal period.

The STOMP model means that women give birth in hospital but receive their antenatal care from the STOMP midwives in two community clinics. Both community clinics are located in early childhood centers, which are readily accessible to women (adequate public transport and car parking options), have appropriate facilities (two rooms for consultation), and are geographically central to the greatest number of childbearing women in the district. In Australia, early childhood centers are where parents take their babies and children aged up to five years to receive care from a child and family health nurse. Before the STOMP model started, antenatal care had never been provided in early childhood centers in this area, nor had midwives and the early childhood nurses worked together. Even if only through a shared co-location of services, this linking of midwives and early childhood was seen as a radical change to service provision.

The clinics are conducted collaboratively, with two midwives attending each clinic time; an obstetrician or obstetric registrar is available if needed. Such collaboration ensures that women with risks associated with their pregnancy can be seen in the community setting and will continue to receive continuity of care from their own, known midwives.

One of the midwives from each STOMP team is always on call for women in labor or to answer questions. STOMP midwives on call carry pagers so the women are able to access one of the midwives twenty-four hours per day. STOMP midwives work twelve-hour on-call shifts to cover labor and birth care in the hospital. Each day, two STOMP midwives cover the twenty-four-hour period. One midwife is on from 0800–2000 hours; she hands over to the second STOMP midwife from 2000–0800 hours.

In the hospital, STOMP midwives receive support from the midwives who normally work in the delivery suite, called "core midwives." Core midwives staff the hospital wards. They don't work in an on-call system but in regular, eight-hour shifts. They also do not attend community clinics for antenatal care. We have learned how important this support from the hospital-based core group is for several practical reasons. Importantly, these core midwives provide STOMP midwives with support and guidance in solving problems. In the event two women from the same STOMP team are in labor simultaneously, the midwives must prioritize and make a decision based on how they will meet the needs of the women with support from their colleagues. Core staff also enable STOMP midwives to take a break when they need to. STOMP midwives continue to provide midwifery care in the operating room for STOMP women who have an elective or emergency cesarean section, usually preparing the woman and her partner for surgery, and receiving and accompanying the baby and the woman's partner back to the delivery suite or, if necessary, the special care nursery (SCN). Midwives at St George Hospital do not scrub or assist in the operating room in any other manner; registered nurses in the operating room fulfill this role.

After the birth, women are transferred to the postnatal ward. They can either choose to remain in hospital for postnatal care, or be discharged early (between four and forty-eight hours) and have community-based care at home with the STOMP midwives.

Every morning shift, a STOMP midwife from each team is rostered for duty on the postnatal ward to work an eight-hour shift. The STOMP midwives predominantly care for the STOMP women in the ward as well as those at home, but they also care for other women in the ward if their workload allows.

The randomized controlled trial set up to test the STOMP model demonstrated very important benefits for women. For example, there was a statistically significant difference in the cesarean section rate between women who had STOMP care and those who did not (13.3% versus 17.8%). Fewer babies in the STOMP group needed admission to a special care baby unit

(Homer, Davis, et al. 2001). Women in the STOMP group reported waiting significantly less time for antenatal visits with easier access to care. STOMP group women also reported a higher perceived "quality" of antenatal care compared with the control group (Homer, Davis, and Brodie 2000) and showed cost savings for the hospital (Homer, Matha, et al. 2001). It seems likely that the relationship that was developed between the midwives and the women contributed to the positive experiences. The way the STOMP antenatal clinics were organized seems to have ensured that they were efficient, ran on time, and thus were less expensive.

The TANGO Caseload Model

In 1990 the hospital opened the Birth Centre in response to a government review that recommended such centers be established where women could have natural childbirth and experience direct care from midwives. At that time, primary care from midwives was not commonplace in Australia; birth centers were seen as a means to provide it. Birth centers were also seen as radical and against the status quo of the hospital system, and so were strongly resisted by some of the obstetricians who worked at the hospital in the early part of that decade. The Birth Centre consists of two antenatal rooms and two birthing rooms (both with baths). The rooms are more homelike than the standard delivery suite. For example, each has a double bed rather than an "obstetric" bed. The Birth Centre is on the same floor as the delivery suite but about fifty meters away.

For about ten years, the Birth Centre model at St George Hospital had a small number of midwives who were rostered to work eight-hour shifts. They often met women in the antenatal period and then provided care for them in labor. This ad hoc system meant that women could not be assured of having continuity of caregiver. The Birth Centre also did not provide any postnatal care at that time. In 2001 we decided to redesign the way the Birth Centre functioned, as our second new model, so that women could get to know their midwives through the continuum of pregnancy, birth, and the early postnatal period—and the TANGO model was born.

The TANGO model evolved over time as we and others learned more and developed the service to become a caseload group practice model. A caseload group practice has fewer midwives than STOMP (each group practice has three midwives, whereas each STOMP team has seven midwives). Fewer midwives per caseload practice means that women are more likely to feel that they know the midwife who attends them in labor. Women give birth in the Birth Centre if everything is normal and they are healthy. If women require medical assistance in labor or consultation and referral to an obstetrician, they are transferred to the delivery suite where their TANGO midwife continues to provide care in conjunction with the core midwives and medical staff.

Community-based postnatal care is now encouraged and supported by all the staff at St George, so the TANGO model also provides postnatal care in women's homes. Women are encouraged to go home soon, often four to six hours after birth, and are visited at home by their known midwife. In 2005 the TANGO model was expanded to include a home birth option. This was the first time in New South Wales (NSW) that women had been offered home birth through the public health system. Developing the home birth model took more than two years of planning and negotiation with the health department and health service administrators. We are delighted that all this planning finally paid off, and the first baby was born at home through the service supported by midwives from the TANGO team in December 2005.

BACKGROUND TO THE CHANGE: GETTING STARTED

In the past, the maternity system in Australia had been characterized by a fragmented service that was usually hospital based and often directed by obstetricians. St George Hospital was typical of such a system. The majority of midwives practice in hospitals, often in one clinical area, for example in an antenatal, birthing, or postnatal ward. Ten years ago, very few midwives in the public hospital system (where most women receive care and give birth) worked anything but shift work organized by the hospital. On-call work, where midwives were at home with pager access if they were needed, was rare, especially in major metropolitan hospitals. Some midwives provided community-based postnatal care in the form of three or four home visits. These were generally not the midwives who had provided the care during the antenatal or birthing periods. Many of us, midwives and a few forward-thinking obstetricians, acknowledged that this system was not making use of midwives' skills in the provision of high-quality care to women. This lack was one of the factors that influenced us to be part of system-level reform that led to the development of the new models of care, some of which we describe in this chapter.

Other factors that led us to make changes at St George included recommendations from a multitude of local, state, national, and international policy documents that reported on women's views about maternity care, and research evidence that was calling for a commitment to improve services. Crucial determinants that influenced the way we undertook reform to develop the models included

1. The need to ensure ongoing sustainability
2. The need for a clear consultation process within the organization
3. The importance of drawing on the experience of colleagues in maternity units in the United Kingdom, where many team midwifery schemes had been discontinued.

We were cognizant of a number of other factors that made a difference to the developments. We knew there were a number of policy statements advocating change that we could draw upon. The research recommending change was also gathering momentum. There was a commitment to promote the visibility of midwifery across Australia and a local commitment to change by improving the system and models of care. We discuss these factors in the next section.

Policy Statements Advocating Change

At the time we were developing our new models of care, a number of state and national government reports in Australia recommended major changes to the provision of maternity services. These included the need to provide opportunities for continuity of care; increase collaboration between midwives, obstetricians, and general practitioners (GPs); and the need to move antenatal care to community settings (NSW Health Department 1989; Victorian Department of Health 1990; NHMRC 1996; NSW Health Department 1996; Senate Community Affairs References Committee 1999), which was reiterated in subsequent documents released by state and federal governments (Senate Community Affairs References Committee 1999; NSW Health 2000; Victorian Government Department of Human Services 2004).

Although many of these recommendations may seem unremarkable to those from other countries, in an Australian setting, where the health system essentially was medically dominated, they were influential and could be used by those of us who wanted widespread change. The recommendations and reports enabled us to demonstrate at every opportunity that what we were proposing was part of a wider strategy and policy direction supported by others. It became increasingly hard for the detractors to argue against "sensible" policy that was responding to women's choices.

One of the earliest Australian reports was most instrumental in our work. In New South Wales, the review of maternity services known as the Shearman Report emphasized certain principles in its recommendations (NSW Health Department 1989). These included providing equitable access to quality care; recognizing the needs of women from non-English-speaking backgrounds; maximizing each woman's participation in decision making during pregnancy, childbirth, and the postpartum period; and promoting cooperation and collaboration among doctors, midwives, and other health professionals. The report recommended that options should be explored to expand and redefine the role of hospital-employed or salaried midwives, and suggested that midwives could be located in community health centers to provide care during pregnancy and childbirth for low-risk women. There were also a number of strategies to meet the needs of women from non-English-speaking backgrounds, including increased funding for interpreter services, care from bilingual GPs, and the establishment of ethnic obstetric liaison officers to provide support and education (NSW Health Department 1989).

Unfortunately, although the Shearman Report was groundbreaking and visionary for its time and context, widespread change in maternity services and models of care did not follow its publication. This dearth of change was one of the driving forces behind our initial efforts to develop new models of care at St George Hospital. The Shearman Report provided a framework on which to base the design of our first model, albeit much later than the writers of this policy document might have expected.

The peak health research body in Australia, the National Health and Medical Research Council (NHMRC) released another important document, *Options for Effective Care in Childbirth*, in 1996. Recommendations included the need to facilitate continuity of care and carer in the antenatal period and encourage the development of small teams of midwives and GP obstetricians. This report stated, "We suggest that a model of joint practice run by midwives and obstetricians providing continuity of care deserves more attention and appropriate evaluation by both professional and health planners" (NHMRC 1996: 26).

Despite all these reports and recommendations, by 1996 very few public hospital maternity services in Australia, including St George, had managed to achieve the changes in the organization of care necessary to introduce the components of continuity of care by midwives and community-based care into maternity services. There are many reasons for this lack of action, including the way the Australian health system is set up and funded. The health system supports a "technocratic" model—a term used to name systems of maternity care that are driven by the ideology and values of obstetrics, which in turn are based on the technological beliefs and values of the wider society (Davis-Floyd 2001). Medicine and medical care are highly valued in the Australian system, and health funding is set up in a way that advantages medical practitioners over other health care providers (including midwives). The funding system also supports medical dominance. Public hospitals and midwives are funded through the state health system, while private medicine is funded primarily through the federal system. Medical practitioners have access to the federal funding system through a universal health insurance program known as Medicare. In order to access this program, "provider numbers" are necessary for the purposes of billing and reimbursement by the federal system. Provider numbers are not available to midwives, and so their capacity to provide private services or even many services in the community is restricted. An example of this is in the provision of antenatal care. Public hospitals are often looking for ways to reduce costs. One way to do this is to reduce the community-based services that are provided by the state system and encourage people to access federally funded services (like private doctors). This can mean that publicly funded antenatal care is increasingly removed from public hospitals, and women have to have care from the GP, who receives federal Medicare funding to provide this service. In many instances around the country, this care will not be free because women will be asked to pay an additional fee to the doctor over and above the government funding provided. This cost-shifting process between state and federal systems creates a continual tension and adds to an inability to bring about widespread change.

There are also significant forces that support the status quo because, a cynic might say, it is sold by vested interests as the "safest" model. Community-based maternity services have no funding base, and as such are not well supported in Australia. Despite all these challenges (many of which still exist today), we were determined to bring about change in the way maternity services were provided in our service.

In addition, we used other national and international reports, particularly from the United Kingdom, to substantiate our model for change. We also applied for research funds to introduce and evaluate our proposals. The principles from the government reports and policy directions that underpinned our work and funding application were based on these documents and incorporated these ideas:

- Providing opportunities for women to have continuity of midwifery care and ready access to care
- Increasing collaboration among midwives, obstetricians, and general practitioners
- Offering maternity services based in the local community and sensitive to community needs
- Recognizing the needs of women from non-English speaking backgrounds
- Maximizing each woman's participation in decision making during pregnancy, childbirth, and the postpartum period
- Promoting cooperation and collaboration among doctors, midwives, and other health professionals

Research Recommending Change

At St George Hospital, we used research both as a strategy and a rationale for the changes we wanted to make. The research framework provided the structure, opportunity, and formal authority as well as the rational basis for introducing, leading, and evaluating change. We used the requirement to conduct research as a platform for the changes, obtaining a high-prestige grant that could not be challenged by the (still-resistant) obstetricians and that overtly included and benefited some others of our medical colleagues, who were included as participants on the grant.

Many of the Australian government and other reports had used evidence on which to base their recommendations. Midwifery continuity of care had been shown to reduce interventions in labor, particularly augmentation of labor, analgesic use, and electronic fetal monitoring (Kenny et al. 1994; Rowley et al. 1995; Waldenström and Nilsson 1997). A small Canadian trial with 200 women demonstrated a significant reduction in cesarean rates (Harvey et al. 1996), and one of the Australian trials reported a trend toward a reduced elective cesarean rates in high-risk women (Rowley et al. 1995). A retrospective cohort study in California also showed that supportive nurse-midwifery care in labor was associated with a reduced cesarean section rate (Butler et al. 1993).

Midwifery continuity of care had also been shown to improve women's experiences (Flint, Poulengeris, and Grant 1989; MacVicar et al. 1993; Waldenström and Nilsson 1993; Kenny et al. 1994; Rowley et al. 1995; Turnbull et al. 1996). In particular, women who had received continuity of midwifery care reported greater preparedness for birth and early parenting (Flint, Poulengeris, and Grant 1989; McCourt et al. 1998), increased satisfaction with psychological aspects of care (Waldenström and Nilsson 1993), and higher participation in decision making (Turnbull et al. 1996) than women who received standard care.

Results from studies available at the time were compelling and influential in the development and design of the STOMP model. By the time the TANGO model was developed, there was considerably more evidence available, including our own evaluation of the STOMP model (Homer, Davis, et al. 2001). More recently, evidence from a report into maternity services in another Australian state has provided additional impetus for change (Hirst 2005).

Promoting the Visibility of Midwifery

Our commitment to developing new models of care at St George also involved a determination to make the profession of midwifery more visible and recognized in the Australian community. For many years, midwifery has been dominated by medicine. Midwifery had also been subsumed under nursing for regulation, professional, and industrial purposes. This meant that nursing leaders often lacked understanding about the actual and potential role of the midwife. It also meant that midwifery was invisible within legislation and was regulated under a Nursing Act in most states and territories. The industrial models were also subsumed within a nursing model, which was antithetical to midwifery continuity of care. For example, industrial leaders could not understand that midwives would want to work in a way that involved on-call work rather than set shift work on a ward. Our determination to raise the status and increase the use of midwives in mainstream maternity service provision was supported by the findings of a national study of Australian midwifery workforce, regulation, and education conducted in 2000 (Barclay et al. 2003). Some of the barriers and current problems in the organization of maternity care in Australia included lack of recognition and support of midwifery autonomy, which was thought to be contributing to a lack of job satisfaction and increasing attrition from the midwifery workforce (Brodie 2002). In this study, it was identified that midwives were unable to fulfill the role for which they were educated, and were losing their skills and confidence. Many reported a lack of support and recognition from nursing managers, which was linked to a general perception that the professional identity and image of midwifery were confused with nursing. Midwives highlighted greater recognition of midwifery work as a key strategy in enabling midwives to contribute effectively in maternity services (Brodie 2002).

Commitment to Change

An important factor in our development of new models of care at St George was the extent of the hospital's commitment to change and willingness to improve the system and models of care. The midwives in the maternity unit at St George Hospital had been committed to improving their service over a number of years, as evidenced by a series of innovations that had already occurred in the maternity unit, such as the 1990 establishment of the Birth Centre, one of only three in Sydney at the time. Despite initial difficulties, including opposition from obstetricians and some midwives, the Birth Centre remains a well-established option for women, and it has shown excellent clinical outcomes (Homer, Davis, Petocz, et al. 2000). Anecdotally, some midwives were opposed to the birth center probably because it challenged their own views and philosophies about birth. Some midwives did not want to work in the way that the birth center model required and felt more comfortable in their familiar setting, which was a conventional labor ward.

The 1995 establishment of a midwives' clinic, which enabled low-risk women to have the same midwife throughout the antenatal period, was another example of the maternity unit's commitment to improved service through greater use of midwives. This clinic was established partly as a result of the Shearman Report recommendations and also in response to a consumer survey conducted in 1994 (Everitt et al. 1995). The survey identified problems we had not yet addressed, such as lack of continuity in the antenatal and postnatal periods, insufficient respect for individual opinions and beliefs, conflicting advice regarding breastfeeding, and problems accessing antenatal care at the hospital. Women from non-English-speaking backgrounds reported difficulties in obtaining culturally appropriate care and accessing adequate information. The STOMP model was developed to respond specifically to recommendations from this survey.

We believe that a number of factors are critical to the development of innovations and these new models of care, including leadership, financial sustainability, and the ability to learn from the successes and failures of programs that had tried similar endeavors. We discuss these factors in the next section.

Leadership as Key

Local leadership was key to the successful innovations. The senior midwifery manager, Jo Wills, was personally committed to changing the system to improve care for women and babies. She was well respected in the maternity unit and had provided many years of leadership during this early time and subsequently. Her dedication to changing the system was integral to our success and has led to the establishment and persistence of the Birth Centre despite active opposition that had previously resulted in the demise of other birth centers.

In 1992 Lesley Barclay, midwife and professor of family health, was appointed to lead research and practice development in midwifery in the area health service where the hospital was located. In the mid-1990s, recommendations from an organizational review of maternity services also led to the appointment of a professor of obstetrics and gynecology—Michael Chapman—as a way to provide leadership in obstetric and, ultimately, maternity care. In conjunction with Director of Pediatrics Tom Grattan-Smith, Chapman provided a shield from many of the negative influences, including threats against and obstruction to the predominantly midwife-led organizational changes we were making. The resistance to change was mainly coming from visiting obstetricians who had little influence, authority, or control over the impending changes.

Soon after the new academic and practice leaders were appointed, the appointments of a staff specialist obstetrician (Greg Davis), midwifery consultant (Pat Brodie), and midwifery researcher (Caroline Homer) occurred. These appointments were targeted and strategic. Positions were awarded to these individuals within a research funding stream obtained by Lesley Barclay as well as from the hospital budget, reflecting high levels of commitment to collaboration between clinical and research leadership. These individuals had beginning track records in clinical and research expertise and an expressed commitment to the vision that was being articulated for St George.

These key people led the innovations and were supported by many others across the health service. What we shared was a commitment to change that would see greater continuity of care and increased use of midwives' skills to improve care for women. The coalition of these individuals was a significant contributor to the success of the models of care. The other important factor was that we all enjoyed working together and respected one another's different capacities, skills, and knowledge. We were able to debate and disagree while ensuring we stayed on track with the vision. Enjoying working together was essential—decisions were discussed and strategies designed over endless cups of coffee.

The trust and mutual respect that these leaders built over time was supported by a number of contextual factors. Sound leadership across professional disciplines and effective preplanning and management of organizational change provided an organizational context for practice. This included shared understanding and enthusiasm for the model of care and the vision for the maternity unit; a culture of learning where we were all encouraged and supported to move beyond our own comfort zones; shared mutual professional trust between members of the team; a commitment to using effective communication skills; a high level of excitement and anticipation about doing something good for the community, health care, and the professions; comfort with, and enjoyment being on, the cutting edge of service innovation; a feeling of mutual respect, with learning and experimentation encouraged and supported; and a recognition that greater midwifery autonomy, interprofessional trust, and effective collaboration were interlinked.

The midwifery leaders in the maternity unit (including managers, educators, researchers, and clinicians) also formed a functional and cohesive group. They were committed to developing an organizational culture that was forward thinking and responsive to consumer needs, government recommendations, and evidence. Central to our collective vision was greater consumer involvement and an enhanced visibility and recognition of midwifery, in particular through midwifery continuity of care models. The shared nature of this vision ensured that the organizational culture change would proceed. Unity was a critical factor—we worked hard to ensure it did not waver.

Financial Sustainability

The maternity unit did not have any additional funds to establish new models of care. Research funds were generated by successful applications; these paid Caroline Homer's salary and the costs of the evaluation, and provided development positions for clinical midwives who were given opportunities to research and share the intellectual work that was required. The new models of care were designed with the understanding that no additional funding would be available for their implementation. Reorganization of existing resources and staff was a challenge but was also essential to enable implementation of the new models of care to proceed. The lack of additional funding had several unexpected positive effects. Implementation within the existing budget meant that the model was embedded in the organization from the outset. We anticipated, and were proved correct, that integration into existing services (rather than a pilot) would make the new model less vulnerable in times of forced budgetary cutbacks.

Learning from Others

Many aspects of the maternity health system in Australia are based on those in the United Kingdom. Organizations often looked there for new ideas and followed patterns that were shown to be useful. For this reason, we looked at the experiences of introducing new models in the United Kingdom to assist our planning and development processes.

The 1993 U.K. report on *Mapping Team Midwifery* (Wraight et al. 1993) was an important determinant in the development of STOMP, and later of TANGO. Of concern was the finding that more than one-quarter of the team midwifery schemes established in the United Kingdom in 1990 had been discontinued by 1991. Discontinuation occurred because of inadequate staffing levels, problems with deployment onto the teams, lack of commitment from midwives and obstetricians, lack of consultation, discontent among midwives, failure to increase continuity of care, and personality clashes within teams. We paid great attention to these factors as we developed the structures and risk management strategies necessary to ensure the new models would survive and prosper.

MANAGING CHANGE AND RISK

Starting Out

In the planning phase, we established a working group to provide a forum for exchange of information and ideas regarding the implementation of the new model. The working group also helped address issues that could not be resolved at a local level. We met every month and had the dates of each meeting decided at the beginning of each year for the next twelve months to maximize attendance and involvement by all members.

Our clinical colleagues who would be most impacted by the new model of care were included from the outset—midwives, managers, educators, obstetricians, and GPs. We engaged with consumers (woman and men) throughout the survey development and evaluation processes. We purposively included those staff that were known or perceived to be unsupportive of the proposed changes. We felt that if these staff members were involved in the process of design and implementation at the outset, they might be "converted," or at least find it difficult to be outwardly obstructive.

Using novel names such as dance styles for our new models was a useful approach, which came from a desire to engage staff informally with the process of change and with the research and evaluation that accompanied the change. We had a light-hearted competition to name the first continuity of care model, which is how the name STOMP was born. After this, we continued with the theme: for example, the Risk Associated Pregnancy Team (RAP) and TANGO. We also extended this approach to naming some of our research projects. A study on routine urinalysis in pregnancy became HULA, or Habitual Urinalysis is a Laborious Activity (Murray et al. 2002). Using dance names meant the projects were easily recognizable, introduced an element of fun, and engaged midwives and other staff in the unit.

Selecting Midwives

Working in a continuity of care model was a new experience for almost all the midwives in our unit. Most midwives in Australia worked in a particular clinical area (for example, antenatal or birthing suite) and were less familiar with working across all areas of maternity care or following women through pregnancy, labor, birth, and the postnatal period. In addition, being on call, even for twelve hours at a time, was an unfamiliar experience for midwives.

At the beginning of our development, we were keen to ensure we had a system that supported all midwives who chose to work in the new models. We decided that having many years of experience as a midwife was not necessarily the best criterion to use when selecting or inviting midwives to work in a new model of care. In our experience, newly graduated midwives are excellent candidates to work in innovative models of care: they have had little socialization into an institutionalized style of care. New graduates are usually enthusiastic and keen, with up-to-date knowledge, which makes them ideally placed to provide continuity of care. In many instances, newly graduated midwives have had some experience providing continuity of care (or learning about continuity of care) during their preregistration education and training.

Clearly, experienced midwives were also important to include in the new models of care. These midwives provided invaluable support, mentoring, role modeling, education, and expertise to less-experienced midwives. However, a midwife with ten years' experience in a birthing room may find antenatal and postnatal care very challenging, and need additional support and education in these areas.

We called for "expressions of interest" in the first new model of care within the unit, STOMP, but first we did a considerable amount of education (formal and informal) about these new models and how they could work in order to ensure that all staff in the unit (midwifery, nursing, medical, clerical, and allied health) understood what was involved. We hoped that this educational process would also refute some of the myths that had arisen—for example, about exactly how much on-call work was involved. Although these efforts were initially successful, we found that we also needed ongoing education about the model, especially with new staff. This was provided by the line managers and also included in orientation programs for new staff.

Preparing the Midwives

Once we selected the midwives, the next step was to ensure that they were well prepared to fulfill their role. There are a number of ways to assess the additional preparation midwives need. We chose a skills inventory or self-assessment process to assist midwives in identifying their own skills that might require updating. This self-assessment process gave midwives an opportunity to address skills and knowledge gaps prior to starting in the new model. With permission, we adapted a skills inventory that had been developed by researchers in the Midwifery Development Unit in Scotland (McGinley et al. 1995). The skills inventory consists of a series of skills that midwives rate using a four-point scale from "I don't have these skills yet" to "I am fully updated." We also included skills relating to consultation and referral because we felt these were also important. More recently, we have worked with the Australian College of Midwives to further adapt this inventory—it has become a Self-Assessment Tool and is available from the Australian College of Midwives.

Information from the skills inventory was used to plan a clinical program to meet the needs of each midwife. We do advise caution in its use. The skills inventory has limitations and should not be the only tool used to assess the learning and development needs of midwives. We realized that some midwives might have good clinical skills but have difficulty working in a team or collaboratively across disciplines. Some midwives may lack confidence in their clinical decision-making capacities or in the way they interact with women and families. These issues may not be identified in a skills inventory, and may require alternative and more than one to one means to identify and address. In particular, each midwife's professional attitude and philosophy of care need to be explicit and shared with other team members at the outset.

Additional research skills and experience were provided through a clinical fellowship program designed and funded under the research grant.

This program released clinical leaders for six months at a time to provide them with opportunities to participate in the research or in analyzing aspects of clinical care. This opportunity was of significant benefit to those who participated, and contributed to building a research and learning culture in the unit.

Developing "Process" Skills

Even though clinical skills are important and necessary, "process" skills are also essential to address with midwives joining the new service. We set up regular team meetings with all the midwives, initially on a weekly basis, as we planned and established better ways of delivering care. These meetings often developed into case reviews and provided educational, professional, and social support for all of us as we embraced the changes. We found that regular meetings are an excellent way to stimulate discussion and debate around midwifery practice and effective ways of working together.

In the development phase, discussions in the group reflected the personal philosophies of the midwives in relation to woman-centered care. Issues around informed choice, control, sharing of information and care during pregnancy, labor and birth, and the postpartum period were some of the issues that were addressed. We explored and further enhanced the listening skills and capacities of the midwives by having workshops and meetings, held in the hospital or in the community centers, to address these issues. We also worked hard to assist midwives to apply evidence in their practice and, subsequently, in their discussions with women. Other topics covered in our meetings included the midwives' knowledge, views, and attitudes toward interventions such as ultrasound, analgesia in labor, and elective cesareans, as well as home birth and community postnatal care. We all developed confidence in collaborating with the medical profession. For example, we actively participated in a multidisciplinary peer review process that we developed as an ongoing professional activity. Prior to starting STOMP, we provided a one-day workshop for the midwives that focused on the all-important interpersonal skills of communication, assertiveness, working in a team, team building, and dealing with conflict resolution.

Since we—Caroline and Pat—were clinical leaders in the unit, we openly and regularly addressed the important process of taking professional responsibility. For midwives in Australian settings of public health maternity, professional responsibility in autonomous midwifery models is significantly different from the responsibility that midwives take in other roles. In models of continuity of care, responsibility to the woman becomes paramount, changing the way many midwives perceive their practice and their relationship with women and other professionals. The changes in allegiances that have been reported by team midwives were discussed with all midwives in the unit.

In the establishment phase of STOMP, and later RAP and TANGO, we had to clarify the characteristics of these models, in particular what they were and were not. Clarification was necessary to ensure that everyone was aware of the issues and considerations that went into the various designs. We found the use of a SWOT (strengths, weaknesses, opportunities, threats) analysis a useful process to engage in that assisted us in clarifying areas of strength and capacity with the new model, while also helping to articulate what might be the limitations and areas of potential weakness. In particular, this SWOT analysis articulated the identification of role boundaries, referral pathways, and acceptance of increased accountability. Discussion around these processes continued with the midwives on an ongoing basis.

Working in a Team

When developing our models, we found it best to focus on building cohesion within the smaller team but also essential to seek out the greater team, which included the larger group of hospital staff or community resource people. It is important to make sure that all midwives feel included in the changes. Setting up new models that exclude some midwives, who then do not feel part of the new model, leaves them feeling isolated, with little support from others, and is unhelpful and unlikely to be sustainable. Regular meetings to build a sense of a team were necessary to establish and sustain the model both for the small groups of midwives forming the teams and also for the wider group across the entire maternity service. Overt strategies of inclusion and recognition of the value of all midwives across the unit were important.

We were mindful of Sandall's (1997) research with midwives in continuity of care models, which identified three important elements that make a group practice effective and sustainable:

- Occupational autonomy (that is, midwives organize their own work and time)
- Social support at home and within the group or team (at work this support is achieved during weekly meetings)
- An ability to develop meaningful relationships with women

We considered these three elements carefully in the initial design of STOMP and incorporated them into all subsequent models. We consider these critical to our success, and we encourage all those looking at improved service delivery to ensure these elements are prioritized and included.

Collaboration

Effective collaboration with obstetric and other medical colleagues was an important part of planning and ongoing implementation. Over the years we have identified a number of practical strategies that may be useful for others to consider and use:

1. *Involve medical colleagues.* We believe that medical colleagues should be involved right from the beginning and see benefit for themselves in participation. In our service, obstetricians who had not received prestigious research funds not only shared in the benefits of our grants but also become far more engaged in research and publication than would have happened otherwise. We invited them to be part of the working group, sent them the minutes of our meetings, raised important issues with them, and made sure that they felt welcome to be a part of the development and ongoing implementation and evaluation of the model. Meeting them individually during the planning phase was also useful. We found that it was worthwhile to be proactive and include in the working party the doctors who were most resistant to change. In this way, they could learn about the proposed model, understand that it has pros and cons (like all systems), and express their concerns and ideas. This process of involvement effectively removes any resistance claims of not being informed or consulted. We found that involving junior medical staff in our discussions and plans was also important. Junior and trainee medical staff members are the obstetricians and GPs of the future, and they are among the people we as midwives want to see involved in sustaining long-term system change.

2. *Communicate.* It is important to actively promote ongoing communication and discussions to maintain momentum and keep the links between midwives and doctors. Communication can be formal and informal, and include "corridor" conversations, meetings, memos, and e-mails, as well as occasional social events. It is often very helpful to raise issues first, that is, to have the conversation even if you think the answer will be no. Sometimes the response will be surprising, and even if it is negative, you will have planted a seed that might bring about change at some stage in the future. Seeing collaboration as an ongoing process rather than an end point is important. We have tried to avoid the issue of "who has the final say." Rather, we have been committed to working through situations with respect and evidence, ensuring that the woman is always at the center of the discussion and ultimate decision.

3. *Develop operational criteria.* We found that you need agreed-upon, clear criteria for recruitment, consultation, and transfer and a plan for evaluation of the outcomes of your model. We would highly recommend this step to others contemplating such change.

4. *Demonstrate and work to develop high-order professional skills.* Working effectively with medical colleagues is a learned skill and one that comes with practice and confidence. Some staff may need initial training and/or support before developing confidence in the area, so have clarity about the issue or problem at hand and address it with professionalism and confidence. For example, if you are discussing the care of a woman with a medical colleague, it is important to have all the facts, present them in a logical order, have some suggestions about the management and outcomes, and be cognizant about the evidence relating to the issue in order to generate confidence, credibility, and strength in your interaction. Ongoing professional education enables staff to grow in their thinking and knowledge, and to be open to further innovations.

5. *Prepare and organize.* It is important to be well prepared and organized—for example, having all of the woman's results and records available at each antenatal visit and not having gaps or unanswered questions about clinical care. If at any time you need to consult or refer to a doctor or another health professional, then all the information will be accessible. This accessibility of information promotes others' confidence in you as well as in the new model.

6. *Integrate innovation—don't just add it on.* Sustainability from the perspective of the medical staff in your unit may be determined by the extent to which the model is integrated into the normal activity of the unit. A model that is well integrated will ensure that activities such as education and training can be included in the development and implementation process.

Leadership

A number of key leadership strategies were developed and adopted as part of an overall change process for maternity care at this hospital. These included our strategy of using the legitimate authority of research and our own research skills and leadership to introduce and evaluate new models of care based on successful models elsewhere in Australia. We were committed to improving and evaluating midwifery practice and maternity care outcomes through the adoption of evidence-based approaches. We also continually reflected, reviewed, and adapted our practice and services in line with consumer feedback and research findings.

We worked very hard to foster interdisciplinary collaboration and the development of relationships of mutual respect and, ultimately, trust based on supporting and enhancing clinical leadership, professional development, and greater visibility of midwives. This meant us sharing responsibility for driving change locally, and promoting and disseminating successful innovations and achievements to other institutions and care providers through seminars, conferences, and publications as well as to the local community through the media. Politically and strategically, we sought out and ensured strong and consistent support and recognition from the heads of the departments in both midwifery and obstetrics, and from health planners and hospital administrators, ensuring continuous communication and feedback through formal and informal channels.

We operated from an assumption that everyone was there to provide the best possible outcome for each woman. We sought to foster an environment and culture of lifelong learning among all health professionals. Communicating effectively, adopting a questioning research approach, and planning to provide the best possible care for the women we served were all overt strategies in our approach to collaboration and providing leadership.

Consultation and Referral Guidelines

Developing guidelines for consultation and referral is an important part of establishing your new model of care. As a basis in Australia, we suggest using *Guidelines for Consultation and Referral,* which are available from the Australian College of Midwives. Other countries have developed similar guidelines that are appropriate for different settings.

Equipment

The type of model and the location of care will guide you in any decisions about equipment. If you are redesigning the system of care so as to improve continuity of care and carer, it is likely that you will not need additional equipment, for it already exists in your organization. For example, sphygmomanometers, stethoscopes, and fetal Dopplers are probably already part of your equipment in the antenatal clinic. If you plan to provide antenatal care from community-based settings, you will need to consider any additional equipment that might be necessary.

When we established STOMP clinics in an early childhood center, we needed to buy portable examination tables. We also bought hand-held fetal Doppler machines, an automated urinalysis device (our evidence-based standard of care includes using an automated machine for urinalysis when it is needed), sphygmomanometers, stethoscopes, and long-range message pagers for all the midwives. One mobile phone was purchased for use when midwives were providing postnatal care in the community. The mobile phone is predominately used for a potential emergency situations or when midwives need to contact women to verify where they live.

Administrative Support

Administrative requirements are important to consider in the planning and implementation phases as well as in the longer term. They include assistance in helping write leaflets and brochures, advertising, and promotion both with the women using the service and with other health professionals. On a logistical level, administrative support assists with filing and paperwork; processing pathology results; lending a hand with writing, photocopying, and sending out minutes of meetings; answering routine phone inquiries; and generally providing assistance with the running of the model.

Administrative support is a key component of successful models and must not be overlooked. Important midwifery time should not be lost in providing these administrative functions. In our early development of models, we did not recognize the importance of administration, and we needed to draw on administrative staff who already had full workloads. More recently, we have tried to ensure that administrative/clerical time is built into the model. For example, this has involved having an administrative assistant rostered onto the specific clinical area for four to six hours a week to assist with filing results, ordering supplies, and other clerical duties. In another instance, a midwife is rostered on for additional hours each week to assist with administrative activities, such as preparing the clinical records of the women for the next antenatal clinic (for example, printing ultrasound and pathology reports to ensure they are easily available at the visit) and collecting the monthly statistics about women booked with the model. These specific, non-midwifery tasks are essential, so time is allocated to them.

Promoting the Model

The development of a leaflet or brochure to promote and advertise the new model was important. We used these leaflets to inform women and also as a resource to explain the model to colleagues and other health care professionals. The leaflet needs to be developed by a group of people that includes women who may use the service. Once the leaflet was developed, we circulated it to all the people who would be involved in the new model. Their feedback helped us edit and refine the leaflet so that it was clear, concise, readable, and woman friendly. Brief translations were also necessary because women in our hospital came from a range of other countries and many did not have English as a first language.

Launching the model was treated as an important event to ensure recognition and a sense of excitement and enthusiasm. We spent time promoting the models of care through the local newspaper and in the hospital newsletter—a useful approach since many women heard about the models through the media.

BREAKTHROUGHS AND BARRIERS

There were a number of breakthroughs and barriers in our quest to achieve an innovative and flexible culture of birth. Breakthroughs included having strong and effective leadership from midwives and obstetricians, developing and then strengthening professional connections between midwifery and obstetrics, attracting talented staff, integrating newly graduated midwives into continuity of midwifery care models, breaking down professional barriers to the women we serve, and increasing our partnership with the women. Barriers included the lack of visibility of midwifery in the highly industrial, professional framework within which Australian midwives work; midwifery shortages; and having a part-time workforce that found it difficult to embrace autonomy and flexible working conditions.

Our firsthand experiences also gave us insight and understanding about the nature of effective and ineffective leadership, the particular attributes of effective leaders, and the environments in which leadership is more likely to occur. We identified a number of key factors needed to address barriers and resistance to new models of care and increased midwifery autonomy. Whether it is the particular traits and attributes of each of the clinical leaders, or the structures, organizational contexts, and collaborative relationships that were developed—or some combination of all of these—that have enabled us to be successful is uncertain. What we do know, however, is that the process of developing the St George midwifery models of care highlighted their capacity to deliver distinct improvements, not only in the care of women but also in the improvement of job satisfaction, professional autonomy, and retention of midwives in practice.

Influence on Policy

The new midwifery models of care at St George have influenced policy and practice and have become a blueprint within Australia for statewide maternity service policy and planning for the future. The research we conducted has been influential internationally. Many of the principles we developed on our journey have been identified as keys to improving the effectiveness of maternity services. The work has been integrated into government policy documents for the planning and delivery of services as well as into midwifery curricula (preregistration and master's degrees). Clinicians and leaders from the hospital are frequently asked to advise and consult with other organizations that are implementing models of continuity of midwifery care, and we regularly speak at conferences and seminars.

Visions for the Future

Our experiences over nearly a decade have confirmed for us that the changes we put in place are worthwhile and important. Women benefit by receiving care from known midwives, and midwives benefit by providing continuity of care. Our own research shows that outcomes are improved—higher satisfaction rates (Homer, Davis, and Brodie 2000), lower cesarean rates, fewer neonatal nursery admissions, and reduced costs (Homer, Davis, Petocz, et al. 2000; Homer, Matha, et al. 2001). The growing confidence and job satisfaction experienced by midwives in the various midwifery models support the ongoing strengthening of the profession. Within a context of widespread health policy change designed to address the costs and morbidity consequences of the current system of medically dominated maternity care, midwifery's capacity to contribute will become increasingly important in Australia. We believe that strong, confident midwives are important in the provision of woman-centered care and in responding to the needs of women. Within this context, enhancing midwifery autonomy can contribute to increased job satisfaction and increasing retention of the midwifery workforce.

We see midwifery as central to sound public health planning. As such, it requires high-level recognition, authority, and support if it is to make an effective contribution to the provision of safe, efficient, and economic maternity services in Australia in the future. If this support is forthcoming in other settings, midwifery in Australia will be well positioned to implement models of care that are reflective of the needs of the local community. These models will be community based, close to where women live and work; they will be collaboratively developed and supported. Midwives will be skilled, competent, and able to provide continuity of care, supporting the woman in her choice of place of birth and ensuring she engages her family and other social support necessary to sustain her into becoming a mother.

Evidence of our vision becoming a reality was given great impetus recently when further expansion of the caseload model was announced. And in what is a groundbreaking innovation for mainstream public health maternity care in Australia, St George is now offering low-risk women the choice of home birth. Such models are rare within mainstream Australian maternity services; we see this development as evidence of increasing acceptance and trust of midwifery models of care at St George.

ACKNOWLEDGMENTS

Sincere appreciation goes to all those individuals who contributed their ideas, fears, vision, and consistent support for midwifery models of care at St George. This was especially important in the early phase of the developments when the models seemed so radical and challenging for many. Others not named in this chapter include Reta Creegan, Louise Everitt, Deb Matha, Tanya Farrell, and Elizabeth Steinlein. Many others quietly worked in the background to make sure the changes went through as smoothly as possible. We thank each of them and share our successes with them.

REFERENCES

Barclay, L., P. Brodie, K. Lane, N. Leap, K. Reiger, and S. Tracy. 2003. *The AMAP Report—Volume I and II.* Sydney: Centre for Family Health and Midwifery, UTS.

Brodie, P. 2002. "Addressing the Barriers to Midwifery: Australian Midwives Speaking Out." *Journal of the Australian College of Midwives* 15.3:5–14.

Butler, J., B. Abrams, J. Parker, J.M. Roberts, and R.K. Larkos, Jr. 1993. "Supportive Nurse-Midwife Care Is Associated with a Reduced Incidence of Caesarean Section." *American Journal of Obstetrics and Gynaecology* 168.3:1407–13.

Davis-Floyd, R. 2001. "The Technocratic, Humanistic, and Holistic Paradigms of Childbirth." *International Journal of Gynecology and Obstetrics* 75:S5–S23.

Everitt, L., L. Barclay, M. Chapman, R. Hurst, A. Lupi, and J. Wills. 1995. *St George Maternity Services Customer Satisfaction Research Project.* Sydney: St George Hospital and Community Services.

Flint, C., P. Poulengeris, and A. Grant. 1989. "The 'Know Your Midwife' Scheme: A Randomised Trial of Continuity of Care by a Team of Midwives." *Midwifery* 5.1: 11–16.

Harvey, S., J. Jarrell, R. Brant, S., Stainton, and D. Rach. 1996. "A Randomised, Controlled Trial of Nurse-Midwifery Care." *Birth: Issues in Perinatal Care and Education* 23.3:128–35.

Hirst, C. 2005. *ReBirthing: Report of the Review into Maternity Services in Queensland.* Brisbane: Queensland Health.

Homer, C. S. E. 2005. "Laying the Foundation: The STOMP Study." In *Midwifery and Public Health: Future Directions and New Opportunities,* edited by P. O Luanaigh and C. Carlson, 129–52. Edinburgh: Churchill Livingstone.

Homer, C. S. E., G. K. Davis, and P. M. Brodie. 2000. "What Do Women Feel about Community-Based Antenatal Care?" *Australian and New Zealand Journal of Public Health* 24.5:590–95.

Homer, C. S. E., G. K. Davis, P.M. Brodie, A. Sheehan, L.M. Barclay, J. Wills, and M. G. Chapman. 2001. "Collaboration in Maternity Care: A Randomised Controlled Trial Comparing Community-Based Continuity of Care with Standard Care." *British Journal of Obstetrics and Gynaecology* 108.1:16–22.

Homer, C. S. E., G. K. Davis, P. Petocz, L. Barclay, D. Matha, and M. G. Chapman. 2000. "The Obstetric Outcomes of Low-Risk Women: Birth Centre versus Labour Ward." *Australian Journal of Advanced Nursing* 18.1:8–12.

Homer, C. S. E., D. Matha, L. G. Jordan, J. Wills, and G. K. Davis. 2001. "Community-Based Continuity of Midwifery Care versus Standard Hospital Care: A Cost Analysis." *Australian Health Review* 24.1: 85–93.

Kenny, P., P. Brodie, S. Eckermann, and J. Hall. 1994. *Westmead Hospital Team Midwifery Project Evaluation: Final Report.* Sydney: Centre for Health Economics Research and Evaluation.

MacVicar, J., G. Dobbie, L. Owen-Johnstone, C. Jagger, M. Hopkins, and J. Kennedy. 1993. "Simulated Home Delivery in Hospital: A Randomised Controlled Trial." *British Journal of Obstetrics and Gynaecology* 100.4: 316–23.

McCourt, C., L. Page, J. Hewison, and A, Vail. 1998. "Evaluation of One-to-One Midwifery: Women's Responses to Care." *Birth: Issues in Perinatal Care and Education* 25.2:73–80.

McGinley, M., D. Turnbull, H. Fyvie, I. Johnstone, and B. MacLennan. 1995. "Midwifery Development Unit at Glasgow Royal Maternity Hospital." *British Journal of Midwifery* 3.7: 362–71.

Murray, N., C. S. E. Homer, G. K. Davis, J. Curtis, G. Mangoes, and M. Brown. 2002. "A Clinical Prospective Study on the Clinical Utility of Routine Urinalysis in Pregnancy." *Medical Journal of Australia* 177.9:477–80.

NHMRC [National Health and Medical Research Council]. 1996. *Options for Effective Care in Childbirth.* Canberra: Australian Government Printing Service.

NSW Health Department. 1989. *Final Report of the Ministerial Task Force on Obstetric Services in NSW: The Shearman Report.* Sydney: NSW Department of Health.

———. 1996. *NSW Midwifery Taskforce Report.* Sydney: NSW Department of Health.

———. 2000. *The NSW Framework for Maternity Services.* Sydney: NSW Health Department.

Passant, L., C. Homer, and J. Wills. 2003. "From Student to Midwife: The Experiences of Newly Graduated Midwives Working in an Innovative Model of Midwifery Care." *Australian Journal of Midwifery* 16.4:18–21.

Rowley, M. J., M. J. Hensley, M. W. Brinsmead, and J. H. Wlodarczyk. 1995. "Continuity of Care by a Midwife Team versus Routine Care During Pregnancy and Birth: A Randomised Trial." *Medical Journal of Australia* 163.6: 289–93.

Sandall, J. 1997. "Midwives' Burnout and Continuity of Care." *British Journal of Midwifery* 5.2:106–11.

Senate Community Affairs References Committee. 1999. *Rocking the Cradle: A Report into Childbirth Procedures.* Canberra: Commonwealth of Australia.

Turnbull, D., A. Holmes, N. Shields, H. Cheyne, S. Twaddle, W. H. Gilmour, M. McGinley et al. 1996. "Randomised, Controlled Trial of Efficacy of Midwife-Managed Care." *Lancet* 348.9022:213–18.

Victorian Department of Health. 1990. *Having a Baby in Victoria: Ministerial Review of Birthing Services in Victoria.* Melbourne: Victorian Department of Health.

Victorian Government Department of Human Services. 2004. *Future Directions for Victoria's Maternity Services.* Melbourne: Department of Human Services, Victoria.

Waldenström, U., and C. A. Nilsson. 1993. "Women's Satisfaction with Birth Centre Care: A Randomised Controlled Trial." *Birth: Issues in Perinatal Care and Education* 21.1:3–13.

———. 1997. "A Randomised Controlled Study of Birth Centre Care versus Standard Maternity Care: Effects on Women's Health." *Birth: Issues in Perinatal Care and Education* 24.1:17–26.

Wraight, A., J. Ball, I. Seccombe, and J. Stock. 1993. *Mapping Team Midwifery.* IMS Report 242 to the Department of Health. Brighton: Institute of Manpower Studies.

Chapter 8

Maternity Homes in Japan

Reservoirs of Normal Childbirth

Etsuko Matsuoka and Fumiko Hinokuma

Hospital birth is the norm in almost all industrialized countries, including Japan, where only 1.2% of births take place outside of a hospital. But the significance of this small number is far greater than it appears, for the potential of normal births achieved in maternity homes and at home is so influential that it contributes to maintaining the quality of the rest of the births in Japan. Moreover, research conducted through a grant-in-aid from the Ministry of Health, Welfare, and Labor in 1999 demonstrated that women who gave birth in maternity homes felt more satisfaction and comfort with their births than those who gave birth in hospitals (Watanabe 1999). Since then, maternity homes have been acknowledged by policymakers and medical communities as a valid choice of birthing place, and the concept of satisfaction has gained acceptance as an important aspect of childbirth for birthing women. This chapter shows that maternity homes in Japan function not only as reservoirs of normal births, but also as training and educational facilities for both young and student midwives. Furthermore, independent midwives working in maternity homes are perceived by other midwives to exemplify how "real midwives" should behave—thereby providing an ideal standard for midwifery practice.

We first describe general attitudes toward childbirth in Japan, contrasting them with those in the West: in Japan, cesarean section is negatively valued, and the use of pain-relieving drugs in labor and delivery is kept extremely low. We then provide a brief history of Japanese maternity homes and describe two of them in detail, along with a vivid depiction of one woman's experience of giving birth in a maternity home. In our analysis, we focus on four features characteristic of Japanese maternity homes in general: the importance of waiting for the baby to be born, the value of labor pain, mothering the mother, and birth as a family event. Finally, we

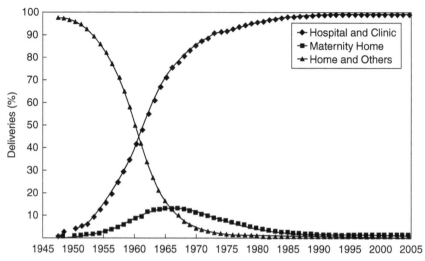

Figure 8.1. Trends in place of delivery.

present the average transfer rates of maternity homes in the pre-, peri-, and postnatal periods to evaluate their overall safety. We are convinced that the maternity home as a birth place is a model that works because babies are born there under healthier conditions than their hospital counterparts. Maternity homes function to keep childbirth from becoming too medicalized and to provide models for optimal midwifery practice.

OVERVIEW OF CHILDBIRTH IN JAPAN

Let's first of all look at where babies are born in Japan. Figure 8.1 shows the yearly changes in the number of births by place of delivery. In 2005, out of 1,062,530 babies born in Japan, 98.8% were born in hospitals or private clinics, 1.0% in maternity homes, and 0.2% at home. Births in the latter two places are conducted by independent midwives who, according to the wishes of their client, deliver the baby either in their client's home or in the maternity home, which they run and which is usually their own home. In Japan in 2006, there were 25,775 midwives: 88% worked in hospitals and clinics, 6% were independent, and 6% were employed at other working places such as universities or government institutions. Independent midwives either own facilities with beds for delivery, or deliver babies at women's homes and have no inpatient facility of their own.[1] In 2005 the number of practicing maternity homes was reported to be 388 nationwide, and the largest number of births taking place annually at one maternity home was around 250.[2] In Japan 47% of babies are born in small, private, doctor-run clinics with fewer than nineteen beds, which means that births are handled, more or less, in small-scale facilities, with the average number of births being about 342 per clinic or hospital.[3] It is estimated that midwives actually deliver about half the babies born in Japan, although government statistics show only 2.8% of births with midwife attendance (Shimada, M. 2001). This inaccurate representation comes from a provision on the birth certificate stating that the doctor has priority to sign her/his name when both a midwife and a doctor are in attendance at the birth—it is usually the case in Japan that a doctor is called in at the final stage of delivery even if a midwife has attended the entire labor and birth.

THE HISTORY OF MATERNITY HOMES IN JAPAN

As shown in Figure 8.1, the history of maternity homes does not go back as early as the pre–World War II period, although there were a few locations that already had in-patient facilities during the war. Why maternity homes increased in number after the war is very clear: until the health reforms initiated by the American occupying force (1945–52), Japanese women delivered at home. Afterward, as part of the health reforms, maternity policy was shifted toward institutional birth modeled on the U.S. system, which was supposed to be modern and superior to that of the defeated country. Hygiene especially was emphasized: American nurses involved in the health reforms believed this was difficult to achieve at home. At the time, there was nothing comparable in America to the Japanese professional midwifery practice based on home birth, which was backed by a highly elaborate educational and organizational system. Thus the American nurses had no means of understanding Japanese midwifery in its proper context. Given the new policies being implemented from above and the poor housing conditions resulting from the bombing during the war, many women began to decide to give birth in hospitals or maternity homes. Some midwives remodeled their own houses to meet the architectural standard for birthing facilities, and the government also built public maternity homes, called "mother-child health centers," in provincial parts of Japan, with the intention of decreasing the infant mortality rate by decreasing the number of home births. The rate of maternity home births peaked at 12.9% in 1965 but gradually declined as hospital and clinic births, including those at small clinics run by physicians, became the modern norm.

The postwar health reforms were very radical in that they reorganized three professions that had had separate organizations—nurses, midwives, and public health nurses—under one new law enacted in 1947. In 1946 the national midwifery association, which had existed since 1927, was dissolved, and in 1948 the educational system for midwives was merged with that for nurses. Prior to that merging, midwives entered directly into professional midwifery schools. After the merger, three years of nursing education were required to be a midwife or a public health nurse. In 1947 the term for "midwife" was changed from *sanba* (*san* = birth, *ba* = old woman) to *josan-pu* (*josan* = help delivery, *pu* = woman). In 2002, it was changed again to *josan-shi* (*josan* = help delivery, *shi* = teacher)—a term with no gender connotation. At that time, it was suspected that this change had been made intentionally to allow men to become midwives and was highly controversial among some independent midwives, who initiated a political movement against this idea as they joined hands with women. The opinions of members of the Japanese Association of Midwives were split concerning this matter.

The immediate postwar period was a prime time for midwives in Japan— they enjoyed professional dominance over normal birth and, with it, high status. The number of midwives peaked at 77,560 in 1951 (this was three times the number of midwives in 2006), but from then on, the diminishing number of home births gradually deprived independent midwives of their jobs. Some survived by setting up maternity homes, others ceased independent practice and went into hospitals, and still others took up family planning and made home visits to care for newborn babies. Since 1976 the number of independent midwives has been less than that of midwives working in hospitals or clinics.

The revitalization of independent midwifery in Japan began with the natural childbirth movement, which came to Japan in the late 1970s, and continued with the postmodern types of practice that emerged in the 1990s (Matsuoka 2001). The natural childbirth movement (Lamaze method) was led by articulate, middle-class women with a sense of feminism; their influence on the media was large because some of them published their birth experiences in books, articles, and photographs. This movement was a stroke of luck for independent midwives, who were on the verge of extinction both in the medical community and in the neighborhoods.

ATTITUDES TOWARD BIRTH IN JAPAN, WITH PARTICULAR FOCUS ON CESAREANS

In Japan cesarean births tend to have a negative image, as delivering by cesarean section implies that a woman was not capable of delivering vaginally. Therefore, it is very uncommon for a woman to request a cesarean when there is no medical indication. The rate of analgesic delivery is estimated to be around 2.1% (Watanabe 1999), and that of cesarean section is reported to be 17.4% in 2005 (Mothers' and Children's Health and Welfare Association 2007). When we consider that childbirth is a human physiological phenomenon experienced by women worldwide, the large differences in cesarean rates among countries, ranging from 15% at the lower end to over 40% at the higher end, implies that cesareans are not conducted for medical reasons alone. The World Health Organization (WHO) recommends that cesarean rates should never be higher than 15%, above which evidence shows that the outcome of birth does not improve (WHO 1985). The publication of the largest prospective home birth study to date in the *British Medical Journal* (Johnson and Daviss 2005) provides a different perspective on appropriate cesarean rates for low-risk, planned home births in the United States and Canada: the cesarean rate for these midwife-attended births was 3.7%, with perinatal outcomes similar to those for low-risk hospital births in the United States. These outcomes suggest that the WHO's estimate has been driven by the reality of high intervention rates worldwide and by a focus on high-risk situations, and not by what happens when normal birth is supported. Japan is one of a very small group of countries, along with the Netherlands and Finland, with low cesarean rates. We suggest two reasons for this phenomenon: (1) the gendered image of women; and (2) the view of obstetrics as a science of human physiology distinct from surgery.

The Gendered Image of Women

First of all, a gendered image of women as the birthing sex that physiologically should be able to give birth vaginally is shared by the general public and by older-generation obstetricians. A woman who demands a cesarean without medical reasons is looked upon as unacceptable, because it is believed that women's bodies are made to give birth vaginally, and the mode of delivery should be decided by obstetricians, not by the women. Women who do not meet this expectation are equated almost with abandoning their gender role. Women who use medical intervention to ease labor pains are also frowned upon, for they are considered to have betrayed the laws of nature. The unpopularity of cesarean section and epidural delivery in Japan originates from the gendered idea that women can and should follow what they are born to do physiologically. Thus, women who undergo cesareans in Japan are made to feel guilty for not delivering in the proper way. There are Japanese websites that talk about couples' experiences with cesareans—many of the writers are upset by unsympathetic comments made by their friends or in-laws, who say things such as "a child who didn't go through the birth canal lacks mental strength to face difficulty," "oh, you had an easy birth," or "I wonder whether one can be a mother without feeling labor pain."

This negative view of cesareans contrasts strongly with attitudes in the West and in Asian countries such as China, Taiwan, Korea, India, and Thailand, where cesareans are equated with modern technology, and the rates are far higher than in Japan. In Korea and China, where we have also interviewed women, the general opinion is that a cesarean was safer for the baby, and women were happy to end up having one. In Japan general attitudes toward cesarean are very similar to those toward an analgesia-assisted delivery, which is thought of as depriving women of a chance to nourish their motherhood. This is very different from what happened in Finland in 1976, when the right to pain relief during birth was demanded by a female physician; her demand brought about a recommendation by the Ministry of Health to increase the number of anesthesiologists to make epidural available in secondary hospitals (Declercq et al. 2001: 15). Of course, strong promotion by anesthesiologists was a key factor in Finland, but the logic that women have the same right as men not to feel pain also gained public acceptance.

In Japan, where the gendered division of labor still pervades all corners of society, the logic of the general public is the other way around: women and men have different gender roles and biological functions; thus, it is not appropriate to treat them equally in every aspect, especially concerning childbirth, where the difference between the two sexes is most clear. In other words, there is an implicit belief that the distinction between women and men has to be constructed culturally and has to be maintained by having women give birth vaginally. Nevertheless, in recent years many women of reproductive age are increasingly taking an interest in analgesic delivery, which is literally called "painless birth" in Japanese, mainly because of the fear of pain. They are looking for hospitals or clinics that provide these services, but at this time, there are only a limited number of such facilities available in Japan. The climate against cesarean section and analgesic delivery is currently undergoing rapid change, and higher rates may soon be seen. However, until now cesarean on demand has been extremely rare, and analgesic delivery is also rare because of the lack of facilities. Our description of this situation does not imply that we, as feminists, want to take labor pain out of birth for the sake of equality between women and men. We will discuss the significance of pain in the context of birth in a maternity home from an anthropological point of view later in this chapter.

Obstetrics as a Science of Human Physiology Distinct from Surgery

The second reason for a low cesarean section rate stems from the reality that in Japan, the definition of obstetrics as a science of the human physiological birth process persisted until the 1970s,[4] although it is also true that American obstetrics was introduced and gained ground in the 1960s and 1970s. Obstetricians practicing before the 1970s took pride in delivering difficult cases vaginally because they believed that these skills created the difference between "obstetricians" and "surgeons." They believed that increasing the list of indications for a cesarean would warp obstetrics toward surgery, the consequence of which ultimately would be denying the existence of obstetrics itself. One obstetrician wrote in a medical journal in 1972, "If you think carefully, the use of cesarean section, even as the last resort, has the potential to deconstruct delivery/obstetrics and to bring it closer to surgery. Thus there is a big contradiction inherent in obstetrics that the more you carry out cesarean sections, the greater the tendency that [obstetrics] will move toward surgery. So future obstetrics should be careful not to move toward cesarean section. We should recognize the true nature of [such a move]" (Kobayashi 1972: 32).

Those who advocated for physiological births shared this view and discouraged the use of unnecessary interventions, which they said would destroy the delicacy of the natural process of giving birth. And the fact that a number of obstetricians and midwives trained under the physiological model of childbirth still practice in the professional community serves to prevent a technocratic model from dominating the scene. The existence of a midwifery system that was not wiped out completely during the period of American occupation after the war also contributes to maintaining the physiological model of childbirth. In fact, the presence of a strong midwifery system as a reservoir of normal birth represents a dividing line between Japan and other Asian countries such as Korea and China (Matsuoka, Hinokuma, and Suganuma 2007). As the older generation of obstetricians retires from the medical community and the number of lawsuits increases, the cesarean rate will undoubtedly rise, signs of which can already be seen in many birthing facilities.[5]

WHAT ARE MATERNITY HOMES LIKE?

Maternity homes are usually found in residential areas: they are ordinary homes of independent midwives. Without a sign announcing the presence of a maternity home, people would not notice that this is where babies are born. The Otani Maternity Home is one such example. Ms. Takako Otani, born in 1934, opened her maternity home in 1967 when she decided to quit working in a hospital as a nurse-midwife. She brought up three daughters on the top floor of this three-story house, and one of them now practices as a midwife in Ms. Otani's maternity home; she wants to practice in Canada in the future since she is married to a Canadian (see Chapter 3). Ms. Otani now delivers about 100 babies a year, with the help of a few other young midwives. When people enter her maternity home, they are greeted by women in aprons instead of white coats and are suddenly reminded that birth can happen in an everyday environment without the need for medical paraphernalia. The same sorts of sofas, bookshelves, desks, and other furnishings found in any ordinary house predominate in the waiting room and in the examining room where Ms. Otani practices. First-time visitors find themselves feeling relaxed and warmhearted in the cozy atmosphere. On the second floor, we find one Western-style birth room, two rooms for postpartum women to stay, and one tatami (traditional) room for multipurpose occasions. The birth room looks like any other room, with an ordinary bed, warm-colored curtains, and a sink for bathing the baby, all of which are surrounded by wooden walls. After the birth, the woman stays in either of the two rooms, one with a single bed and the other with twin beds, both of which are big enough for mother and baby to sleep together.

Ms. Otani performs antenatal and infant checkups and gives preparatory classes for expecting couples on different days of the week. A pregnant woman can bring anyone she wishes with her, so on those days, children, friends, grandmothers, and husbands fill the maternity home. Because Ms. Otani lets women use the extra tatami room for yoga classes, cooking classes, childcare activities, and study groups, her maternity home functions as the place for exchange of information for many women from different backgrounds.

Another maternity home is Mohri Maternity Home, situated in Kobe. It was founded in 1959 by Taneko Mohri, a nurse-midwife trained after World War II. Her daughter, Taeko, trained as a nurse-midwife but soon left the hospital to work in the maternity home with her mother. Both mother and daughter reside on the top floor of the maternity home. The Mohri Maternity Home was destroyed in the earthquake that devastated the city in 1995, but the whole community participated in rebuilding it. The first floor consists of a large room that serves both as a community library full of books on birth, parenting, and breastfeeding and as a living/dining room. The large table in the center is where macrobiotic meals, cooked in the shiny kitchen nearby, are served to maternity home clients and guests. All interior walls are covered with wood paneling that provides a rich, warm effect. The birthing room on the second floor is equipped with a futon, a large birth tub, a pole for pulling on during upright birth, and sound absorbers, which ensure that birthing women can make any noises they want without being heard by the neighbors or others in the building. There are three attractively decorated rooms for mothers who want to remain for a week after the births, with futons on the tatami floors for mother and baby. Those who choose to stay for a while are pampered and fed the home's delicious macrobiotic food, and visited by family as often as they like.

A woman who gives birth in a maternity home experiences it almost as a place where her own mother resides, which she can go back to at times of difficulties. As we will illustrate later in the chapter, the characteristic of most Japanese maternity homes as contrasted with birth centers in other countries is that they are truly the homes of a mother figure, the midwife, where she lives with her own family. Very often these maternity homes are handed down to the next generation, usually to a daughter or daughter-in-law. This traditional type of maternity home may, in the future, give way to a postmodern-style midwifery practice not organized around family ties but based on group practice or other flexible relationships between independent midwives (Matsuoka 2001).

EMIKO'S BIRTH[6]

The Takizawa Maternity Home in Tsuruga City, Fukui Prefecture (central Japan), is where Emiko chose to give birth. Ms. Takizawa, the midwife who owns the home, has been practicing here since 1975, when she took it over from her own mother, who had opened this maternity home in 1947. It has been serving the community for more than fifty years, and currently 16% of the babies born in this city are delivered there, which is extremely high considering the national average of 1% maternity home births. Ms. Takizawa worked as a nursing teacher in primary schools and in high schools until 1975, but even before then, she helped her mother deliver babies, especially from 1955 to 1965, when the maternity house was extremely busy. The rooms for parturient mothers, where they stay for four to five days after giving birth, have Japanese-style tatami floors. In the waiting room, photo albums of many women from early pregnancy to birth are laid out to be seen by other pregnant women and families, who are expected to grow within them images of their own babies. Ms. Takizawa considers birth to be a family event and invites not only the husband and children but also the parents of the pregnant women to attend antenatal checkups so that they can familiarize themselves with the baby while it is in the mother's uterus. Another of her firmly held views is that the baby decides when and how it wants to come into this world; the convenience of health professionals or of mothers should not outweigh that of the baby.

Emiko, a thirty-year-old primipara, became pregnant after going through infertility treatment. She chose this maternity home, and her choice was supported by both her husband and her parents. Her contractions had started three days previously, but she waited until they became stronger before coming to the maternity home.

After Emiko entered the room, the light was dimmed at her request. She leaned against her husband in a half-sitting position, with her husband sitting behind her on thick cushions. Her husband stayed with her all the way through, giving her a massage and supporting her emotionally and physically. Emiko ate rice balls and went to sleep between contractions. Her parents and younger sister talked casually. The atmosphere was quiet and peaceful, with the sound of laughter every once in a while, which gave

TABLE 8.1 Emiko's labor time compared to the hospital average

Date	Time		Emiko's Time in Labor	Average Time for a Primipara
25 July	7:10	Labor starts	Phase I 12h40m	10h–12h
	14:20	Arrival at maternity home		
	19:50	Fully dilated		
26 July	1:40	Baby's head appears slightly	Phase 2 6h35m	1.5h–2h
	2:15	Crowning		
	2:20	Baby's head out		
	2:25	Whole body out	Phase 3 15m	5m–30m
	2:40	Placenta out		

Emiko comfort and helped her relax. Midwife Tazikawa stayed by Emiko's side, giving her a massage. She said to Emiko, "Breathe out deeply and relax your body, so you won't push hard all at once." Knowing the baby's head would be seen soon, the midwife told Emiko's husband to go behind his wife. The midwife put a mirror at Emiko's feet so Emiko and the others could see the baby's head. When the baby's head became more visible, the midwife encouraged Emiko and her family to touch it one after the other so that they could feel even more intimate with the baby. At the crowning stage, the midwife said, "Don't push any more. Dad, have mom breathe out while saying faah, faah, faah slowly. Let the baby decide when it wants to come out. Don't push, even though you feel like doing so." She asked Emiko's husband to hold his wife's wrists in his hands and to hold her arms wide apart (evoking the famous scene of the hero and heroine on the prow of the ship in the movie *Titanic*).

This posture was to prevent Emiko from pushing too hard. Then the midwife said to Emiko's family, "Have a chat; the baby will like it." When the baby's head moved some more and half of its body came out, they said one after another with excitement, "Oh, it's moving, it's crying, it's a big baby!" "You've worked really hard, well done!" The midwife encouraged Emiko to pull the baby the rest of the way out herself saying, "Hold here, and don't let it slip out of your hands." As Emiko pulled out the baby in her hands, everybody clapped saying, "Congratulations!" The baby's hearty cries resounded. "Thank you for coming to us. We have all been waiting for you," Emiko said as she held the baby in her arms while her husband supported her from behind.

Table 8.1 shows the time spent for Emiko's birth compared with the average time for primiparas. The time for phase 2 (from being fully dilated to the time the baby's whole body comes out) was extremely long for Emiko, especially the time between the head being seen slightly and crowning. This took thirty-five minutes, and the time from crowning to the head coming out took five minutes. If this birth had taken place in a hospital, the time for this phase would have been curtailed by attendants urging her to push out with all her might. But in the maternity home, the baby decides when to be born, and the people present at the scene of the birth are expected to follow its pace.

In the following sections, we will discuss some primary characteristics of maternity home births and their significance.

THE IMPORTANCE OF WAITING FOR THE BABY TO BE BORN

In a maternity home, waiting does not mean so much time wasted or the time of just enduring pain for a birthing woman. It is a meaningful time, shared by the birthing woman, her family, and the midwife together all in one place. Everyone is involved in one thing, namely "waiting for the arrival of the baby." The baby's journey into this world is considered to be the time necessary for the family to get ready for this new member, which is thought of as the time of maturation needed for family members to metamorphose into their new roles of parents and grandparents. Thus, shortening this time is not thought to produce any good results; rather, sharing these powerful moments together can help build strong ties among those present. It is well known from our daily experiences and from the anthropological literature that those who share difficult times together are bound by strong ties thereafter, which work to surmount any hardships encountered—for instance, in childrearing by the new parents in the future.

Waiting also means to respect a woman's physiological process of birth by giving her as little injury and discomfort as possible. For instance, as in Emiko's case, Ms. Takizawa did not encourage pushing hard, so the pelvis opens slowly and the perineum stretches out well, thereby avoiding the need for an episiotomy. In one study conducted in Japan comparing a group of maternity home births and hospital births, the rate of episiotomies for births in maternity homes for primiparas was 5% and for multiparas it was 1%; in the hospital, the rate of episiotomy for primiparas was 88% and for multiparas 41% (Matsuoka 1995).[7] Another study found that the mood of women after birth is significantly correlated with the bodily pain and discomfort they feel three to seven days after birth. The prevalence of maternity blues and postnatal depression was much less for women who gave birth in maternity homes than in hospitals, because bodily damage and pain are experienced much less in the former (Matsuoka et al. 2005).

Furthermore, waiting drives women to give birth with their own strength. The sense of accomplishment felt by women after birth leads to a newly found confidence in their bodies and selves—an important motivating force for childcare. This is why Ms. Takizawa encouraged Emiko to pull the baby out by herself instead of delivering the baby and handing it over to Emiko. Women whose babies are born with a great deal of medical intervention tend to be grateful for what was done to them but do not gain confidence in their own ability to give birth. But the midwives who operate maternity homes think it very important that women grow into motherhood by accomplishing birth by themselves, which they believe is made possible by allowing time for the baby to be born spontaneously.

THE METAMORPHIC VALUE OF LABOR PAIN

Those who advocate for analgesia argue that enduring a painful birth is an outmoded idea, and women should give birth happily with smiles on their faces, their pain taken away by drugs (Shimada, N. 2000: 516). But in maternity homes, labor pain is considered to be an important element in childbirth. Independent midwives think that women can handle labor pains if they are not left alone but are supported by a mother-like figure. Moreover, they believe that labor pain is a necessary process for a birthing woman as she grows into motherhood—to face her own self through the experience of pain. Here, we will discuss the sociocultural meanings of pain that are recognized by independent midwives through their experiences of assisting in birth, even though they are not usually discussed openly in any structured way.

First of all, independent midwives believe that a woman reflects and talks to herself during labor, as pain makes her look into her inner world and contemplate herself more deeply. Midwife Komatsu Toshiko, owner of the Megumi Maternity home in Saitama Prefecture, explained in an interview:

> A birthing woman thinks of many things when she is in pain. I once delivered the baby of a 19-year-old woman. She was unmarried and said she would leave her baby in a foster home. After the birth I let her breastfeed the baby. The next day she said to me, "Do you think I might be able to bring up the baby myself?" I said, "Why?" She said, 'Because the pain was far too much—after such pain I want to raise the baby by myself; otherwise the pain I had endured had no meaning." In pain people contemplate. . . . We have an expression for referring to your own child: "a child (born) after pain in the abdomen." Having pain is the utmost proof of being a mother. If you overcome a big pain, you can overcome anything. If you work extremely hard to get it, you don't want to lose it. I remember there was even data that the longer a labor takes, the stronger the bonding is to your baby.
>
> Having said that, I don't think post-partum pain means anything, so I give women medication for it.

As this midwife explained, pain makes one reflect upon oneself and provides an occasion to change oneself. Labor pain is not seen as futile in

Japan. It is pain to produce something invaluable—a baby. So this young woman felt that after having made such a big effort to endure pain, to reject the outcome of it, her baby, would almost equate to nullifying what she had tried so hard to do. The experience of pain, which is also the experience of looking at her inner self, has made her stronger both mentally and physically to be able to accept the reality she faces. The baby in her arms is decisive evidence that she could overcome the pain and is now a mother with a responsibility to look after her baby. The pain played a big part in making this transformation possible—it is an explicit marker that something unusual is taking place, and things are not the same as before.

One midwife writes that labor pain is not an absolute pain; it is rather a regular pushing of the uterus trying to empty its content, which affects the muscles, tendons, and organs surrounding it. The effect of all these movements is felt as pain in a secondary sense. If a woman is not relaxed, her bodily muscles become tense and tight, including those of her vaginal canal, and her pain will be even stronger. Women who are relaxed during birth often comment afterwards that labor pain was "such a pleasing sensation," or it was "like swells of the cosmos coming and going," or they "could feel the bodily sensation of the baby coming down inside" (Suganuma 2007).

The effect of pain has been used in many cultures in various rites of passage, especially in initiation rituals. Although for some of us many of these rituals may be difficult to comprehend, since they inflict pain on those to be initiated, they are not represented here in a negative way. These rituals are described to show how pain is used in some cultures, especially during times of transition. In Bali for example, initiates' teeth are ground down, while incisions are traditionally made in the skin of Native Americans performing the Sun Dance. In these rituals pain is used both as a device to bring about change in people psychologically and as a symbolic marker to announce their change in status to the public. Although pain itself, when taken out of context, is given a negative meaning in highly industrialized societies, it becomes tolerable when it is embedded in local cultural contexts. Such is the role of pain in human metamorphosis: societies around the world have used pain in various forms and extents to bring about role transformation. Of course, labor pain is a physiological pain and not the same as cultural pain created in the aforementioned rituals, but both can cause profound change in those people who experience them, allowing people to see themselves from a different perspective. Thus, many independent midwives in Japan believe that to nullify labor pain by medication is unwise.

In Europe and the United States, the rate of epidural delivery is high, and women insist that denouncing the use of pain-relieving drugs is a prejudice against women based on the biblical sentence to painful childbirth (Showalter and Griffin 1999). Even though women and men should be treated equally, they are not biologically equal in this matter of birth. In fact, one feminist psychologist in Japan writes sarcastically, "For boys sexual experience always accompanies pleasure, whereas for girls menstrual pain, pain of breasts becoming large, first sexual intercourse, pain of abortion, sickness during pregnancy and labor pain all give pain to women. Where is the equality between men and women?" (Ogura 1999: 46). In maternity homes, the significance of pain is positively evaluated, and midwives help women go through pain rather than offering to take it away from them. Whether taking pain away from delivery contributes to equality between men and women or whether it is just a form of medicalization is a difficult question to answer. A woman can take a central role in the birth if she decides to do it all by herself, whereas an epidural delivery will put anesthetists and obstetricians in the center, diminishing the autonomy of the birthing woman. Also, in Japan, taking on the new role of motherhood is considered to be an important aspect of childbirth, of which labor pain is a part.

MOTHERING THE MOTHER

Granting that pregnancy and birth are physiological phenomena, independent midwives agree that midwifery does not consist of providing medical treatment but of providing care to a healthy woman. What is care to a healthy woman? One independent midwife says it is an attitude of accompanying a healthy birthing woman and not of instructing or educating her, nor of trying to manage her birth. She mentions three things to describe what she specifically means by "accompanying a woman": (1) to give a woman assurance by touching her somewhere on the body all the time during birth; (2) to stay by her side and not leave her alone; (3) and to accept whatever a woman says or does, by saying for example, "Yes, it is painful, isn't it!" or "It's okay for you to urinate or defecate during birth—don't worry" or "It's all right to call out or scream" (Yajima 2002: 176–77). Independent midwife Morhi noted, "'A woman whose birth and postpartum period were well taken care of passes her happiness on to others and to her family. In this way the positive cycle goes on and she becomes a mother who takes her childcare responsibilities seriously even in times of hardship'" (quoted in Takahashi and Ishimura 2005: 549).

These examples illustrate that midwives look after birthing women as if they were their mothers and think of what they do as "mothering the mother." Consequently, in Japan women expect mother-like attention from their midwives during birth. In other words, a maternity home is the place where a mother-like figure provides mothering care to women giving birth.[8] This is why many independent midwives object to allowing males to become midwives. They think that men are unfit for midwifery practice, and that only a female midwife can accompany a woman's journey to becoming a mother.

The relationship between an independent midwife and a birthing woman is very different from that between an obstetrician and a patient. An obstetrician often defines the relationship as professional versus lay and thinks it his/her duty to disseminate proper knowledge and treat morbidity by discovering it. Furthermore, most obstetricians are men, and birthing women are 100% female. Thus, in hospital births, triple hierarchical relationships are played out: professional/lay, male/female, and healthy/morbid. This hierarchy is completely different from the relationship between an independent midwife and a birthing woman in maternity homes, where the relationship is based on mutual affection and respect.

BIRTH AS A FAMILY EVENT

In Japan childbirth is considered to be a family matter. In other words, childbirth is a rite of passage not just for a birthing woman but also for her partner, siblings, and the parents of the couple. A midwife's job is not only to deliver a baby but also to have all those involved take on a new role, so that the baby can find its position easily in the family. Accordingly, Emiko's midwife invited family members to antenatal checkups so that they could develop intimacy with the baby before it arrived and look forward to its arrival. Also, during the delivery, the midwife encouraged the grandparents and siblings to touch the half-appearing head of the baby to facilitate bonding with the baby as early as possible. In this way, independent midwives pay attention to family members as a whole and try to involve all of them from the beginning of the pregnancy: the midwives believe the baby is born not just to a woman but to the family as a whole.

HOW SAFE ARE JAPANESE MATERNITY HOMES?

As we noted above, maternity homes have gained recognition as a choice of birthing place since government research showed that women gained more satisfaction from births in maternity homes than in hospitals (Watanabe 1999). But the *safety* of maternity homes relative to hospitals is yet to be officially recognized. The medical community prefers to allocate "safety" to the hospital and "women's satisfaction" to the maternity home, saying that hospitals should also accommodate satisfaction in order to meet women's needs. But are maternity homes really not as safe as hospitals? If a healthy woman has a satisfying and relaxed birth, there is a better chance that the outcome will be good for both the mother and the baby. This means satisfaction and safety are likely to go together. It depends on how you look at birth: If it is defined from a medical perspective, the availability of medical interventions looks crucial to guarantee the safety of the birth. If it is seen as a physiological process, a woman's relaxed mind and body will help labor progress smoothly and result in a good outcome. It is well known among midwives and some doctors that unnecessary medical interventions often upset the physiological birth process and cause problems rather than solving them (Davis-Floyd 2004; Introduction, this volume).

Now let's look at the outcomes of births conducted by independent midwives to evaluate their safety. Government data only represents the completed number of births at the final place of delivery. However, the Japanese Association of Midwives (JAM) is interested in knowing the transfer rates from both maternity homes and women's homes to evaluate how well independent midwives are performing, and also to demonstrate how safe it is to give birth at either of these places. Data are collected retrospectively every year by JAM. However, the numbers obtained by JAM are not the same as the government figures obtained from birth registrars[9] since some independent midwives do not have time to hand in their data to the association. According to data collected by JAM from 388 maternity homes, there were 10,526 births conducted by independent midwives in 2005, 1,295 of which took place in women's homes—and some maternity home midwives also attend home births (see Note 1) (Yamada et al. 2006). However, government statistics reported 10,676 births at maternity homes, not including home births, which those statistics indicate as 2,184. If we consider that some home births are unplanned with no midwife attendance from the outset, it would be reasonable to calculate the response rate of data submission from independent midwives by basing it only on births occurring inside maternity homes, which would be 10,526 minus 1,295 = 9,231, or 86% of the number provided by the government.

According to data obtained from JAM, the number of women who planned to deliver in a maternity home or at home was 11,676 initially.[10] Out of these women, 707 (6.05%) and 443 (4.03%) were transferred in the antepartum and the intrapartum period, respectively. Out of the 10,526 women reported by independent midwives to have actually completed giving birth in a maternity home or at home, 51 women (0.48%) and 196 babies (1.86%) were transferred postnatally. The total number of antepartum and intrapartum transfers was 1,150, and the ratio of this number to the initial 11,676 women who planned to give birth either in a maternity home or at home is 9.8%, which means that *more than 90% of women who planned to deliver at home or at a maternity home completed their birth according to their initial wishes.* Furthermore, it must also be stated that not all transfers were emergencies. Only 13% (97 out of 707) of antepartum transfers, 65% (290 out of 443) of intrapartum transfers, and 72% (37 out of 51) of postpartum maternal transfers were emergencies.

In decreasing order, the reasons for all antepartum transfers were these: pregnancy induced hypertension, signs of preterm birth, infection in the mother, being past the due date, breech position, and others. For all intrapartum transfers, the reasons were these: weak contractions, premature rupture of membranes, failure to progress, and others. The highest number of emergency maternal transfers occurred in the postpartum period. The main reason was hemorrhaging, followed by fever and then perineal tears. Moreover, what is interesting is that if we consider the transfer rates in the antepartum (3.9%) and intrapartum (3.2%) periods for home births, we can see that they are lower than those from maternity homes, which were 6.3% and 4.2%, respectively. In sum, whether giving birth at home or in maternity homes, more than 90% of women planning to give birth in either place did so successfully.

These national statistics, compared with birth center data in the United States and home birth data in Holland, illustrate that the intrapartum transfer rate of 4.03% from both Japanese maternity homes and home births and the 3.2% transfer rate from home births alone are very low. This implies that screening of low-risk cases during the prenatal period is done strictly enough in Japan to produce low transfer rates during the intrapartum period. In the National Birth Center Study in the United States, for example, Rooks, Weatherby, and Ernest (1992a, b) found that 12% of women were transferred during the intrapartum period; De Vries (Chapter 1, this volume) notes that in the Netherlands, 9.4% were transferred during the intrapartum period from home to hospital in Holland in 2002; and the Johnson and Daviss (2005) study of planned home births in the United States shows an intrapartum transfer rate of 12%. There is always a small percentage of births that do not progress as planned, making it almost impossible for the transfer rate in the intrapartum period to be zero for any out-of-hospital place of birth.

A prospective study in Japan that compared two groups of low-risk women, those intending to give birth in maternity homes (1,107 women) and those in hospitals (1,320 women), who were screened at sixteen weeks' gestation, showed that the morbidity rates for the following items were lower in the maternity home group than in the hospital: perinatal mortality rate (PMR):[11] 1.8 and 3.8 per 1,000 total births for maternity homes and hospitals, respectively; newborn birth weight of less than 2500 g: 3.9% and 5.8%, respectively; cesarean section rate: 1.17% and 6.97%, respectively;[12] preterm birth of earlier than thirty-seven weeks' gestation: 2.2% and 4.3%, respectively; hemorrhage > 500 cc: 4.3% and 16%, respectively; and neonatal morbidity rate: 4.16% and 8.9%, respectively (Matsuoka 1995). In this study the transfer rate in the intrapartum period from the maternity homes was 2.72%, which implied that the screening out of high-risk cases had been done properly.

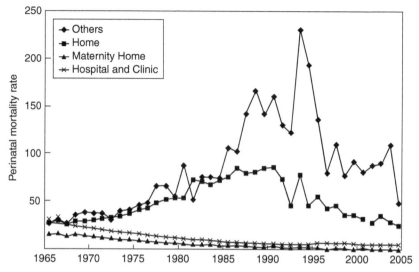

Figure 8.2. Perinatal mortality rate (per 1,000 total births) by place of delivery for Japan.

One final piece of evidence for the safety of maternity homes is shown in Figure 8.2, the PMR by place of delivery in Japan. It shows that the maternity home has always had the lowest PMR since the start of data collection.

From the above it can be concluded that low-risk births attended by independent midwives, whether at home or in maternity homes, are as safe as or even safer than births in hospitals. In other words, midwives deliver babies of healthy women in a healthier way, which results in healthier outcomes.

THE SIGNIFICANCE OF MATERNITY HOME BIRTHS

It is important to know that the maternity home is not just a place for giving birth, but also one that satisfies women's varied needs throughout their lives and influences the wider health care delivery system in Japan. Here we will discuss three functions that we think the maternity home fulfils in Japan.

First, maternity homes act as a breakwater in Japan to prevent childbirth from becoming too medicalized. In any society, there are plural modes of delivery. Even though some societies strongly discourage giving birth outside of hospitals, there are always small numbers of women who give birth at home or in other places, either intentionally or unintentionally. In this sense, there are plural maternity care systems in any society: hospitals, birth centers, small clinics run by GPs or family physicians, a midwife's house, or a woman's house. In Japan, theoretically, women can decide where to give birth and can move from one place to another, although in reality, most of them regard the hospital as the only possible place for birth because the hospital is culturally imbued with the most legitimacy and power. But if, for example, a woman does not want to have a cesarean for a breech position, she can consult an independent midwife and try to reverse the breech position, which may include external cephalic version or exercises aimed at reversing the position of the baby. (In some instances women still consult independent midwives to try to have a vaginal delivery in this kind of case, but this does not comply with the recently introduced guidelines set out for what independent midwives can do.) Experienced independent midwives used to deliver and still have the skill to deliver vaginally "difficult" cases such as breeches, twins, vaginal births after cesareans (VBACs), and women over forty years of age.[13] There are women who also choose to deliver in maternity homes to avoid episiotomies, to deliver in a position they like, or to be able to stay with their babies twenty-four hours a day. The maternity home gives women an alternative choice for their place of birth—one that suits their values and allows them to take refuge from unwanted medicalization. Equally for midwives and obstetricians working in hospitals, maternity homes assure the existence of alternative ways of giving birth and exemplify optimal care, which can cause medical practitioners to reflect on their own ways of carrying out birth in hospitals.

Secondly, the maternity home is considered by most midwives to represent how midwifery *should* be: a source where the midwifery model of care prevails and can be pursued. For example, when a midwife wants to become independent by opening her own maternity home, she almost always begins with an apprenticeship in an experienced midwife's home for a year or so. She regards the independent midwife as a role model, the archetype of the midwifery profession, and she knows that she needs to become socialized to a different model of care. She considers achieving an identity as an independent midwife as important as acquiring the skills necessary for independent practice. Although many hospital-based midwives believe that midwifery should be different from nursing because it involves working with healthy women, they find it difficult to maintain that perspective in actual dealings with pregnant patients in hospitals because of the pressures in the hospital to treat patients in medicalized, interventive ways. Maternity homes are recognized by many midwives as the places where midwives can go back to rediscover their identities and be reminded of what is the essence of midwifery practice.

Thirdly, the maternity home provides midwifery students with a place to observe normal births. Midwifery education requires practice, which can be done in hospitals, clinics, or maternity homes. Students at nursing universities carry out their practical studies at university hospitals, which are far from suitable places to learn about normal birth because of the overuse of high-technology medicine. To develop a balanced image of midwifery practice, student midwives need to have a chance to observe and actually attend normal births. Yajima Maternity Home in Tokyo, for instance, which has one of the largest numbers of birth per year (about 250), accepts students from twelve different midwifery schools and universities (Yajima 2002: 176). Ms. Yajima also accepts midwives from other countries for observation and training as well as those who want to open their own maternity homes. In other words, the maternity home is a sanctuary of normal childbirth, where midwifery students and midwives from both inside and outside Japan can train themselves by observing normal birth.

CHALLENGING TASKS FOR THE FUTURE

Despite their lower morbidity rates, the safety of maternity home births has long gone unrecognized. The greatest concern about the maternity home felt by the general public is that in an emergency, additional time is wasted for transfer to a hospital. In Japan the medical law states that every maternity home in which births are attended needs to have a backup physician. However, a maternity home, in the case of an emergency, usually transfers women not to its backup doctor, who is usually a doctor in a private clinic, but directly to a big hospital where neonatal intensive care unit (NICU) facilities and cesareans are always available. In fact, the law that requires registering a backup doctor for each maternity home with an in-patient bed does not serve any practical purpose any more: the level of medicine employed in a private clinic is not much superior to that in a maternity home, though it is true that a doctor can use some amount of medical intervention but a midwife cannot. Indeed, the medical law was passed right after World War II when there were not yet big hospitals in many parts of Japan. In this sense, the provision is outmoded and works now as a hurdle for many midwives when they want to open a maternity home because finding backup doctors has been very difficult. Yet a revision of the medical law was made in 2006, and enacted in April 2008, which states that a maternity home should not only have an ob/gyn as the backup doctor but also an affiliated hospital or a clinic with an ob/gyn. This revision has raised the hurdle even higher for most maternity homes that already had difficulty finding backup doctors who, until March 2008, could be doctors of any specialty. In fact, some maternity homes are said to have been forced to close because of their inability to meet the two provisions required by this amendment. Furthermore, having hospitals accept emergency transfers has always been a difficult task for a maternity home because hospitals tend not to welcome any transfers and usually blame women for having chosen to deliver in a maternity home—a situation typical of hospitals in many countries (see, for example, Davis-Floyd 2003).

So it is of utmost importance to build regional referral systems that include maternity homes and private homes as viable places of delivery in order to gain the trust of the public for maternity home births. Midwife Yajima writes, "Our biggest wish as independent midwives is to have a referral system built which makes safe and assuring birth possible, wherever and in whichever way a woman chooses to give birth" (2002: 178). The maternity policy should be made to cover all women irrespective of their place of delivery, so that their right to life in case of an emergency would be protected. At present, the rights of those women who choose to give birth outside of hospital are not treated equally.

Furthermore, Ms. Yajima says that requesting an extension of the scope of midwifery practice in case of emergencies is absolutely necessary. There are times when a normal birth takes a sudden turn, in which case a certain amount of medical intervention, such as an episiotomy or injection, should be allowed to be performed by midwives. Defining boundaries among health professionals is at issue here, but the best interests of the mother and baby, not of the health professional, should come first (Yajima 2002). Legally in Japan, in case of complications, midwives are required to call a doctor and not give any medical treatment unless it is an emergency. But how much emergency is a real emergency has always been a matter of contention: the boundary between normal and abnormal is unclear and has to be negotiated. Thus, the autonomy of a midwife tends to be easily impaired. In practice, many independent midwives ask permission to give injections or medications from a backup doctor over the telephone and thus do so technically under "supervision"—a clear limitation of their autonomy that can interfere with their ability to act rapidly. But the law binding them turns a blind eye to this double-standard situation, a situation Ms. Yajima believes must be officially mended. Extending the boundaries of legal midwifery work to allow some medical measures to be applied at the midwife's own judgment, and including these in midwifery education, are beneficial to women and thus should be seen as ethical.

As Wagner (1988: 31) notes, "Governments must ensure that the woman and family have the right to freedom in having the experience of their choice, free of coercion (even subtle coercion) and with full respect for the integrity of the person, during one of the most important events in their lives, pregnancy and childbirth." We affirm that Japanese midwives should be given their proper position as caretakers of normal births, and that the Japanese government should adapt a neutral stance toward a woman's decision about place of birth. Maternity homes in Japan have played a significant part in ensuring women's choice in birthing place and have broadened Japanese views about the different ways women can give birth. They have also contributed to increasing women's confidence during birth by providing them with warm and empowering midwifery care. Their excellent outcomes and high quality of care make them birth models that work *par excellence*. Their continued existence is essential to a viable future for birth in Japan, and we highly recommend their replication in other countries.

ACKNOWLEDGMENTS

We express great appreciation to Emiko and her family, and to Ms. Takizawa, Ms. Otani, and Ms. Mohri, who kindly gave us information and inspiration for future models of midwifery. And we are very thankful to Robbie Davis-Floyd for giving us the opportunity to contribute to this fascinating book and for her gentle waiting attitude and careful editing.

NOTES

1. Some midwives do not own facilities with beds because they prefer to deliver babies at a client's home, or they give only breastfeeding counseling, postnatal visits, and similar support. Such midwives, once they start working independently, give their midwifery practice names such as XXX Maternity Home—in other words, a "maternity home" can mean both a birthing facility and a midwifery practice without "in-patient" beds. A midwife who owns her own facility usually employs other midwives for help while she takes the leading organizational role. In Japan, a group practice where several midwives cooperate on an equal basis is not yet common.

2. Because this figure is based on self-reported cases, there could be some maternity homes that did not report but actually had attended births.

3. A recent survey by Japan Society of Obstetrics and Gynecology showed that as of December 1st 2005, there are 3,063 hospitals and clinics that actually handle births in Japan, excluding maternity homes (Asahi Shinbun 2006). Since the total number of babies born in 2005 was 1,062,530, of which 1,049,345 were born in either hospitals or in clinics, the average number of babies per facility was around 342 per year. This small number per clinic implies a decentralized policy for birth in Japan, but currently the Japanese government is shifting its policy away from decentralization to centralization so that there can be more than one obstetrician at any birthing facility to ensure safety and relieve the burden on the medical staff. Behind this shift is a shortage of obstetricians resulting from long working hours and liability for lawsuits, which has currently caused obstetric wards in many parts of Japan to stop delivering babies. Consequently, women in provincial areas, in particular, do not or cannot deliver in their hometowns, either because there is no birthing place nearby or because they prefer better facilities in urban areas.

In Japan the number of medical lawsuits is still small, around 1,000 cases per year, but is increasing rapidly. It is possible but very rare for a hospital midwife to be sued because she is not recognized as having full responsibility in situations where medical intervention becomes necessary. On the other hand, an independent midwife can take full responsibility in dealing with a normal delivery and thus has more possibility for lawsuits when birth takes a sudden, unfortunate turn. Nevertheless, lawsuits against independent midwives are rare.

4. In Japan the whole population is covered by government health insurance, which reimburses 70% of medical costs to medical facilities; patients pay the remaining 30%. However, in Japan a normal childbirth is not covered by this insurance, because birth is not defined as a disease. Consequently, if a woman has no complications, she pays the full fees for childbirth out of pocket, the amount of which is freely set by birthing facilities. But later she receives a lump sum of 350,000 yen (about US$2,950) directly from the government, whether the birth ended normally or needed some medical intervention. Only when births require medical interventions such as episiotomy, suturing, or cesarean section do they come under insurance coverage. Seventy percent of the amount specified by the insurance system goes to medical facilities. This implies that (unnecessary) medical interventions with proper diagnosis attached can bring profit to hospitals and clinics—an attractive incentive for owners and managers of private clinics but not for hospital-employed doctors, who are paid a regular salary every month.

5. In Japan the nationwide cesarean rate is not calculated every year. It is estimated by collecting data from the month of September each year and from each birthing facility every three years.

6. One of the authors (Fumiko Hinokuma) had already developed a good relationship with the staff in this maternity home by participating in antenatal checkups and family classes as a midwife before she started to do this observational research. She received written informed consent from Emiko and her family during her pregnancy after the aim and the method of research had been explained to everyone concerned.

7. By law Japanese midwives are not allowed to perform episiotomies nor suture except in case of emergency. Even though it is very rare that an episiotomy is done, this research shows that independent midwives do perform it on occasion.

8. It is also possible to interpret the relationship of a midwife and a woman as an equal partnership rather than as that of mother and child. But the majority of independent midwives are above fifty years of age, which makes it easier to assume a mother-child relationship with a client during the vulnerable time of birth. In Japan people say the experience of good and spontaneous birth changes a woman into a mother, whereas in Holland the experience of a good birth is described as liberating women (De Vries et al. Chapter 1, this volume).

9. The government data are collected from birth registrations submitted to each municipal office by parents. This registration specifies the place of delivery of each baby.

10. The data collected here on transfer cases are based on reports from independent midwives. So if a midwife categorizes a case as antepartum, it is included in the antepartum period. Normally antepartum ends and intrapartum begins when contractions start every ten minutes as self-reported by a laboring woman and ends when the placenta has come out. The reasons given for the transfer in each period are also defined by independent midwives, so depending on how a midwife sees the transfer case, it is classified either as antepartum or intrapartum; for instance,

premature rupture of membrane can be classified as a reason for antepartum transfer when contractions have not yet started but as intrapartum when they have.

11. In 1995, when this research was published, the PMR was calculated as death between twenty-eight weeks gestation and fewer than seven days after birth. Now the PMR has been changed and is calculated from twenty-two weeks gestation.)

12. The cesarean section (CS) rate was based on the five hospitals that participated in the study. CS rates vary greatly from hospital to hospital, and the national average was 17.4% in 2005.

13. According to guidelines issued by the Ministry of Health, Welfare, and Labor in 2002, prospective clients who want to give birth in a maternity home are divided into three categories: those who can deliver in the maternity home, those who should be monitored by the maternity home and by obstetricians together, and those who should be handled by obstetricians. These guidelines state that women who are younger than sixteen or older than thirty-four need shared care, and those who have had a previous cesarean section, twins, and breech should give birth with obstetricians. But most experienced, independent midwives attended such cases before the guideline came into effect.

REFERENCES

Asahi Shinbun. 2006. "Bunben shisetsu jittai wa 3000 kasho" [Delivery units only 3000 places]. *Asahi Shinbun*, June 15.

Davis-Floyd, R. 2003. "Home Birth Emergencies in the U.S. and Mexico: The Trouble with Transport." *Social Science and Medicine* 56.9: 1913–31.

———. 2004. *Birth as an American Rite of Passage*, 2nd ed. Berkeley: University of California Press.

Declercq, E., R. De Vries, K. Viisainen, H. Salvesen, and S. Wrede. 2001. "Where to Give Birth?" In *Birth by Design: Pregnancy, Maternity Care, and Midwifery in North America and Europe*, edited by R. De Vries, C. Benoit, E. Van Teijlingen, and S. Wrede, 28–50. New York: Routledge.

Johnson, K., and B.-A. Daviss. 2005. "Outcomes of Planned Home Births with Certified Professional Midwives: A Large Prospective Study in North America." *British Medical Journal* 330:1416–22.

Kobayashi, T. 1972. "Sanka no shorai to teiou-sekkai" [The Future of Obstetrics and Cesarean Section]. *Sanhujinka no Sekai* [World of Obstetrician] 24.10:29–32.

Matsuoka, E. 1995. "Is Hospital the Safest Place for Birth?" In *Curare: Gebären-Ethnomedeizinische Perspektiven und neue Wege*, edited by W. Schiefenhövel, D. Sich, and C. Gottschalk-Batschkus, 293–304. Berlin: Verlag für Wissenschaft und Bildung.

———. 2001. "Postmodern Midwives in Japan: The Offspring of Modern Hospital Birth." *Medical Anthropology* 20:141–84.

Matsuoka, E., F. Hinokuma, and H. Suganuma. 2007. "Kankoku ni okeru ripurodakushon no hensen [Reproduction Changes in Korea]. *Asahikawa Ikadaigaku Kiyo* [Annual Report of Asahikawa Medical College] 23:71–85.

Matsuoka, E., N. Kanou, N. Masataka, R. Tsuchikura, and S. Takahashi. 2005. *Ripurodakushon to ikuji o naritataseru Shakai-bunkateki bunmyaku o meguru kenkyu*

[Research on Sociocultural Contexts of Reproduction and Childcare]. 2002–4 Grant-in-Aid for Scientific Research (C) No 14510330, Asahikawa Medical College.

Mothers' and Children's Health and Welfare Association. 2007. *Maternal and Child Health Statistics of Japan.* Tokyo: Mothers' and Children's Health and Welfare Association.

Ogura, C. 1999. *Onna no Sugoroku* [The Woman's *Sugoroku* Game]. Tokyo: Chikuma Bunko.

Rooks, J., N. Weatherby, and E. Ernest. 1992a. "The National Birth Center Study Part II: Intrapartum and Immediate Postpartum and Neonatal Care." *Journal of Nurse-Midwifery* 37.5:301–29.

———. 1992b. "The National Birth Center Study Part III: Intrapartum and Immediate Postpartum and Neonatal Complications and Transfers, Postpartum and Neonatal Care, Outcomes, and Client Satisfaction." *Journal of Nurse-Midwifery* 37.6: 361–97.

Shimada, M. 2001. "Shussei shomeiosho ni okeru bunben kaijoritsu to jittai." *Josanpu* 55.3:45–50.

Shimada, N. 2000. Masui bunben ni taisuru josanpu kyouiku no hitsuyou-sei [Necessity of Education to Midwives of Anesthetic Delivery]. *Shusanki Igaku* [Perinetal Medicine] 30.4:514–16.

Showalter, E., and A. Griffin. 1999. "Commentary: All Women Should Have a Choice." *British Medical Journal* 319: 1401.

Suganuma, H. 2007. "Sutekina osan wa anatamo dekiru" [You Can Do a Wonderful Birth, Too]. In *Umu Umanai, Umenai: Onna no karada dokuhon* [Give Birth, Not Give Birth, Cannot Give Birth: A Book for Woman's Body], edited by E. Matsuoka, 133–56. Tokyo: Kodansha Publishing Company.

Takahashi, Y. and A. Ishimura. 2005. "Ninpu ni yorisou osan ha koushite umareta" [This Is How We Came about Birth That Accompanies Women]. *Josan zasshi* [Japanese Journal for Midwives] 59.6:548–52.

Wagner, M., 1988. "The Public Health versus Clinical Approaches to Maternity Services: The Emperor Has No Clothes." *Journal of Public Health Policy* 19.1:25–35.

Watanabe, N. 1999. *Riyosha no tachibakara mite nozomasii shussan no arikata ni kansuru kenkyu* [Research on the Better Childbirth from the Point of View of Clients]. Grant-in-Aid for Scientific Research. Tokyo: Ministry of Health, Welfare, and Science.

World Health Organization (WHO). 1985. "Appropriate Technology for Birth." *Lancet* 326.8452:436–7.

Yajima, Y. 2002. "Nihon no josansho ha dou kawaruka" [How Will the Japanese Maternity Home Change?] *Shusanki Igaku* [Perinatal Medicine] 32, Suppl.:176–81.

Yamada, M., S. Kamiya, K. Noguchi, M. Miyashita, A. Murakami, T. Kato, and T. Ishii. 2006. "Heisei 17 nen 1 gatsu–12 gatsu zenkoku bunben kensu oyobi tenin kensu shukei ni tsuite" [Nationwide Statistics of Birth and Transfer from January to December 2005]. *Josanshi* [Journal of the Japanese Midwives' Association] 60.3:109–12.

Chapter 9

The Northern New Mexico Midwifery Center Model, Taos, New Mexico

Elizabeth Gilmore

After a truly disheartening round of discussions with our local hospital's administration and nursing staff, pediatrician Charlie Anderson took me and Tish Demmin, my midwifery partner, aside and said, "If you want family-centered care, you're going to have to start your own birth center." That was the winter of 1977 in Taos, New Mexico. With those words, we began to create a "working model" for a midwifery practice adventure. Our model is always a work in progress, and we've progressed, regressed, reorganized, remodeled, renewed, restructured, and are about to embark on yet another remodeling of the "model that works."

What did we mean by "family-centered care"?[1] We meant that the mom got to stay in the labor room to give birth (no getting moved to the delivery room). She didn't have to use any drugs she didn't want—no more twilight sleep and being strapped wrist and ankle into the bed because of hallucinations produced by scopolamine and Demerol. (Yes, they were still doing that in New Mexico as late as 1977!) The mother could use breathing techniques or hypnosis or any other technique for pain relief; she didn't have to have her pubis shaved, nor have an enema; she could ask questions about what was going on, and everyone had to ask her permission if they were going to do anything to her or the baby. She got to walk around and eat and drink fluids in labor; dad and her mom and her sisters got to keep her company during labor and birth as long as she wanted them—no more pacing in the waiting room. Kids got to visit the new sibling in the room—no more peering through the window from the parking lot. Mom got to room in with baby, and nurse as much as she wanted—no more having to beg someone to bring the baby to her from the nursery, no more sugar water and formula supplements. If she wanted to, she could refuse to sign the circumcision permission; she could have her birth photographed;

she could listen to her favorite music; she got to hold the baby while it was getting any tests or shots, and she got to have additional support with her—us midwives, for instance.[2]

OUR HISTORY

We were radical in those days.[3] Tish had been living in a commune in the Huerfano Valley of southern Colorado where she and others, like Lenya Reese, a physician assistant and licensed midwife (retired from a very busy midwifery practice in Santa Fe that spanned three decades), had been assisting Dr. Mai Wah Ting to deliver the community babies. (Dr. Ting still practices today in Santa Fe.) Community members were teaching and learning from each other how to reduce health risks and maximize quality of life. I had come from Chappaquiddick Island, off the coast of Massachusetts, where four friends and I had been the local childbirth class teachers. We had a study group every week and taught childbirth classes on Wednesday nights in the basement of the Episcopal church, starting in 1969, all thanks to an open-minded family practitioner named Dr. Hoxsie. When Fran Greene and I had our first babies three months apart, in the winter of 1970–71, we ended up giving birth in the Oak Bluffs Cottage Hospital because there was no one who could help us birth at home. We each had stayed home as long as we could, but when a seemingly inordinate amount of labor time had gone by (thirty-two hours in my case) with no babies, we had gone to the hospital after all. Both of us had given birth within a short time of arriving. Dr. Hoxsie handed little Anna over to me immediately, and he was amazed that she could nurse right away. Before Fran and me, he'd never seen an unmedicated baby and mother interact. "You should teach other mothers how to do that natural childbirth," he said. "That was real nice!"

That's how Fran Greene, Peg Goodale, Bronwyn Hill, Lee Fierro, and I started the Martha's Vineyard Education for Childbirth Association in 1970 (no longer in existence), and ended up accompanying over 400 families over the next seven years—either in the hospital or in their homes—and observing the extreme contrasts between home and hospital birth. We only had two emergency transfers from home during those years: the first was for a postpartum hemorrhage; the second was for one of our own babies—our first shoulder dystocia. Bronwyn discovered what had occurred by looking it up in *Williams' Obstetrics* (the most widely used American obstetrical textbook). Little Courtney wasn't breathing, and at the time we hadn't been trained in cardio-pulmonary resuscitation (CPR). Because mom was on her hands and knees, we placed baby on mom's back and massaged baby's chest while doing gentle mouth-to-mouth. That was a sensation I'll never forget as long as I live—that feeling of resistance against my breath as baby Courtney began to breathe!

During the first half of the 1970s, scopolamine and Demerol were still the order of the day in the hospital. The hallucinations caused by these drugs were such that moms had to be strapped hand and foot to the bed, which was fitted with leather leg restraints and wrist cuffs with buckles. I remember one mom giving birth in the hospital, babbling on about how she could smell coffee and felt like a toaster was coming out her bottom. Another repeated "cans of tuna fish, just cans of tuna fish," over and over. Despite Grantly Dick-Read, who was the inspiration for my mother's natural birth attempts in 1947, 1949, and 1952, natural childbirth continued to be a new phenomenon in 1970.

The contrast between home and hospital boiled down to this: fear was the operative mode in the hospital. When I began standing next to doctors while they were delivering our childbirth class clients, my initial impression of the reason for the way they treated moms and birth was that they just hated women. But after awhile, it dawned on me that they didn't hate anyone. They were afraid—afraid of birth, afraid of death, afraid of not doing enough or of not doing the right thing. They truly did not believe that the baby would come out if they didn't "do everything." After awhile I realized that most of these docs didn't hate women at all: they cared about them very much, only from our point of view, they had a strange way of showing it.

Meanwhile, at home, 1970s parents had decided to take their lives into their own hands; many of them said, "I'd rather die at home than go to the hospital." These were the hippie parents, determined to choose each moment of their own living and dying, who grew their own food, chopped their own wood for the fire, hauled water from the well for bathing, made their own soap and candles and all their baby's clothes and toys, used cloth diapers, slept on mats on the floor covered with paisley, believed in peace and love and authenticity, and thought it was really cool to get a film of the actual birth so that the kid could see it later. They made beautiful, hand-made items for sale and started eating only organic food—no more Tang (a powdered sugary orange drink), even if the astronauts *had* taken it to the moon. They milked their goats instead.[4] I came to their births as the child-birth teacher/birth coach and took the movies and photos. If there was a cord around the neck and the dad asked, "Elizabeth, what should we do?" I would put down the camera to see how tight the cord was, and if it was loose, I would say, "It's okay; the baby will come through it." If it was too tight, I would say, "Here, clamp the cord here and here and cut between the clamps; now unwind it so the baby can be born." And when other parents had heard how I'd been at Suzie's birth and had "saved" the baby with the cord around the neck, I got an undeserved reputation for knowing more than I really did—for being a "midwife," not a label that I yet applied to myself. In those days, I always said I was a "childbirth educator."

I declared that "education is the key to freedom," and in keeping with this sentiment, studied midwifery with a passion; started the Vineyard Montessori School on Martha's Vineyard, Massachusetts, in 1975 with other parents so that our children could get a piece of that "educational freedom"; and taught childbirth classes every Wednesday night with my co-teachers.

Our childbirth students asked us to accompany them to the hospital and during their home births. When the doctors at the Oak Bluffs Cottage Hospital heard that we had been attending home births, they said, "This is not good, but since it's happening, we're going to point some things out to you when you come into the hospital as a labor coach. If you ever see these things happening at home, bring the mother in."

This was my training from 1969 to 1977: our childbirth teachers' study group, going to home births, having my own babies, delivering my child-birth co-teachers' babies, going to hospital births, reading every obstetrics and natural childbirth book there was, going to conferences and work-shops held by the International Childbirth Education Association and the National Association of Parents and Professionals for Safe Alternatives in Childbirth, subscribing to the La Leche League newsletter, visiting nurse-midwife Christina Kielt in Boston and taking classes in subjects like pel-vimetry from her, attending a week-long, intensive course from midwifery educator Shari Daniels, and on and on. I was like a sponge—I soaked it all in and thought I knew exactly how everyone should give birth and nurse their babies, and was quite happy to be very opinionated and directive toward my childbirthing charges. It took years of trying to get everyone to do it my way for me to finally realize that it was much more fun if the moms and families and the other budding midwives could do it their own way, whatever form that should take.

Starting the Birth Center in New Mexico

I had started with a "my model is best," and eventually graduated to "what-ever form it takes," which was why Tish and I believed Dr. Anderson when he said we needed to start our own birth center when our family moved to Taos in 1977. Right away, we went looking for a building. We had been renting space in La Clinica, in Ranchos de Taos, a free clinic started by Drs. Rosen and Kilgore to take care of hippies and others who needed free care in the 1960s, and staffed primarily by medical students from the University of New Mexico to this day.[5] Every Tuesday we would meet our home birth clients there to do their prenatal care. We could test their urine and check their hematocrits, take their blood pressures, listen to the babies, and assess the babies' positions and growth in the cozy comfort of this tiny facility.

In 1978 we formed the Taos Midwives Group Practice, PC (Professional Corporation). This was our first "model." We charged $4 per visit and gave half to La Clinica as a thank-you. We would then go to the mom's house for the delivery, but there were the inevitable transfers, and we wanted family-centered care at the hospital so that the moms would have a hospital experience that would more closely address the reasons they had wanted a home birth in the first place. We taught childbirth classes to home birthers and hospital birthers and wanted both to be able to access a family-centered experience.

When we found the building we wanted to turn into our birth center, the neighbors refused to give us a variance, asserting that it meant the ambulance would be making lots of noise on their street, not to mention the horrible smell that would waft from our backyard incinerator. (What did they think we would be burning?) Also, there was a strong showing from those who believed all babies should be born in the beautiful, clean Holy Cross Hospital, with access to all the modern technology and the wonderfully trained doctors and nurses, as was their "American birthright." But there were also those who had been born at home, and those whose parents had been born at home.

In 1979 Dr. Ashley Pond, the most senior of our community physicians at the time and president of the New Mexico Medical Society, came to testify at the public hearing sponsored by the New Mexico Department of Public Health to determine if midwifery should be outlawed beginning in December of that year. We midwives were trying to get approval for modernizing and preserving New Mexico's midwifery regulations. Speaking on behalf of adopting the proposed regulations rather than abolishing midwifery, Dr. Pond testified that midwifery was a tradition in Taos, where only one generation had not had access to home birth, as a result of World War II. He explained to the hearing officer that at that time, there had been a midwife in every *barrio* (Hispanic neighborhood), who would deliver the local babies. These midwives would call on one of the doctors to come to the house to assist them if they encountered a problem during a birth. Beginning in the early 1920s, the New Mexico Public Health Department had developed a training program for New Mexico midwives, had equipped them with basic supplies in little suitcases, and had taught them how to fill in the birth certificates. In exchange for midwives' participation in the training program, they gave these midwives annual physical exams.

During World War II, all the doctors except one—Dr. Pond himself—got called away to the war. Finding himself the lone physician in the community, he put an announcement in the local newspaper requiring all moms to come to the hospital to give birth: there was no way he could be away from the hospital to assist with home deliveries. That was how the model of hospital birth for everyone had come into being in Taos—in response to the exigencies of wartime. But there was still plenty of positive community memory of, and desire for, access to home birth. Our regulations were approved and promulgated in 1980, and to this day, we owe Dr. Pond our deepest gratitude because we continue to be sheltered by, and supervised by, the Department of Public Health, with modified regulations based on the very ones at issue that day.[6]

Before 1980, the state midwifery regulations were very simple, including such basics as clean cord cutting, hand washing, and birth registration. Our new regulations were very detailed regarding the "modern" scope of care; reasons for consulting and transferring; apprenticeship requirements; written, oral, and practical registration exams; statistical reporting, and more. We continue to update these regulations in collaboration with the Department of Public Health. More and more, we are focusing on reducing maternal and infant risk rather than protecting the territory of the "practice of medicine." Sadly, these modern regulations required passing a written exam, in addition to an oral and a practical exam. This requirement meant an end to the original *barrio* midwives, the Mexican-American *parteras* in every community. Jesucita Aragon, a renowned traditional midwife who had been practicing for decades in Las Vegas, New Mexico, couldn't pass the test in 1983, and only *parteras* Elsie Sanchez from Albuquerque and Emma Estrada from Gallup remained among us. Jesucita was honored by the Midwives Alliance of North America (MANA) with their Sage Femme Award in 1986. Emma joined us in Taos for IV and neonatal resuscitation classes, but died before she could be honored, and Elsie received MANA's Sage Femme Award in 2005, at age ninety.[7]

In 1978 we found another place to house our birth center, right across the street from the hospital. This time the neighbors objected less strenuously and the ayes rather than the nays won. We stayed in this building until 1997. The Northern New Mexico Midwifery Center, Inc., a 501(c)3 (nonprofit) birth center and midwifery education facility, was born. We had an opening party August 13, 1981, and a baby boy was born there that day, so we celebrated especially joyously. We delivered babies at home and at our center, and we took on students so that we would not be "the last of the midwives." This was our next "model."

Family-centered care looked just like whatever the parents wanted it to look like. Would we be at home or at the birth center, or in the back of the truck where baby was conceived? Did they want to give birth standing up or squatting or side lying, outside in the warm sunshine or in the tub of warm water, with the dad and the children helping to catch the baby, or with mom catching it herself, or just let it land gently on the bed and she be the first to touch it? Did one of the family or the mom want to tie and cut the cord? Would that be right away or after the delivery of the placenta? Who would get to announce the sex of the new baby? Would all the family members be at the birth or only a small number? Would there be prayers, lighting of candles, playing of music, drumming and dancing, Buddhist meditations, Hindu or Muslim chanting? Would there be reciting of the rosary in English or in Spanish, and would we be eating chicken-head soup to celebrate and give the mom strength afterwards, or take-out from McDonalds? There might be calls of "thank you Jesus for the pain" to help get through the contractions, Lamaze breathing, walking to the river, pacing the aisles in Wal-Mart, or making the rounds at the Taos Gems and Minerals Shop, and rides on bumpy roads to increase the contractions in low-riders, VW combis, pick-up trucks, or convertibles. The parents might bring their own special blanket or pillow for the children so they could feel at home in the center and sleep on the mats around their mom's bed. Caring for the children might be grandma or a friend. Would the parents be treating the baby's eyes for gonorrhea and chlamydia, and administering vitamin K as prophylaxis against newborn bleeding? Would they be bathing the baby afterward and dressing her in frilly bonnet and organdy dress with patent leather shoes to go home, or wrapping her naked in a sheepskin? Would the baby be sleeping with them in bed, in a gingham-decorated bassinet, a flannel-lined basket, or a top drawer in her mom's bureau? Would mom be eating grapes in labor, raspberry tea frozen into ice cubes, yogurt, *frijoles*, *atole*, or *horchata?* Would there be videos during labor to make the time fly?—like the time the family brought *Pumping Iron, Lassie Come Home,* and *Dracula,* which seemed to make labor come on really strong.

The Teaching Model at the Northern New Mexico Midwifery Center

From the start, we had people who wanted to learn from us. Our model for teaching our students went like this:

> I am already a midwife, I'm already happy. You are becoming a midwife for your own sake, not for mine, so you need to be clear on what the midwifery requirements are in the state in which you intend to practice, on the academic material and clinical skills required, and clear about what you need from me. When you are ready to perform a skill, tell me you want to do it, and I'll say okay. Anyone can deliver a baby, so you will be catching babies right away with the dads and whoever else in the family is helping. As you get more expert, you will reach the point where you can be the charter (the one who does the charting) who has eyes in the back of her head—eyes that know if a little one needs the potty, if a mother-in-law needs to be sent on an errand, if the midwife caring for the baby needs to be handed the warmed baby blankets, or if the oxygen needs to be turned on. The charter knows how long

pushing has been happening, when the heart tones were last taken—she's the one who has the handle on the normalcy (or lack thereof) of labor progress. She is in charge of the safety of the mother and baby, of the family, of the midwives, and of the entire environment of the birth.

Remember that you are not doing the mom a big favor by caring for her or going out of your way to help her; rather, she is doing you a big favor, letting you learn from your experience with her. We teachers never want to hear "after all I've done for her, now she doesn't want me at the birth," from any student. Sometimes the chemistry isn't right—it has happened to all of us. We midwives have to take in stride that we cannot be all things to all moms.

We are committed to our students, so as soon as you are ready to do the history and physical exam, we will have you perform the intakes on our moms so that they will bond with you. We will sit in the background and supervise. We will work in teams of at least 2 or 3 students with the midwife so that there are always enough hands to keep the birth calm and orderly, even during an emergency. In addition, we will not let the mom choose just one midwife—she will get to know all three of us so that whichever midwife ends up at her birth is someone she knows. This policy helps to avoid midwife burnout, so that we can meet our family commitments and obligations, and can be good models for our moms, who admire us. They need to see us taking care of ourselves and of our families as well as of our clients. Sometimes midwives who are the "be all and end all" exclusively for each client for years reach a certain critical point of maximal stress and quit due to burnout. By then, they are usually highly experienced, so their quitting is a huge loss to the community. We've decided to work in teams to help us last longer; we feel we are kept young at heart and enthusiastic by a constant cadre of committed students.

At the first midwifery conference that included all types of midwives ever held in the United States, which was put on in El Paso in 1978 by pioneering midwife Shari Daniels, we discovered the model of using midwifery meetings as our specific teaching and learning arena. In the past, we had been attending childbirth education, breastfeeding, and consumer-oriented conferences to learn from our peers and to make contacts and friends. Suddenly, we realized we could have our own national midwifery conferences. In 1982 we found ourselves in Boulder, Colorado, talking about organizing the Midwives Alliance of North America conference for 1983.[8] But later there was scrambling for control of the organization; eventually, I stopped going to these conferences for some years because I didn't like the strife between the midwives (see Davis-Floyd and Johnson 2006). Looking for another place where I could learn from midwives, I went instead to the National Association of Childbearing Centers (NACC) conferences.[9] These were primarily for nurse-midwives because they were the population most actively participating in the birth center model. Because theirs was an "out-of-hospital" environment, I found it sympathetic and relevant. I learned from their model the discipline that charting proves that while I was with this mother/baby, they were well, and if they were not well, I responded promptly and correctly according to the midwives' and my medical community's standards of care.

In 1980 we were primarily clinical midwifery instructors at the center, using Wednesdays to teach on a particular issue of interest that had come up during the course of care. The model was that students would undertake their own academic tutelage and preparation for the licensing exam, just as we had done. The New Mexico Department of Health provided the tests, written by the nurse-midwife who was the project manager for the Maternal Child Health Program in charge of regulating and licensing nurse and lay midwives. As the years went by, we began to notice that our students were having an increasingly difficult time passing the exam on their first try. So in 1984 we decided to provide a more formal academic component to our apprenticeship program, including preceptor-led studies of the course of a woman's care from antepartum to intra- and postpartum; newborn and well-woman differential diagnosis, and management in normal cases. Our model was to cement all the variations of normal into our apprentices' tools for management and to teach them the cardinal signs for differentiating a condition requiring consult. The politics of regulation and interactions with local medical, lab, social services, and emergency resources inevitably wove their way into our discussions, along with trends in parenting techniques and changing models of preparation for childbirth and breastfeeding. The progress of the midwifery movement, the rivalries between those who supported apprenticeship training and those who believed in formal schooling, the "bliss ninnies" versus the "mainstream," the unattended home birthers versus midwives who thought that was awful, the diversity of the religious and sexual identity of midwives, the pros and cons of the licensed versus the unlicensed practice—we incorporated all of these political and philosophical issues into our academic offerings along with our clinical trainings.

Politics, Funding, and Becoming a Change Agent in the State

During the early 1980s, the bulk of the funding for our building and start-up costs came from my inheritance and from my family. My family had promised the entire cost of the building but was only able to come up with one-third. This was my first lesson in fundraising: even people who love you the most won't always be able to come through, so fundraising will be a continual work in progress. In 1980 the town of Taos had a population of only 5,000; the entire rural county of Taos in northern New Mexico had only 25,000 total. So we knew from the start that we would not be able to raise the operating funds from fees for service alone. There were fewer than 350 births in the county per year. Of those, our newspaper survey results showed we could probably attract one-eighth. The majority (over 80%) of our citizens had no health insurance.[10] The local indigent fund paid facility costs only, not provider fees. At times we were able to contract with one or two insurance companies, such as Prudential or Blue Cross and Blue Shield, for reimbursement of our care.

It would be almost a decade before we tried to qualify as Medicaid providers. (Medicaid is the United States' public medical assistance program for persons unable to obtain health insurance because of poverty.) There were chunks of two years here and there where we were able to buy malpractice insurance. Except for those rare years, we "went bare" (without malpractice insurance) until the late 1990s. Thanks to the persistent and tireless efforts of Janice Trinin, president of the New Mexico Midwives Association, we were reimbursed by Medicaid for our services plus $50 per birth as our facility fee from 1989 to 1997. By that time, the system had even graduated to being able to accept our billing online, and we were doing better financially: our clientele had grown to about one-fifth of all the births in Taos County.

In 1997 the New Mexico Department of Human Services, which runs Medicaid, decided to contract with three health management organizations (HMOs) to manage state Medicaid funds in order to "reduce medical costs."[11] The HMOs immediately cut us off with the excuse that there were enough midwives delivering babies in hospitals (28% of New Mexico's births are attended by nurse-midwives in hospitals), so they didn't need us. It took us two years of persistent and heartbreaking work with politicians and bureaucracies to qualify again as providers, during which time we continued to take care of our Medicaid moms (82% of our practice by then) without getting paid. We did fundraising, but a more important saving grace was that two ob/gyns, Heidi and Rudy, started at the center as our employees. They brought in the majority of the income that kept us afloat during those two years.

I had put up the remainder of the cost for the building and land in 1978, and because we couldn't buy liability insurance at the time, my husband and I signed a sole and separate property agreement to ensure that I would have no assets. I gave up all my property for the privilege of being a midwife, so that if I got sued or went to jail (for injuring a mother or a baby), my family would continue to benefit from my assets rather than lose them. My mom had been especially worried about my choice of career. How could I justify putting my entire family at risk just so I could practice some dangerous, nonmainstream, nonprofessional, hippie midwifery? (Don't worry—she declares she's proud of me now!) My husband, Carl, staunch midwifery supporter, was our landlord, and we paid him rent. The model was that if we were just a poor little midwifery center with no assets, we'd be less of a target for lawsuit. So far, the Northern New Mexico Midwifery Center has not had any suits against it.[12]

That was how I began a life of paying to work, rather than being paid. I donated my salary to the nonprofit to help defray the start-up costs of paying my partner, Tish, and the other overhead of running the center. We hired a secretary/receptionist to answer the phone and greet clients. Her presence gave us the freedom to go to births and do home visits while maintaining a presence in the center as you would in any regular business with hours. This was the next model we tried.

Tish is one of those people who can clearly visualize and articulate how what we do now will affect our future. She convinced me to join the National Association of Childbearing Centers pilot project in 1983. She said if we didn't participate, they might come up with regulations that prohibited registered lay midwives like us from having a birth center. So off I went and joined all the round-table-style meetings of the pilot project, where the rules for responsibly running a birth center were hammered out. I loved it! I was the only non-nurse midwife; I found myself surrounded by nurse-midwives, doctors, nurses, childbirth and breast-feeding experts, advocates and consumers, all of whom loved the idea of being able to have their own facilities where they could provide family-centered care; quite a number of them attended home births as well. The leadership had developed the Maternity Center in New York and had a great deal of experience with midwifery.[13] As a bonus, they articulated the history and traditions, the triumphs and the heartbreaks of the midwifery experience in the United States. I had found peers in a group that I had imagined would be hostile to the culture of birth that I represented. That was how I became a student of the birth center model. Our birth center qualified for NACC accreditation and has gone through the process every three years to this day. One time our accreditation was denied. It was scary. Our site visitors did not recognize some of our paperwork because it was so different from the mainstream forms and record keeping. The accrediting body, therefore, thought we did not meet several of the required accrediting standards. We appealed. Sister Angela Murdaugh was sent to do our appeal site visit. Our accreditation was reinstated, to our great relief.

Despite the great financial burden of accreditation, we have continued our efforts to maintain it. Accreditation linked us to other birth centers and to the leaders of the birth center model, giving us the ongoing opportunity to monitor our financial, planning, clinical facility, record-keeping, and other aspects of the practice. It also provided our medical community with some sense that we were not without oversight.

Registered lay midwives (now called licensed midwives) in New Mexico have always practiced autonomously. Although New Mexico midwives are not required to have physician backup for their practices, we connect each mother with a physician to enhance her opportunity to obtain a second opinion and to have a physician who knows her in advance should she have problems.[14] The only other formal oversight is provided by the Department of Health in the case of receiving a written complaint about a midwife. At the Special Use Permit hearing before the Zoning Board in Taos that reviewed our request for permission to start our birth center in 1977, and again in 1978, an audience member asked who would be overseeing us to make sure we were not "burying babies in the backyard" or "incinerating dead babies" in our outdoor garbage incinerators. Between 1993 and 2002, we experienced increasing hostility from a Taos obstetrician. He reported us to the New Mexico Licensed Midwives Advisory Board for practicing medicine when we ordered ultrasounds, and he tried to have us investigated for starting the National College of Midwifery. Not always, but often, he would tell the mothers whom we had transferred into his care because of an emergency that "the midwives almost killed you." In 1981, one of the family practice doctors who actually was our advocate told me that he was sure we were going to end up with several dead mothers and was surprised that it hadn't happened yet, a sentiment he repeated when there was a maternal death at the hospital for one of the family practice docs! (We have never had a maternal death.) At a hospital in-service, one of our favorite family docs commented that "having a home birth is like letting your child cross the street without holding his hand. Usually you can get away with it, but every now and then—the accident!" These are examples of the reasons why we were comforted by our accredited status. We saw it as evidence for our community that our practices were aboveboard, reasonable, and part of an acceptable culture of birth in our country.

During the late 1980s, we were integrating more into the health provider network in our community by participating in an organization called Taos Agencies Working Together, and a Centers for Disease Control (CDC) initiative called the Planned Approach to Community Health.[15] This initiative included a huge survey of our community's health problems and led to the formation of the Taos Maternal-Child Health Council, followed by the Community Wellness Council and the Taos CARES Coalition (www.taoscommunitywellnesscenter.org). We've participated in these incarnations of health promotion in our county, taking leadership roles and administering grant monies in order to participate in the community's efforts at reduction of risk. We have brought our students to these meetings to introduce them to this public health aspect of midwifery responsibility so that they could grasp the impact that midwifery interaction with community health leaders can have on the families we serve.

Our Birth Center and Educational Model Develop and Expand Beyond Taos

In 1982 we began to see our vision going beyond our borders. Vicki Penwell, a midwife from Alaska who had been inspired by working and studying with us in Taos that year, took our New Mexico licensing model back to Alaska, and took the birth center model a step further by hiring her own physician, who could provide expert assistance and act as a liaison with the hospital there. Eventually, she also took this model overseas to the least fortunate communities she could identify in the Philippines, where, supported by her church, she could provide much-needed midwifery care to the poorest of the poor, offering food programs, orphanage services, and midwifery training to local and international midwifery students. In her model, she eventually turns over these birth centers to the local midwives, and goes on to start a new one. She added primary care to the scope of midwifery care to help reduce risk, and continues to develop these centers in the Philippines to this day (www.mercyinaction.com/midwife_index.php, and see Chapter 12, this volume).

In 1984 I wrote a presentation on Successful Rural Lay Midwifery for the International Confederation of Midwives meeting in Sydney, Australia (Gilmore 1984). Our model was expanding its communication to the international arena. What an amazing experience as I traveled to Sydney with members of the American College of Nurse-Midwives and listened to midwives from all over the world talk about their efforts to reduce maternal and infant mortality and morbidity. I brought this message home, and our model began to articulate the reduction of maternal and infant mortality as a primary goal. It had been quite a shock to learn at this conference just how badly the United States compared with other industrialized countries in the area of maternal and infant care. At that time, the United States was twenty-second in infant mortality, and our maternal mortality was going up, not down. Equally compelling was the revelation that the industrialized countries where midwifery was incorporated into the health care team had the best outcomes. Bringing this message home to Taos helped us increase support for our integration into the medical team, an issue we struggle with to this day.

THE MODEL OF CARE AT THE
NORTHERN NEW MEXICO MIDWIFERY CENTER

Free pregnancy testing is our initial draw for the public. Our core schedule of midwifery care consists of office visits every month for the first twenty-eight weeks, childbirth classes for eight weeks, one visit every two weeks until thirty-six weeks and every week until birth, the birth, a twenty-four-hour and a third day home visit, two- and six-week postpartum visits, and well-woman visits. Prenatal visits include comprehensive discussion of whether out-of-hospital care is desirable given the mother's condition and her and her family's inclination; signing up the new client, first with the MANA statistics project and then with CPM2000, a research project to investigate care given by Certified Professional Midwives (CPMs) in the year 2000 (Johnson and Daviss 2005); and using the Understanding Birth Better database (www.understandingbirthbetter.com) to complete our data, because we believe strongly in the importance of midwives keeping their statistics to show the quality of their care. We analyze women's diets routinely according to their height, weight, activity levels, and physical and psychological stress factors to ensure moms are getting enough of the right stuff. We draw and order our own lab work; we order our own ultrasounds as needed and use our microscope to check for certain vaginal infections and for the presence of amniotic fluid when mothers think their bag of waters has broken and there are no contractions or the pregnancy has not reached the required thirty-seven weeks of gestation. When needed, we offer referrals for counseling, housing, food supplementation, transportation assistance, medical consultation, breastfeeding classes, addiction management, family violence counseling, education, and peer group and play group gatherings. (You can visit the center's website at www.midwiferycenter.org.)

Our favorite births are home births: anecdotally, we have fewer transfers from homes than from the birth center, and home births take us out of our indoor environment and culture into someone else's, which is most welcome after days of filing charts and completing phone follow-up; cleaning and getting the center's laundry all washed, folded, and put away; sorting equipment into needed packs; ordering supplies; rescheduling appointments; and teaching classes—all mostly indoors at one location. At home births we can relax from our day-to-day chores and enjoy the family, especially their children and extended family members and pets. We are constantly astounded by our clients' talents. Everyone in our community is doing something interesting—there are artists of all kinds, musicians, sewing geniuses, mechanics, farmers—the abundant creativity refreshes and inspires us! It's always fun to participate in finishing a bassinet or a baby quilt, or in making a meal with the family while we're waiting for the baby. They include us in their family routines, and we include them in the birth care. We teach interested family members to take blood pressure, listen to the fetal heart rate and count it, write these in the chart, give mom a back rub or a foot rub, take her for walks, help her in and out of the tub, think of ways to vary her activities so she doesn't get antsy (American for "restless"), and of course, we assist the family members the mom has chosen to assist with the actual catching of the baby (her partner, sister, mother, or another)—unforgettable for them and satisfying for us. Our students do much of the teaching and in the process cement their own learning, with the preceptor looking on and adding her own contributions.

As our model of birth-center-and-school grew, we realized that we needed to provide not only childbirth classes for our parents, but also CPR and first aid classes, space for battered women to meet and sheltering facilities for them, English classes and GED classes for immigrants and young parents, and parenting classes for all parents, including teen parents—not to mention home visiting for all our families. Our model incubated all these services, and many went on to become independent 501(c)3s (federally recognized not-for-profit charitable organizations) of their own. Taos now has a women's shelter (www.taoscav.org), a home visiting program, a *Mujeres en Progreso* (Women in Progress) group for Spanish-speaking immigrants, and parenting classes and facilities in the high school. There's a teen pregnancy prevention group, and a *Puentes* (Bridges) group for young mothers to help them obtain college degrees and to provide mutual support. (For descriptions of these programs, see www.taoscommunitywell-nesscenter.org.)

The College-without-Walls Model

Around 1986 Tish became president of the Midwives Alliance of North America, and we convinced the state of New Mexico to identify us as "licensed midwives" instead of as "registered lay midwives." I became the chair of the New Mexico Midwives Association (NMMA) Education Committee, a position I've held continuously and now share with licensed midwife Ruth Kauffman, who in 2005 started a birth center with another licensed midwife, Terri Simmons, focusing on undocumented immigrants in the South Valley of Albuquerque. Ruth is also a registered nurse working in the University of New Mexico Hospital Obstetrics Department. In 1985 the NMMA gave me the responsibility of exploring the provision of a route for the education of New Mexico midwives that could result in a degree in addition to a license. New Mexican apprentices and preceptors were looking for a way to provide more academic consistency from apprenticeship to apprenticeship. That's how it came about in 1985 that as the education chair of the NMMA, I contacted the New Mexico Commission on Higher Education for the regulations on licensing postsecondary institutions in New Mexico (www.hed.state.nm.us). With these regulations as a template, the members of the New Mexico Midwives Association helped me to develop an associate of arts in midwifery (AAM) degree as the entry level for licensing, a baccalaureate program for already-licensed midwives who wanted to contribute a clinical research paper and receive case management mentorship for a year, a master's program for midwives who wanted to concentrate on coursework and research focused on positively impacting the health of the community they served, and a doctoral program for midwives who wanted to concentrate on coursework and research that would have a large impact on practice.

The model looked like this: candidates for the associate's degree would apply to the New Mexico College of Midwifery, a nonprofit 501(c)3, with their preceptors, agreeing to undertake the required course of academics and clinical experiences based on the requirements for licensing in New Mexico (listed at www.health.state.nm.us/programsandservices/midwives). To save money on rent, light, heat, water, phone, copying and administration, my colleagues and I housed the college—a federally recognized, state-licensed, nonprofit entity—at the Northern New Mexico Midwifery Center. The New Mexico Midwives Association supplied members for the board of directors and often helped with file updating during the first few years. They also provided the womanpower to review research proposals for the upper division and graduate programs.

The beauty of the "college-without-walls" model was that students could stay in their communities and study with their preceptors to avoid the expense and disruption of traveling to live in another town or state. Later, with the addition of several science, English, and math college courses, we developed an associate of science in midwifery (ASM) degree, designed as a three-year equivalent that could be undertaken at the pace appropriate to the student, the preceptor, and the practice catchment to which they had access. If the student already has transcripts for required courses, the program can be finished in as little as a year, or it can take as long as five years if needed.

The student is required to apply to the college with her clinical and academic preceptors to ensure that she will have access to the required clinical and academic resources. Therefore, students and preceptors apply as a team. Sometimes one student will apply with as many as nine or ten preceptors to be sure that she will have enough clinical experiences and academic support. Preceptors must be either state licensed or state or nationally certified, and must disclose the number of clinical experiences they can guarantee the student in the proposed time. Preceptors must also agree in writing to meet regularly with the student, to provide and receive written feedback, and to participate with the student in course planning on a trimester basis.

Because students were often in a one-on-one apprenticeship, the New Mexico Commission on Higher Education required that the exit exam be an outside exam, not one provided by the college, to reduce the chances of cheating or favoritism. Thus, in order to graduate from the associate's program, a student must pass either a state licensing exam, a state midwifery association exam, or a national certifying exam administered by the North American Registry of Midwives, the American Midwifery Certification Board, or the equivalent in a foreign country. Should the student who has successfully completed all courses with the required 80% grade choose not to take the outside exam or fail the outside exam, the student graduates with a certificate in midwifery instead of a degree. Upon furnishing proof of passing the outside exam, the student receives the associate's degree.

For the upper-division and graduate degrees, the college model is based around the need for clinical research by and for midwives. The college offers a baccalaureate of science in midwifery (BSM) program to mid-wives who have either completed the associate's degree or have been state licensed or nationally certified. This program requires a year of additional mentoring, where the student reviews her care and outcomes with her pre-ceptor in a guided chart review. In addition, the student writes a clinical research paper with the approval and supervision of her preceptor and of a research oversight committee selected from the college faculty advisory board; that committee reviews the research proposal and approves the final draft of the completed research. The resulting document is placed in the college library.

The master of science in midwifery (MSM) program requires that the candidate be a licensed or certified midwife and have a bachelor's degree. It was built around obtaining thirty credits based on a community development model, with courses that facilitate the midwife's competent grasp of her own community's health strengths and challenges, as well as facilitating the midwife's ability to have an impact on the reduction of her community's infant and maternal mortality and morbidity. Her master's research project is based on clinical community data. For the PhD, the midwife and her supervising committee would design a sixty-credit course of studies to support the midwife's research, culminating with the publish-ing of the research and presentation before a national or international midwifery conference.

In the early 1980s, the New Mexico Department of Public Health Maternal Child Division had required licensed midwifery applicants to submit papers outlining the correct course of care for each of the categories of antepar-tum, intrapartum, postpartum, newborn and well-woman care, as well as for childbirth preparation, to the director of the Maternal Child Program (usually a nurse-midwife, although a registered nurse who was also a licensed midwife had the job for a period of a few years). In addition, a clinical preceptor had to attest in writing that the student midwife had acquired all the requisite clinical skills and clinical experiences. To assist with the achievement of these requirements, the college would supply a book of comprehensive learning objectives to the AAM candidate and her preceptor, covering all required areas, to lead the student and the preceptor through the required academic details. How the student and the preceptor accomplished this was their business—they would undertake the learning process at their own pace, with five years allowed for completion, and report their mutual evaluations and the apprentice's grades and clinical experience accomplishments at the end of each trimester. Upon passing the New Mexico licensing exam, the student would receive her AAM degree. This last was a requirement of the Commission on Higher Education as a quality control measure.

In 1997, however, we realized that the college had to offer additional college-level courses to ensure that the candidate not only was a competent midwife but could also communicate effectively, read and understand materials, analyze relevant research, be culturally sensitive and competent, understand the basics of starting and running a business to ensure greater practice stability, be able to analyze conditions in her own community, and participate in bettering maternal/child health in her town, state, and nation. Although our initial associate's degree model had been based solely on the state midwifery licensing requirements, our later model added college-level English, math, statistics, cultural issues, business communication, midwifery literature and art, and other courses.

This model had the student paying the college an administrative fee and paying her preceptor separately. In addition, the student and preceptor could accomplish the requirements in their own setting, never having to travel to headquarters in Taos for any courses. These policies helped keep the cost low: because the college was not the middleman between the student and her teachers, there was no building filled with classrooms to pay for, and no travel and relocation away from home needed to accomplish schooling. Content for courses that are not about midwifery, such as English, math, statistics, or chemistry, can be borrowed from the college library. These video-based courses with texts and workbooks are designed by such companies as the Annenberg Foundation. The student also can pick these up at her local community or other college.

Once licensed or certified nationally, by her state, or by her state midwifery association, the new midwife would qualify to enter the college's bachelor's program. In 1992 requests from members of the National Coalition of Midwifery Educators caused us to broaden the college's scope to include students from around the country and those studying in midwifery settings abroad. We added the general education requirements (mentioned above) to the midwifery courses, and broadened the learning objectives for the midwifery courses to match the Midwives Alliance of North America's *Core Competencies for Practicing Midwives* (available at www.mana.org), and we added the skills list developed by the North American Registry of Midwives (www.narm.org) as soon as it became available. In 1995, to reflect this newer, broader population of students we were reaching, we changed the name of our college from the New Mexico College of Midwifery to the National College of Midwifery (NCM). (You can visit our website at www.midwiferycollege.org.)

The college was licensed by the New Mexico Commission on Higher Education in 1991. Until my retirement from the birth center in 2001, I ran the college from the Northern New Mexico Midwifery Center, using the center's staff, facilities, phone, computers, copiers, paper, and students to support the college's burgeoning activities. The biggest obstacle was providing a $5,000 bond, which had to be made out to the commission, to be used as a fund from which to reimburse students in case of the failure of the institution. I donated the original bond in the form of a Certificate of Deposit made out to me and to the Commission on Higher Education. It was a great day when in 1999, the college became successful enough to pay me back for the original bond. And the college has paid for itself ever since. It is now housed in my home, in the back office I shared originally with Beth Enson, co-college conspirator and visionary dean of students, supported by Registrar Lisa Brown, who tracks students' accomplishments and keeps them on task with the paperwork. Since this writing, Beth has retired from the college to participate more in the home schooling of her daughter and to continue her poetry writing career (she is a published author). Emily Gemmel, CPM, a graduate of NCM through Vicki Penwell's program, took Beth's place during our transition and is now pursuing an academic degree of her own. Anna Khamsamran, my daughter, has joined us to revamp our database and to handle our website design and the new format for the CDs we send to incoming students. She is now our administrative dean.

Our upcoming model is this: we want to reunite the college and the midwifery center in the same building so that we are not separated from our beloved clinical midwives, their students, and the staff at the Northern New Mexico Midwifery Center. We are in the process of refinancing the birth center to improve cash flow, and exploring the possibilities of either selling the facility and building a smaller, more suitable one on our acre next door to house us together, or figuring out how to convert the present space to house us together in a way that will generate enough cash flow to meet our debt obligations. Ideally, we would sell the building for enough profit to become debt free. However, we are debating the practicality of the "owning assets" model, which would make us a bigger target for frivolous lawsuits. The model of renting a facility, having to fundraise constantly, and having no malpractice insurance is safer from a frivolous-lawsuit perspective. However, being able to be paid as Medicaid providers has required us to have malpractice insurance. The debate over caring for our now 85% Medicaid contingent and how much we get paid (or don't) to do so, continues. Should we give up our malpractice insurance (now costing us

$54,000 dollars annually and promising to increase), we could still take care of our Medicaid mothers but would not be reimbursed, or else would be reimbursed very little.

Starting an Accrediting Agency

In the late 1980s I started realizing that an unaccredited college was not an optimal model for our midwifery students. In 1990 the members of the National Coalition of Midwifery Educators, including myself, were noting the lamentable lack of decent accreditation options for our certificate- and degree-granting midwifery schools that were independent vocational schools, not university-based programs. The coalition asked the Division of Accreditation of the American College of Nurse-Midwives to consider accrediting our programs—a request they turned down. (Nurse-midwives in the United States have a long history of valuing only university-affiliated programs; see Davis-Floyd and Johnson 2006; Chapter 15, this volume.) So, based on my experience with the development and implementation of the accreditation of freestanding birth centers through the National Association of Childbearing Centers (NACC), I suggested that we form our own accrediting agency. Therese Charvet (then director of midwifery education at the Seattle Midwifery School) and I wrote the first draft of the proposed Standards for Accreditation, based on the American College of Nurse-Midwives' Department of Accreditation model for accrediting programs of midwifery within larger institutions.

I agreed that my midwifery partner, Melissa Bauer, LM, and I would spearhead the incorporation of the Midwifery Education Accreditation Council (MEAC—pronounced "meek"), obtaining our nonprofit 501(c)3 status in 1991 in New Mexico. (You can learn more about MEAC at www.meacschools.org.) MEAC was another child of our birth center model, and as such, the center housed and fed it for several years. In a nine-year-long process, the National Coalition of Midwifery Educators' accreditation subcommittee developed standards to fit the federal Department of Education's criteria for accrediting agencies, and by 1994, the coalition became subsumed into MEAC.[16] We supplemented our fledgling project with our membership payments, in addition to paying our own way to our meetings, which we held in our houses to save money. Thanks to connections through the North American Registry of Midwives, we were the recipients of some small grants that paid for our pilot project to accredit midwifery schools. The first school to reach accredited status was Maternidad La Luz, in El Paso, Texas, run by Deborah Kaley. (See www.maternidadlaluz.com.)

Alas, though this accreditation model was succeeding, it was not working for the National College of Midwifery! The conflict of interest caused by housing the college and its accrediting agency in the birth center's offices, all run by me, prevented the college from qualifying for accreditation. A new home for MEAC was needed. It was a happy and auspicious day in 1996 when Mary Ann Baul, in Flagstaff, Arizona, agreed to house MEAC in her Woman Care Midwifery Service office. Mary Ann served as MEAC's executive director for many years, retiring in 2007; Joanne Myers-Ciecko, former director of the Seattle Midwifery School, currently (2008) holds that position.

Getting More Connected with Obstetricians

Imagine our surprise, our suspicion, and finally our delight when in 1994 we began to receive visits at our little Northern New Mexico Midwifery Center from physicians looking for a birth center in which to practice! Outstanding among those who showed up were a family practitioner with his nurse-midwife wife, an obstetrician with her nurse-midwife partner, and two obstetricians married to each other! How was our birth center doing, they wanted to know? We were always about $60,000 behind and having to do major fund-raising to keep us going, and I was continuing to pay to work. Then the president of our board of directors, Steve Kenin, spearheaded a fund-raising campaign involving art auctions and dances, which two years in a row brought in enough to begin to pay me and Melissa Bauer. Between 1994 and 1996, the center had also managed to effectively bill Medicaid. We were doing one-fifth of the births in Taos.

These physician visits spurred us into conceiving of a new model, wherein one set of these very cool physicians would become employees of our nonprofit birth center. What heaven to have our own obstetricians so that we wouldn't have to depend upon the very hostile current obstetrician incarnation in our town for advice and hospital care. This guy's attitude toward me was, "Haven't you been burned at the stake yet?" and my attitude towards him was, "Yes, but I'm back for your benefit!" Such was the brand of humor with which we attempted to hold each other at bay.

Our model envisioned the guarantee of a full-time-equivalent salary for the first two or three years of our obstetricians' employment, and paying their malpractice and life insurance. In return, the income they generated would help reduce the center's deficit. Our board was thrilled, and conceived the idea of buying land to house a "health campus" that would include the birth center, with its valuable doctors and midwives, a day care facility so that all our kids would have a great place to be cared for while we were working—maybe we could even coax the pediatric practice to move to and build on our campus, and how about a *curandera* center, where traditional New Mexican healing arts and herbs could be fostered?

"Build it and they will come!" The excitement of the vision prompted Heidi Rinehart and Rudy Fedrizzi—married ob/gyns, parents of young

Julianna and nursing baby Peter, and experienced home birthers themselves (their first birth took place on The Farm in Tennessee—a renowned midwifery haven [www.thefarm.org/midwives] and their second in Phoenix)—to leave the great metropolis of Phoenix, Arizona, when Rudy had completed his service debt by working as an ob/gyn for the Air Force. (Heidi had been working part-time for a private ob/gyn service in Phoenix.) Commuting to and from work would be a burden they wouldn't have to put up with in Taos. This was their bargain with us: if we would buy the land out by the new hospital and build a birth center on it before they came, and if we would allow them to buy land for their new house from us at the same low rate the seller was offering as support for this endeavor, then they would become employees of the nonprofit, just like us. They would be guaranteed their first year's salary: it was a pittance, we knew, but they were willing to sacrifice for the cause.

The days of the model in which all employees of the center, from the midwives to the receptionist, were deemed equally important and received equal pay, came to an end. We raised the midwives' salaries, promising to give the physicians one-third of any profit above and beyond operating expenses; we happily went $500,000 into debt; bought eight acres and sold three of them on the spot to the physicians at the same rate at which we bought them; got $200,000 in matching grant moneys; and raised $130,000 in one afternoon with a professionally run Tuscan lunch fundraiser at a former Playboy Bunny's exotic Taos home. With Heidi's articulate help, we had gotten the land and pulled off the fancy lunch mega-fundraiser!

We built the required new birth center. It was beautifully designed with birthing tubs in each room, a kitchen/living room with a striking sculpture in it for families, a place to rest and shower for the midwives while they did laundry resulting from the births, and a huge storage room for supplies. Office hours we held in our old birth center, with Heidi and Rudy now occupying our beloved old birth rooms as their offices.

The practice took off. Soon our old birth center was full of wonderful new clients, delighted to see the new ob/gyns, who with their hospital privileges, their kindness, and their expert and evidence-based practice soon took most of the clients from our old nemesis, who subsequently left Taos. We started doing business as the Women's Health and Birth Center to reflect the broadened scope of care. Heidi and Rudy brought the obstetric service at the hospital to a new standard, lowering the cesarean rate from close to 35% to 15% with excellent outcomes! As far as we midwives were concerned, these accomplishments alone made Taos the Camelot of birth.

The little old birth center became so crowded that plans to build new offices onto the new birth center in five years were immediately moved up, and by 1999, we were completely moved into the most gorgeous new facility we could ever imagine. But Camelot was far from perfect. The billing system we had bought to deal with the enlarged practice was in its startup phase, with accompanying glitches. Our midwives, who had been promptly reimbursed via an electronic billing system by Medicaid in 1997, got dropped as providers the very October day Heidi and Rudy started: as I mentioned above, the New Mexico state government was convinced that using HMOs was the way to reduce skyrocketing medical costs; the HMOs decided there were enough nurse-midwives, and so they didn't need us. Suddenly, we were bringing in one-tenth of the income we had before Heidi and Rudy arrived. As a result, the one-third of the profits that were supposed to go to our new physicians never materialized. The development person we'd hired to help us promote and grow the practice had to be let go.

Even so, the babies were coming, the students were humming, the practice clicked along, and NACC granted me its Professional Achievement Award in 1999. We applied for and received recognition as Safe Motherhood providers from the World Health Organization (WHO) in 2000,[17] the same year our Chamber of Commerce recognized us as the best nonprofit health service in Taos. And ours was the first birth center to be recognized by the Coalition for Improving Maternity Services (www.motherfriendly.org) as "Mother-Friendly" in 2001.

Our model was an inspiration, but it was not without its challenges. A power struggle arose between the board and the staff as differing agendas for providing the center with leadership personnel surfaced. We fired our board of directors, struggled to assemble a new one, and adopted the consensus model for running the center. We worked hard to cut spending wherever we could, and Rudy took over the billing to ensure that we billed the maximum and in a timely way for every procedure. We bought health insurance and retirement accounts for the entire staff in this new model. I retired from the birth center in 2001 to focus on administering the college, and the physicians had an opportunity to run the center themselves. I remained on the board as the founder to give my support. Running the birth center was challenging, but Heidi and Rudy were able to hang in there for two more years.

Two years before they left, we had decided to hire helpers for them, and so we advertised and recruited for another full-time ob/gyn. Our model was going through a restructuring with the hope that by adding another position to the mix, some of the clinical pressure would be lessened for Heidi and Rudy, each of whom had been on call every other day and barely had time to visit each other or play with their children. Although their salaries had increased, they still were insufficient for their family needs. We hoped to relieve their exhaustion by the addition of Scott Reznick and Shanti Mohling, an ob/gyn couple from Colorado about to give birth to their first child and planning a cesarean due to placenta previa. Their arrival and contribution to the center's capacity was much anticipated. It was really fun to invite them to see their first water births in the center, and to have their particular medical areas of expertise to complement those of Heidi and Rudy. But differences in expectations and working styles resulted in conflict between the two ob/gyn couples.

In response, the midwives wanted to continue working with the physicians in the same building but separate the midwifery practice once again. They wanted the physicians to start their own business but rent from us. Shanti and Scott thought about leaving Taos completely, but in a surprise reversal, Heidi and Rudy decided to leave. Later, Shanti and Scott did leave our employ and the physical location of the birth center, and started their own Women's Health Institute in Taos in another building. They continue to this day to back the midwives, and Shanti sits on the birth center's board, spearheading our big annual art auction and fancy dinner fundraiser.

Joan Norris, one of the center's midwives, took on the role of director when Rudi and Heidi departed. The center has continued to thrive under her kind and competent direction, both as a clinical facility and as a teaching program. The midwives and their students continue to provide loving, attentive, and excellent care to one-quarter of birthing mothers in Taos, and persist in seeking a better solution to the financial crunch that characterizes any practice primarily serving Medicaid recipients. Joan was instrumental in helping forge a statewide agreement with Medicaid that allows home birth midwives to be reimbursed for their services whether or not they hold liability insurance. The center is currently the only direct-entry midwifery practice in New Mexico that holds liability insurance, which has become prohibitively expensive in the past few years. Joan also oversees the center's annual fundraising campaign, which must secure the operating funds to fill the substantial shortfall created by low Medicaid reimbursement rates. The midwives' annual art auction and dinner is always a highly anticipated and successful event.

Heidi and Rudy's departure was the end of our beautifully low community cesarean rates. How we loved to get Rudy's statistical report at the end of each year! At that point, the midwives were attending one-fourth of all 364 annual births in Taos County. Our cesarean rate was 4% (the community's was 13%), our antepartum transfer rate was 24%, and our intrapartum transfer rate was 12%.

Our Present Working Model

In addition to lowering cesarean rates, another huge gift from the "midwives and physicians together" model had been the 501(c)3's ownership of the large birth center building and land. Now that the hospital is no longer our tenant, we are hoping either to sell the current center and use the profits to build on our remaining adjoining acre, or to come up with a way to convert the present extra office space into a self-sustaining center and college combination with a real teaching space.

We have talked to the nurse-midwifery program faculty at the University of New Mexico, who tell us that 60% of their students would like out-of-hospital experience while in school, which is unavailable to the vast majority of nurse-midwifery students in the United States.[18] Ruth Kaufman and Terri Simmons of Luna y Sol Midwifery are starting a birth center in Albuquerque to serve the immigrant population there. We are imagining a collaboration in which nurse-midwives and licensed midwives train their students side by side, in home, center, and hospital so that we can grow the number of midwives in New Mexico by working collaboratively.[19] We imagine increasing the numbers and the variety of sites of access to midwifery care for New Mexico families. We've talked to a family practice physician who had a home birth and wants all moms and families to have the wonderful, amazing experience she had. She'd like to start a birth center, too. We want to retain our Mother-Friendly status and also qualify as a Baby-Friendly facility.

The college started a relationship with Ticime, a Mexican nonprofit organization promoting midwifery (see http://www.parteras.org/what_is.htm) and focusing on Tepoztlan, in the state of Morelos, where we worked with midwife Lucila Garcia Sanchez who runs a *Posada de Nacimiento* (birth center) there. (For a description of Lucila's training and practice, see Davis-Floyd 2001.) For two years we brought midwifery students down to study with her and her midwifery colleagues for one or two months, providing the students with intensive Spanish and academic study if they wished. In return, we funded our Morelos midwife friends to come and visit us at our center so that we could experience a real exchange of ideas, helping each other reduce maternal and infant risk while improving our care and our lives through these new, transnational relationships. We went to Tepoztlan three times a year: January–February, May–June, and September–October. We were hoping these activities would also help mitigate the current campaign in Mexico to phase out midwives in favor of hospital births. We had to suspend this program unexpectedly when program director Juanita Nelson's mom became seriously ill, and she was needed at home.

At this writing in April 2008, the National College of Midwifery has graduated 169 students: 159 ASMs, 9 BSMs, and 1 MSM. Currently 159 are enrolled (134 ASM, 23 BSM, and 2 MSM), and we have 137 preceptors.

To date the Northern New Mexico Midwifery Center has served over 5,000 families for births, well-woman and prenatal care, and postpartum home visits; our midwives attend 21% of Taos County babies annually. Since 1981, the total number of births we attended at home was 438; the total number of births at the center was 1,027; and the number of transfers to the hospital during labor was 348—a transport rate of 19%. We recognize that this rate is higher than that for CPMs, generally at about 12% (Davis-Floyd and Johnson 2006)—many of these transfers would probably have done well in any case. Our population is demographically varied, and in addition, we tend to be overcautious in the interests of maintaining good relationships with our community physicians, who ask us to transfer early because they get upset with us when the transfer is an emergency.

Community savings is $24,000 per year thanks to cesarean prevention. Breastfeeding rates at six months are more than double (88.6% compared to 39%) the rate for the general population in New Mexico. The cost savings for breastfed infants is $752.94 per infant per year to WIC (the Women, Infants, and Children program, which helps needy families obtain supplementary food in New Mexico) and $1,435 per infant per year in medical claims. (Breastfeeding numbers and cost savings were provided to us by the New Mexico Department of Health, WIC Department, August 2005.)

Current statistics for the Northern New Mexico Midwifery Center include provision of well-woman care for an average of 78 women per year and pregnancy care for just over 200 women per year. We currently attend an average of sixty-five births per year, about thirteen at home and fifty-two in the birth center. We transfer an average of three mothers intrapartum. The one maternal death associated with our center was a hospital client of our physicians who had had three cesareans and was planning a fourth. Her placenta grew through her scar and into her pelvic vasculature, causing a fatal hemorrhage during a miscarriage at nineteen weeks. We have experienced nine perinatal deaths during the last twenty-nine years: two fetal demises within one week of their due dates from placenta abruptio, two fetal demises within one week of their due dates from unknown causes, two anencephalics who couldn't survive after birth, one SIDS death, one gastric volvulus at four days of age, and one fetal demise during precipitous delivery.

The 2000 results for our birth center were sent to us by the CPM2000 study authors (Kenneth C. Johnson and Betty-Anne Daviss). During that year, when our physicians were part of our practice, and including all mothers who began care with the midwives and were transferred in labor to our physicians and the hospital, compared to "all singleton vertex births in the USA at 37 weeks +" (Johnson and Daviss 2005), our center's

1. Electronic fetal monitoring rate was 22%, compared to 84.3% nationally
2. Induction rate was 4% compared to 21% nationally
3. Labor stimulation rate was 3% compared to 18.9% nationally

4. Episiotomy rate was 3% compared to 33% nationally
5. Forceps and vacuum extractor rate was 4%, compared to 7.4% nationally
6. Cesarean section rate was 9% compared to 19% nationally

There's an empty billboard outside Taos. I've been fantasizing the following sign: "Welcome to Taos, Home of the Northern New Mexico Midwifery Center"!

ACKNOWLEDGMENTS

Louis and Helen Stephens, my mother and father, the foundation of my caring

Carl Gilmore, my husband, core of my love

Anna Khamsamran, Ezra Depperman, Jan Gilmore, Jang Khamsamran, Logan Gilmore, children and grandchildren, giving me reason to live

Daniel Depperman and Judith Reynolds, co-parents of Anna and Ezra, enduring family

Charles, Louis, Alice, James, and their spouses, children, grandchildren, my siblings, my "pack"

Fran Greene, Bronwyn Hill, Peg Goodale, Lee Fierro, Martha's Vineyard daring co-beginners

Dr. Hoxsie, physician who delivered my first baby, confirming that we should teach conscious childbirth

Drs. Pond, Rosen, Deveau, Kilgore, and Knudsen, community physicians who did everything that was needed

Tish Demmin, founding partner of the center, visionary

MeLissa Bauer, clinical center midwife and administrator for the founding of MEAC, sustainer

Kate Trieschmann and Molley McCracken, laughter, more laughter, and girl stuff

Joan Norris, Kiersten Figurski, Bobbi Boyd, and all the center's midwives, the pearls encircled

New Mexico Midwives Association, founding partners of the National College of Midwifery, sisters

New Mexico Department of Health Maternal Child Health Program, regulating and protecting midwifery

Larry Schrieber, Taos family practitioner, original physician on the center's board of directors, pioneer

Charles Anderson, Taos pediatrician, inspiring the birth center, selfless dedication to the children

Loretta Ortiz y Pino, Taos pediatrician, caring for the babies, hand of true friendship

Heidi Rinehart and Rudi Fedrizzi, ob/gyns, saving lives through a c-section
rates lower than ever before or after
Shanti Mohling and Scott Reznick, ob/gyns continuing to back mothers
who choose our care
Holy Cross Hospital and nursing staff, caring for those mothers and
babies who need to be transferred
Town of Taos, County of Taos, continuing to support families who want
midwives
Beth Enson, tireless, inspiring, first college dean of students
Lisa Brown, calm college registrar
Anna Khamsamran, administrative dean, taking the college to a whole
new service level, my very own darling daughter
Center board of directors, staunch, loving supporters
MEAC board of directors, faithful to midwifery education
NCM faculty advisory board, intrepid college preceptors
NCM board of directors, shepherding us through thick and thin
All the midwifery students, keeping us young
All the Taos mothers and babies and their families, asking us to their
births

NOTES

1. For the origins of the concept of "family-centered care": www.icea.org/
mem.htm.

2. For a description of the Midwives Model of Care: www.cfmidwifery.
org/mmoc/.

3. For perspectives on being "radical," see Arms (1975).

4. See Ina May Gaskin's book *Spiritual Midwifery* for a deeper description of this
generation of home birthers.

5. For a current photo of the La Clinica sign: www.state.nm.us/hsd/pdf/
TaosResources.pdf.

6. To view the New Mexico Department of Health midwifery regulations
for both licensed midwives and certified nurse-midwives: www.health.state.
nm.us/programsandservices/midwives.

7. For a wonderful documentary on the history of the *parteras* in New Mexico,
see Felina Ortiz's video, *El Espíritu de las Parteras,* http://www.unm.edu/~market/
cgi-bin/archives/000431.html.

8. Visit the MANA website for an in-depth look at their documents and for an
update on the next conference: www.MANA.org.

9. NACC has since changed its name to American Association of Birth Centers
(AABC). To see AABC's philosophy and for an update on their next conference:
www.birthcenters.org.

10. For more information on the economic and social health of Taos, New
Mexico: www.taosba.org.

11. To learn more about the New Mexico Medicaid service: www.state.nm.us/hsd/mad/index.html.

12. For an interesting article in the *Harvard Forum* about malpractice suits in cases of collaboration between midwives and physicians: www.rmf.harvard.edu/files/documents/forum_V19N5.pdf.

13. For the history of the Maternity Center Association in New York: www.binghamton.edu/womhist/wccny/doc11.htm and www.childbirthconnection.org.

14. For a discussion of the physician back-up requirement for nurse-midwives, see Hartley (1999), "The Influence of Managed Care on Supply of Certified Nurse-Midwives: An Evaluation of the Physician Dominance Thesis," *Journal of Health and Social Behavior* 40.1:87–101. For a look at the California law that governs licensed midwives requiring physician backup: www.socalbirth.org/school/midwiferylaw.htm.

15. To find out more about the CDC's PATCH program: www.cdc.gov/nccdphp/publications/PATCH/index.htm.

16. To learn more about the federal Department of Education's requirements for accrediting agencies: www.ed.gov/admins/finaid/accred/index.html.

17. For information about the Safe Motherhood Awards: www.comminit.com/awards2005/awards2005/awards-1074.html.

18. For more on the University of New Mexico's nurse-midwifery program: http://hsc.unm.edu/consg/CNM_About.shtml.

19. Ruth Kauffman can be contacted at Luna y Sol Midwifery: 505-243-1875.

REFERENCES

Arms, Suzanne, 1975. *Immaculate Deception.* New York: Houghton Mifflin.

Cunningham, F. Gary, Kenneth J. Leveno, Steven L. Bloom, John C. Hauth, Larry C. Gilstrap, and Katharine D. Wenstrom. 2005. *Williams Obstetrics,* 22nd ed. New York: McGraw Hill Professional.

Davis-Floyd, Robbie. 2001. "*La Partera Profesional:* Articulating Identity and Cultural Space for a New Kind of Midwife in Mexico." *Medical Anthropology* 20.2–3:185–243. Also available at www.davis-floyd.com.

Davis-Floyd, Robbie, and Christine Barbara Johnson (eds.). 2006. *Mainstreaming Midwives: The Politics of Change.* New York: Routledge.

Dick-Read, Grantly. 1959. *Childbirth without Fear: The Principles and Practice of Natural Childbirth.* New York: Harper and Row. Originally published 1994.

Gilmore, Elizabeth. 1982. "When Should a Midwife Say No?" *Mothering* 22:72–77.

———. 1984. "Successful Rural Lay Midwifery." Abstract of oral presentation for the International Confederation of Midwives Conference Proceedings, Sydney.

———. 1986. "The Malpractice Crisis." *Mothering* 4040:76–83.

Hazell, Lester D. 1976. *Commonsense Childbirth,* rev. ed. New York, NY: Berkley Books. Originally published 1969.

Johnson, Kenneth C., and Betty-Anne Daviss. 2005. "Outcomes of Planned Home Births with Certified Professional Midwives: Large Prospective Study in North America." *British Medical Journal* 330:1416–1422.

Lee, Anita. 1986. "Northern New Mexico Midwifery Center." *Mothering* 38:66–71.

"The Taos Midwives." 1981. *Mothering* 20:74–86.

FURTHER READING

Chester, Penfield. 1997. *Sisters on a Journey: Portraits of American Midwives.* New Brunswick, NJ: Rutgers University Press.

Huston, Allegra. 2006. "Catching Babies in New Mexico." *Mothering* 136. http://www.mothering.com/articles/pregnancy_birth/midwives_doulas/catching-babies-newmexico.html. Accessed December 3, 2008.

Taylor, Catherine. 2002. *Giving Birth: A Journey into the World of Mothers and Midwives.* New York: Perigree.

PART THREE

Local Models in Developing Nations

*Traditional Midwives, Professional Midwives,
and Obstetricians Working Together*

Chapter 10

Teamwork

An Obstetrician, a Midwife, and a Doula in Brazil

Ricardo Herbert Jones

INTRODUCTION

My name is Ricardo Herbert Jones, and I am an obstetrician. I live in a city in the extreme south of Brazil named Porto Alegre, in the state of Rio Grande do Sul, and I graduated from the Federal University of Rio Grande do Sul in 1985. I work in private practice; that is, women pay out-of-pocket for my services. My cesarean section rates are low, and I work on a sliding scale. All my clients are middle class; they are the women most likely to have a cesarean in the care of any other doctor in my region. This chapter describes my individual paradigm shift and the options that this shift has created for the women in my practice. This "birth model that works" is a replicable model of simplicity: a doctor, a midwife, and a doula attending births in a setting of the woman's choice.

AWAKENING

My initiation into the humanization of childbirth occurred in 1986 when an event in the emergency room of the hospital where I worked as a resident directed my attention (and afterward my whole life) toward the critical questioning of medical assistance at birth. During a weekend shift as a first-year resident, I was called to the emergency room to attend a patient in heavy labor who had walked in from the street. When I opened the door, I saw no one on the table, and I started to scold the nurse for calling me unnecessarily. But she said, "Doctor, please open the door further," and then I saw the woman squatting on the floor in the corner of the room. My immediate reaction was fury. I yelled at her, "You clumsy woman, what are you doing? You cannot give birth on the floor! Can't you see how dirty this is? Get up on the table!" But she gave me no heed; she looked not at me, but right through me, as if I were made of glass. I lifted her skirt and saw the baby's head emerging. I had no time even to put on gloves, and for the first time in my life, I felt the odd sensation of a wet, bloody body in my bare hands. I handed the baby to the nurse as quickly as possible, all the while still yelling at the mother, who was further dirtying the floor with her placenta.

The orderlies got the mother onto the stretcher and whisked her away. The baby, of course, was sent to the neonatal intensive care unit (NICU) because it was "contaminated." Afterward, the nurse said to me, "Doctor, thank goodness you were there! What would have happened without you?" I spent most of the rest of the day feeling annoyed and angry at that woman, and asking myself, "Yes, what would have happened without me?" And then, hours later, the terrible answer hit me: Without me, the birth would have been just fine; in fact, it would have been much better! I had done everything I possibly could to ruin that birth and then had congratulated myself for helping. I felt devastated.

My attitude during this "emergency" was driven by the philosophy and ideology transmitted to me during my medical education, which had not taught me to take into account the human dimension of assistance. This birth showed me how much I was separated from a medicine centered on the individual and from what (I later discovered) was the scientific evidence showing the importance of respect for the patient's subjectivity. The shame I felt ended up obliging me to study and practice alternative forms of birth assistance. I began changing the position of my patients at the moment of birth, encouraging them to adopt vertical positions like that woman in the ER, because it became clear that this position was the most effective physiologically and the best for attending to women's needs. I began slowly to get rid of "standard obstetrical procedures," which later, thanks to the work of American anthropologist Robbie Davis-Floyd (1987, 1992), I came to perceive as rituals, unsupported by scientific evidence. In the years that followed, I abandoned enemas, shaving, artificial rupture of the membranes to speed labor, the electronic fetal monitor, routine IVs, the separation of the woman from her partner and family, episiotomies, fasting, and other rigid, standardized forms of attending birth. That simple woman in the emergency room of the university hospital had given me one of the more important lessons that I have ever had in my entire life, and she did that without saying a single word.

INITIATION

A book that I discovered in the late 1980s, called *A Good Birth, a Safe Birth* by Roberta Scaer and Diana Korte (1992), showed me for the first time the parallels between the physiology of sexual response and childbirth. For me, recently graduated from the traditional medical school (the puritanical keeper of the patriarchal values of our society), this book was a real find. The great secret was unfolding before my eyes: birth and sexuality presented the same set of psycho-organic responses. The second chapter of the book is called "The Pleasure Principle"; it describes how the physiologic adaptations of labor and birth amazingly and surprisingly resemble those of the sexual encounter, like images that get closer in a mirror. There was no way to escape the evidence that was becoming incontestable: sex and birth are physiologically parallel events, but are interpreted as entirely separate. There lay "the best kept secret of the universe," as Ina May Gaskin would tell me a decade later.

Some years ago, I had the opportunity to personally thank Roberta Scaer for this book, and to tell her how much it had helped me understand the erotic dynamic of birth. As soon as I realized the hidden sexuality behind the events that surround birth, I understood that the repercussions of this "new" vision of birth could be nothing but traumatic for the established order. It would no longer be possible to see birth as a mechanical event, artificially controlled by the variables that were taught to me in medical school: fetus, birth canal, and contractile strength. It would be necessary to completely change our perception of birth as transcending the domain of the profane and entering the realm of the sacred. This radical vision made it impossible for me to keep seeing human birth as I used to: sexuality clearly surpasses the boundaries of corporality. As in sex, there's much more in human birth than you can find in the measurements of the body. A new dimension in birth was opened to me—the impossibility of dissociating feeling and emotions from the known physiological aspects of labor and birth. Women showed me though their births the most profound abyss of contemporary medical discourse: the weakness of its concept of "subject." When sexuality emerges with such strength during childbirth it is impossible not to see the uniqueness of the psychological and physiological responses to this event: body and mind inextricably connected.

I realized that many women were unable to have their babies in a more natural way because something *beyond physiology* stopped them. I also began to realize that the degree of pain itself was clearly connected to the way women relate to the experience of labor. Far more subtle (but no less powerful) elements than the cells, tissues, and organs come into play during both sex and labor. It would be our responsibility as maternity care practitioners to discover these other "hidden forces" that, as in sex, were embedded in deeper layers of consciousness.

But how to discover these elements? How to question the positivist pillars of our biomedicine, placing birth at the same level as sexuality, with all its mysteries and taboos? It would be impossible to perceive birth in this way without honoring women and "the feminine," because these events occur in the intimacy of women's bodies. Facing birth as we face sex would oblige us to a special reverence to which we are unaccustomed. To perceive labor and birth, with their sounds and gestures, as movements filled with erotic meanings seems disruptive to one steeped in Western notions; it might lead us to question our own sexuality.

Panic!

It's impossible to enter this new universe opened by understanding the sexual dimension of birth without putting at stake all the authoritarian structures that rule human birth. It would be impracticable to introduce a conceptual change of such magnitude without causing great turbulence, because it challenges the very structure of our patriarchal society. The scars of the contemporary technocratic paradigm related to health care can be seen in the aseptic and cold manner that we manage birth in hospitals. We go deep into tissues, to the dark hideouts of the cells, down to the nucleus and its atoms to dodge the sight of the evidence of the eroticism that sparks from the face of a woman laboring without drugs, refusing to notice how very much she looks like a woman who is making love. We deafen our ears to the moanings, the screams, and the ecstasy of life that ultimately blossoms from the vagina's humidity. For us, it seems unbearable to think that life emerges from such intensity of sensation, in the writhing of a body that twists in the twilight that blurs pleasure and pain. We stop ourselves from seeing this reality by covering the writhing bodies with sheets and drapes, hiding behind our instruments, and putting into flesh the scalpel that ultimately rectifies us: There is nothing that escapes my senses, we think. There is nothing besides the blood that taints my gloves. We breathe in relief, but only till the next woman gets closer to us and shows us on her face the enigmatic smile that hides the secret. Then the wound of the deep knowledge, that we refuse to acknowledge, will bleed again.

This overwhelming discovery of the erotic dynamic of birth obliged me to enter another sphere of comprehension of the parturition phenomenon. I begin to translate every single event during labor, birth, and the puerperium as filled with sexual meaning. I started changing the way I talked to my patients, but I still lacked a real understanding of how to help these women, how to offer them ways to realize their potential. My hope was to discover a key that could open the energies that I noticed were put to sleep by the imposition of rules, protocols, and prohibitions, most of them favoring institutions and the work of doctors and not helping childbearing women. That key took years to emerge, but eventually I found it by putting aside my prejudices and accepting the teachings that circumstances graciously offered me.

MIDDLE-CLASS BIRTH IN PORTO ALEGRE

Sadly, Brazil used to be known as the "Word Champion of Cesareans," a title that has no meaning now because many other countries have cesarean rates that are as high or higher, but that still is widely quoted and still permeates the thinking of many health professionals throughout the world. Nevertheless, Brazil does remain a prime example of interventionism in birth: the amount of money spent on cesareans is unquestionably high, and our cesarean rate, presently at 42.9% (DATASUS/SINASC 2005), is almost three times the maximum rate recommended by the World Health Organization (WHO) of 15% (World Health Organization 1985). The highest rates are found in our private sector: some private hospitals have cesarean rates as high as 99%, and most range between 70% and 90% (DATASUS/SINASC 2005). The rate in the public sector is approximately 28.6% (RIPSA 2007; ANS 2008), but these births still routinely involve disrespect for and objectification of the woman, and many scientifically unjustifiable interventions; in public hospitals, institutional violence against women is the norm. Birth assistance in private hospitals is certainly more gentle and respectful, but the odds of achieving a normal birth are very low.

In my city, Porto Alegre, the odds of a middle-class woman having a vaginal birth are less than 20%. In other words, her chances of cesarean are four out of five. When I ran across women in the mall carrying babies, I used to ask them "Where was your c-section?" When they replied, "How do you know I had a cesarean?" I would smile and say, "Well, you are in a shopping center, a place visited by the middle class. I see your car keys in your hands, and that reinforces me the idea that you belong to the middle class. In this city, your chances of having a vaginal birth were 1 out of 5, so it was easy to guess that you had a cesarean." On the rare occasions when I was wrong, it was always because the woman in question had undergone a tremendous struggle to have her birth the way she wanted to.

My city is well known as one of the most traditional and conservative in the country. The medical model cannot be different from the structure and characteristics of the culture in which it is embedded (Davis-Floyd 2004). We have a clearly technocratic view of health. The local universities are dominated by the positivist and Cartesian paradigm of medicine. The local obstetrical system produces important directors of national associations of obstetricians, all of them linked to the interventionist model. The medical meetings are completely sponsored by the pharmaceutical industry, a phenomenon that works to block discussion of any model of assistance not strongly connected to a drug-oriented understanding of pathologies. We have not created an effective counterpoint to the economic power of the industrial conglomerates and hospitals.

Another important characteristic of my city (and state) lies in the professional groups related to birth assistance. We differ from all the other states of Brazil in not allowing nurse-midwives to attend low-risk births, even though nurse-midwives have been recognized as primary birth assistants in all the other states for many years. In the obstetric wards of private hospitals in Porto Alegre, it is almost impossible to find a birth without intervention. Most of the few vaginal births are conducted with shaving, enemas, lithotomy position, pitocin, epidurals, and episiotomies. When I read *A Good Birth, a Safe Birth* at the end of the 1980s, there was as yet no space in my city for a discussion about evidence-based medicine. The very mention of birth as sexual would sound indecent and heretical. Human birth was—and still is—understood as a medical event to be technologically conducted, full of dangers and risks and likely to produce mutilation and death if not controlled with skill and ability and . . . only by doctors.

It was in this medical and cultural context that I first realized the idea of "birth as a part of a woman's sexual life," words that Michel Odent would say to me later. This discovery, as I mentioned above, became fundamental to the path I decided to take. It was no longer possible to look at a birthing woman with the same eyes. Women continue to surprise me at each birth, each blossoming of life. And despite all the attacks I receive from my colleagues for my rebellious attitude, I continue to treasure the deeply feminine smiles on their sweaty faces. As a man participating in a women's secret circle, my attitude could only be, from the moment I discovered the mystery, one of reverence and respect.

THE MYSTERY OF PAGE 130

Brazilians tend to think of Buenos Aires as a city where we can "breathe civilization." The civilized behavior of the people from that city always delights us. In return, Argentinians see our happiness and spontaneity as our best qualities. I was studying in the charming capital of Argentina in 1993 in the Paschero School of Homeopathy, and my colleagues and I spent the nights discussing our new lessons while walking in the well-lit *calles*. This is a city where one can walk safely late at night and find an elegant coffee shop and some marvelous secondhand bookstores. The downtown, different from the big capitals in Brazil, is a living organism during the evening. The clean sidewalks, the elegant people, and the blondish women give us the vivid sensation that we are in Europe as we watch the couples heading toward the theaters and tango houses.

It was in one of these Buenos Aires bookstores that I suddenly found the book on a bookshelf—a used Spanish edition. On the tattered cover I could see a doctor holding a woman, helping her have her baby in a squatting position. I could see her only from the waist up, and her face carried an intriguing expression. She appeared not to be in pain. Her chin pointed toward the ceiling; her mouth was open. She appeared to be smiling, but there was something really strange in the way that woman was expressing herself.

I was immediately galvanized by the cover, and skimmed the pages, filled with black and white pictures, with intense curiosity. At that time I was already assisting squatting births in my city, and my path as a doctor "outside the box" was well established. Some years before, I had read *Learn How to Birth with the Indians* by the Brazilian obstetrician Moysés Paciornik (1997), and the idea of a *parto selvagem* ("savage" or "wild" birth) was a well-established concept for me. I still lacked a more profound comprehension of the strategy needed to bring forth the strength that women have in birth, but, step by step, I was building a more complete image, adding little pieces made of experiences, stories, and concepts to the gigantic puzzle of human birth.

Before my friends could complain about my delay, I bought the book, not knowing at the time that it would open new doors of perception for me about "the miracle of birth." The book was *Nacimiento Renascido*, the Spanish edition of the remarkable book *Birth Reborn* (1984) by the French doctor Michel Odent—a decade later it would be translated into Portuguese. It described his experience with childbirth in a small city near Paris called Pithiviers.

I devoured the pages of that book. I could barely wait to show everyone what I had discovered. It was becoming clear that the humanization of birth was an issue that involved people from different latitudes. Odent's vision was so close to the ideals I pursued that it gave me hope that my ideas as an obstetrician might someday be understood, too. But in addition to confirming the philosophies and practices I had nurtured in lonely isolation for years, that book showed me something I didn't expect: a limit, a boundary, a dead end. On page 130 there was a picture that shocked me more than any other in the book. It possessed strength and an impact that made the others look like ordinary images. Breech birth, water birth, birth assisted by the woman's partner were already familiar in my modest experience, but that picture has never left the wall of my warmest memories. It was a picture of intimacy, harmony, closeness, and compassion.

In this picture, Dominique, a Pithiviers midwife, holds in her arms a naked woman on the floor on the obstetric ward. Their bodies connected, their arms interwoven, and their heads down and touching showed a bond of empathy and communion, a union of bodies and spirits, the like of which I had never seen between patient and caregiver, *and could never achieve.* That was the limit; that was my shock. That picture shed light on a personal mystery: Why did my cesarean rates reach a certain point and then stop going down? Why couldn't I overcome some of the inexplicable obstacles in the conduct of birth? Why, even practicing as humanistically as possible, did I keep performing more interventions than I wanted to? The answer came to me synthesized in the rawness of that picture, in the touch, the closeness, the affection, and the intimacy I could witness. Things now started, slowly, to make sense, and this new discovery was accompanied by the sadness of my unbridgeable barrier. It would be useless to deny that my condition as a man in a Latin culture would prevent me from having the kind of intimacy shown in the picture. The contact that Dominique provided to her patient was out of my reach. The limits of propriety determined by the culture and society I live in prevented me from that kind of deep, physical intimacy with the women I attended.

Where you stumble, there your treasure lies. I decided to face the picture on page 130 as a challenge to creativity, and not as a barrier, and a new and stimulating dimension opened before my eyes. I realized that the presence of the feminine component could facilitate the free flow of the sexual energies present at birth. I found, if not a complete answer, a truly seductive clue. Women present at birth *as women,* and not as obstetricians or other kinds of professionals who hide behind technology, could add what I lacked in my lonely work as an obstetrician and might actually be accepted by the obstetrical community.

Obstetrics is an intense, socializing force that works to obscure the natural femininity of female obstetricians, and thus their presence at birth could not add feminine elements that could make a positive difference. The rates of interventions and cesareans among the female obstetricians in my area were even higher than those of my male colleagues, showing that the fact that they were women did not work to humanize their care. Female obstetricians clearly perceived that their acceptance by the medical community could be achieved only through their incorporation of the specific masculine values of medical practice. Without that, they would be seen as fragile and weak, incompetent to deal with the toughness and complexity of medicine.

It seemed to me that a door was being opened in front of me. To add femininity to childbirth through the incorporation of women in birth was a seductive idea. But how to achieve it? How to make this change? What today seems obvious, over a decade ago in Brazil seemed insurmountable. At that time, I had never encountered the works of Klaus and Kennell, and I had only just read Michel Odent's first book.

How to make this change?

A "PROTOCOL FOR HUMANIZED OBSTETRIC ASSISTANCE" (PHOA)

From 1989 to 1993, I did obstetric shifts on the periphery of the Porto Alegre, in a hospital in a very poor area—as it turned out, one of the best apprenticeships possible for learning about the reality of birth in my country. There I saw the problems, the violence, and the destructive nature of the maternity care system for poor women in Brazil. At the same time, I was working as an obstetrician and gynecologist in a small military hospital in the city of Canoas, just a few miles away from Porto Alegre. In this hospital I was working with two other obstetricians. One of my colleagues and I were interested in creating a better way of working—based on actual evidence, supporting normal birth, and respecting women's agency. The third colleague was a dyed-in-the-wool interventionist, who did not accept the principles of humanization because he deeply believed in the biological inferiority of women. One day, during breakfast in the hospital cafeteria, I noted to my sympathetic colleague that the two of us composed two-thirds of the medical maternity assistance at that hospital, and that a profound change in obstetric outcomes there depended solely on our initiative. At that time, although we were assisting no more than twenty low-risk births a month, our small maternity unit had the shameful cesarean rate of 45%. We couldn't convince our colleague to work our way because he didn't accept our values, so we decided to create a protocol that the two of us could use to decrease the cesarean rate. This protocol consisted of four simple points:

1. Every indication for a cesarean should be discussed with a colleague.
2. Women should be encouraged to give birth in upright positions.
3. Patients should have the right to the companion of their choice.
4. Practices would be based on scientific evidence.

Only the two of us used this model, while our colleague continued to use his traditional way. With two-thirds of births based on this simple protocol, in two months our hospital's cesarean rate dropped from 45% to 22%; probably the lowest rate in our state. What results might we have obtained if all three of us had been using this protocol? This simple initiative showed the power of individual decisions—in this case made by just a couple of doctors—to produce significant change, albeit on a small scale. Unfortunately, because this model depended completely on our personal (and not an institutional) initiative, it ceased to exist after I left the hospital, for my colleague needed support and could not carry it on alone. Nevertheless, the exciting results of this initiative stimulated me to make a fundamental decision about my private practice, which I opened during this period. The births that I attended in this incipient private practice served as a counterpoint to what I witnessed in the public hospital where I worked on shift. These few, humanized births were the source from which I drew the hope of building a better and more integrative model.

My only companions were the books, the medical journals that came from other countries, and the benevolent ears of my wife. In part to better understand my anxieties, she decided to study nurse-midwifery during this period. Her decision turned out to be an amazing help for the rest of my life. From 1986 to 1998, I had no other doctors with whom to dialogue about nonviolent practices in childbirth. The few colleagues that dared to listen to my words discouraged me with responses like "That only works for Indians; civilized women can't squat for birth" and "This is just a romantic and naïve approach; get over it!"

Despite such criticisms from my colleagues, my former teachers, and even some of my patients, my determination and obstinacy didn't allow me to stop. I knew that doctors' attitudes toward birth were profoundly embedded in their core values (Davis-Floyd 2004). I understood that the repetitive violence that I witnessed was not coincidental: it was determined by a belief system grounded in our social unconscious. We were rude and insensitive to pregnant women because society acted in the same way toward women and feminine values. My actions as an obstetrician, like someone receiving a special cultural assignment or role, maintained and disseminated these values. I was equally responsible for a reality that was unfair, violent, and unacceptable. Something had to be done to change the situation: it seemed to me that if we could change the way we conduct human birth, it would be possible to produce a cascade effect that would reverberate in the whole social structure. Many years later, I would listen to Michel Odent's words, "To change society it is necessary to change the way we are born"—words that confirmed what I had been intuiting.

In the face of these ideas and the need to produce something concrete in relation to medical conduct during labor and birth, in 1990 I created a "Protocol for Humanized Obstetric Assistance" (PHOA), a list of basic principles that would guide my professional obstetric practice from that time on. It contained five points:

1. *Appropriate environment.* This meant a cozy room without interruption from strange people, no sound of machines or instruments, with music if desired, low lighting, and above all an environment privileging the intimacy that an event of a sexual nature deserves. Obviously, this could not be achieved without causing some degree of conflict in the hospital. At the time I created this protocol, I also established the routine of asking the nursing staff to knock on the door every time they wanted to enter the labor room, because I understood that this moment of intimacy should not be abruptly broken. Even this simple request caused conflict with hospital personnel, who complained that they were being "constrained in their daily routines." No step toward humanization would be easy.

2. *Emotional support.* This meant my constant presence in the hospital with the mother from the beginning of labor to the end. I followed one of the aphorisms that I found in the writings of Balint (1957) that "the doctor's best prescription is himself": the doctor's presence is a fundamental part of the treatment because of its calming effect. (Doctors can be more than iatrogenic!) Beyond that, the presence of family members, mostly the husband, was encouraged, because I noticed the calming effect of his presence and its benefits on labor progress. A recent study of women's response to pain showed that during an artificially stimulated pain,

a woman's stress response was significantly lower if she was holding her husband's hand—a question of common sense now backed up by scientific measurement (Coan, Schaefer, and Davidson 2006). At this time and still today, it was common for doctors to stay at their private offices for as long as possible while the nurses cared for their laboring patients in the hospital, with orders to call them only when pushing began. The nurses, already overwhelmed with paperwork, had little time to stay at the bedsides of the many patients in the obstetric ward. The obvious result was that women were isolated and alone, which put them into the vicious cycle of fear-tension-pain described by Grantly Dick-Read (2004) so many decades ago.

3. *Restricted use of drugs during labor.* The multiple interactions of drugs can negate the action of endogenous (natural) oxytocin, adrenalin, and endorphins. The principle is not to interfere by using drugs unless a serious enough problem warrants their use. To meet the demand for attention to pain, and lacking the resources that I would acquire only later on (like doulas and water), I created a pain relief protocol with six levels:

- Emotional Management—The constant presence of the doctor, conversation, explanation of the stages of labor, reassurance, and encouragement
- General Measures—Hot baths, walking, massages done by the woman's companions, stretching exercises, hot packs, acupressure
- Homeopathy—Homeopathic remedies applied to specific individuals under appropriate circumstances (homeopathy is a highly individualized form of care)
- Analgesic Drugs—Acetaminophen
- Opiates—Pethidine
- Epidural analgesia

I used this list in descending order, applying the next thing on the list only if the previous one was not sufficient. So only when I failed with emotional and general measures did I resort to homeopathy, and so on down the list. With this protocol, the vast majority of my patients didn't reach level 4, and almost 100% didn't go past level 5 (use of opiates). In 1,612 births, I used an epidural with only one patient, in spite of the fact that this resource was available to almost all of them.

4. *Upright positions preferable.* I came to determine that the standard for birth assistance should be the position that privileged the physiology of birth. My determination was strongly influenced by Drs. Cláudio and Moysés Paciornik, who studied Brazilian indigenous tribes and the advantages of upright birth (a term I use to mean that the patient is in a vertical position—squatting, sitting, standing, or sometimes on hands

TABLE 10.1 Comparison of outcomes in private and public hospitals
for births attended by Ricardo Jones
(percent of all births)

Variables/Protocols	Traditional: 1980–1990	PHOA: 1990–1998
Cesareans	23.9	15.7
Forceps	21.7	6.9
Acute fetal stress	4.4	1.2
Episiotomy	72.5	24.7

and knees) (Paciornik 1990). Of course, my patients could choose to lie down if that was their desire, but I stopped using the lithotomy position routinely because I noticed the various problems that it created for the mechanism of birth. Upright birth produces repercussions that go far beyond the enlargement of the passage for the fetus and the unquestionable benefits for the physiology of both mothers and babies. It symbolically inverts the birth hierarchy: now women are "on top" and thus in control (Davis-Floyd 2004). Their agency and position as the central protagonist in birth is assured, thus creating a new balance of forces. A woman in an upright position has much more control over the environment and all the other actors, and this postural change has repercussions for her psyche.

5. *Restrictive criteria for use of interventions and maneuvers.* This means a firm and continued questioning of the obstetric routines/rituals used indiscriminately in hospitals (Davis-Floyd 2004; Wagner 1999), such as episiotomy, forceps, shaving, enema, fasting, epidurals, surgical masks, routine IV, electronic fetal monitoring (EFM), and the language used (like "sweetie" instead of the woman's name), among others. This is one of the most difficult protocols to apply in hospitals because these nonreflexive and non-evidence-based practices are firmly attached to the work of caregivers in obstetric wards, and not even the most rational arguments are able to stop their endless repetition.

After I attended my fifteen hundredth birth in the year 1998, I gathered the statistics for all the births I had assisted with under my humanized protocols, and I did an evaluation of the outcomes. The numbers were compelling and significant, essentially because they compared *the same obstetrician* working under two different protocols. The first group began after my graduation from medical school, from 1986 to 1990. More than a change in the application of specific techniques, the change in my way of assisting birth emerged from a change in my *attitude* toward childbirth. The principal outcomes that I collected from my own data are presented in Table 10.1.

In addition, I noted that with the adoption of a restrictive protocol in relation to episiotomy, one-third of my patients had intact perinea after birth, and 64% had vaginal tears that were less damaging than an episiotomy would have been. These data agreed with the data I found in the international literature (Woolley 1995) and indicated, each time with more emphasis, the value of a conservative attitude toward the perineum (Carroli and Belizan 1999). This correlation reinforced my conviction that the episiotomy doesn't represent any advantage for laboring women and is routinely used only as an initiation ritual comparable to clitoridectomy in traditional Islamic societies (Wagner 1999; "Episiotomy" n.d.), or as tonsillectomy and circumcision in modern Western cultures (Bolande 1969).

Another piece of data that emerged from my analysis was the 57.6% rate of VBACs (vaginal birth after cesarean) observed in the PHOA group that was similar to the results seen by some other researchers, who showed VBAC success in two-thirds of the patients, but below others that showed more than 80% positive results (Agency for Health Research and Quality 2003).

I defined acute fetal distress as when the decelerations were intense enough to indicate a cesarean. The use of upright positions and not using routine fetal monitoring (which requires immobilizing the woman) made my incidence of acute fetal distress fall dramatically from 4.4% to 1.2%.

Meanwhile, my struggles continued in spite of the dramatic enhancements produced by my adoption of the PHOA. It was no longer possible for me to see birth as a dangerous and fickle process; on the contrary, I could see the grandeur that was sleeping in its hidden essence. The writings that began to come to my hands from Marsden Wagner (1994), Ina May Gaskin (1975), Henci Goer (1995, 1999), Michel Odent (1990, 2000), Janet Balaskas (1989), Brigitte Jordan (1993), Emily Martin (1987), Elizabeth Davis (1993), Wenda Trevathan (1987), and principally Robbie Davis-Floyd (2004, 1987, 1998) showed me a much more open path and a completely different direction from the narrow box of contemporary medical thinking. Slowly, I began to perceive the *ultrastructure* that governs human birth under a belief system that goes far beyond our rational comprehension.

The evidence captivated me but at the same time brought me anxiety. My most troubling concern was why my work as a humanistic doctor stopped at a specific point without going beyond. My cesarean rates seemed stuck around 20%. Why? I continued accumulating failures that I did not understand, even though my overall intervention rates were much lower than those of the other doctors around me, and were very close to the WHO recommendations. At the same time, I could not accept the diagnosis of "failure to progress" or even CPD (cephalopelvic disproportion) in babies of less than 3.5 kilograms (7 pounds). There was something beyond my comprehension that was acting in the unfolding of these births and producing a barrier to their success, by which I mean a physiologic birth with little or no intervention. The years after the end of my residency, from 1986 until 1997, were a period of silence, introspection, solitary study, and professional isolation.

CRISTINA

She came to my office very pregnant, bringing her story under her arm, mixed with a few copies of the results of prenatal exams. She told me that her previous birth had been in Rio de Janeiro, and that she had been supported by a yoga teacher with the odd name of Fadynha (little fairy). Her baby ended up being born into Fadynha's hands because the doctor did not arrive in time, and Fadynha was the only person present who had some birth experience. This story immediately reminded me of my own personal birth mythology as recounted by my mother. She said I had come to this world in a hurry, with the speed of "one who cannot wait." I was born into the warm hands of a midwife—at that time, midwives still worked in the hospitals of Porto Alegre—because the doctor was delayed, and there was no time to wait. My foundational myth, my birth legend: I was not born on demand; I established for myself my moment to arrive in this world, breaking barriers and disobeying. I believe that, much more than the reality of this fact, my conceptual interpretation of my birth can explain much of my personal history and the paths I followed in this life, even the profession I chose and the direction I took inside that profession. I used to joke that my birth established a profound debt with midwifery, and that I married a midwife as a way to pay a part of this debt.

Cristina continued her description of her birth. She told me that she had moved to Porto Alegre after a divorce, and that the baby she was now pregnant with was from a new relationship. Her big green eyes were looking for a place to hang her hopes. She gazed at me with firmness, as if she knew that what she was asking me was her own choice. "I found an interview with you in an alternative magazine. In this article, you talked about squatting birth and the possibility of having a 'birth without violence' in the Leboyer style. Can I count on you to attend me?" I said yes and told her that the fact she already had had a previous birth according to her desire, and with whom she wished, was a strong indication that she could do it again. We agreed on the presence of her mother, on the idea of having music in the birthing room, on surgical intervention only if absolutely necessary, and on the squatting position for birth. I continued to attend her through the prenatal period until the birth of her son, Miguel, who came into the world through a normal hospital birth.

The story of Cristina could stop there, and I would still be searching for an answer to the mystery of page 130. But much to my good fortune, she returned to my office after a few weeks for a routine postnatal visit, holding her chubby son, Miguel, and made a statement that still echoes in my ears. "I am a doula, Dr. Ricardo. Do you know what that is?" I said no; I had never heard this word at that time. This was 1998, and the works of Klaus and Kennell (see Sosa et al. 1980) had not yet come to my attention. Cristina looked into my eyes and continued: "Doulas are women who help women in their births. They give emotional and physical support to women in labor. They are not midwives; they don't perform medical procedures; they don't interfere with the work of other professionals. They don't listen to the fetal heart tones or take the blood pressure. Their focus is the well-being of the woman. I am a doula; I was born to do this work. And we are going to work together."

She spoke simply and straight to the point, inviting me to work as a team with her. In a way, *she* was hiring *me*. Her proposal was to offer her work to my patients as a pregnancy yoga teacher and a doula (she was also a physiotherapist). But what was this "doula thing"? What could this add to my work as an obstetrician? Would it produce positive results to have another person in the birth scenario?

Cristina continued explaining to me what she had read about the role of these professionals. It turned out that up until this time, she had never actually worked as a doula; she had only recently discovered this calling. Like other doulas that I met later in working for the humanization of birth, she felt that working together with laboring women was a spiritual calling. When she first read about doulas, she thought to herself, "That's what I want to do for the rest of my life." Later, Debra Pascali-Bonaro, an American doula from New Jersey, told me a similar story about her awakening to the doula calling—as a woman who helps women—and she said the same about the countless other women who ask to take her doula trainings: "Women get magnetized by the magic of birth." Robbie Davis-Floyd said something similar when she described the awakening of traditional midwives: they, too, feel a call, a strong spiritual force that drives them to a "mission" of midwifery. It's as if these women look for birth to absorb the tremendous energy that emanates from birth, and through this force, they nourish themselves and spread this feminine energy wherever they go. Many doulas I have met throughout the world speak jokingly of their work as an "addiction," something that you can't stop doing once you have started. (For more information about doulas, see www.dona.org/mothers/index.php.)

For a medical professional to "work in a team" most of the time means sharing actions over the body of a patient with other professionals. The pneumologist treats the lungs of the sick person, asking his nephrologist colleague to check on the kidneys while the surgeon takes out a tumor. The system is dissociative. It understands human beings as machines composed of relatively separate compartments, each of which has its own medical specialist, reserving little attention for the whole. This system is conventionally called "multidisciplinarity"—a group of professionals acting autonomously, portioning out the body according to their knowledge and skills.

Cristina was proposing something different. She wanted to work together with me, collaboratively and integratively, without rigid hierarchies or separation of body parts while acknowledging each others' differing competencies. Cristina didn't want to be my "helper," not even my "assistant," but to work side by side with me to offer our patients the support that would facilitate for these women a more complete experience of birth. Her proposal was horizontality in opposition to hierarchy.

My initial contact with Cristina made my curiosity grow. I began to search for literature on this subject and soon found the works of the American doctors John Kennell and Marshall and Phyllis Klaus. In this way, I discovered the history of doulas, their origin and cultural meaning. I came to know the epic story of Wendy in Guatemala, who subverted a medical research project by staying at the side of laboring women. The data showed that her presence had a positive effect on their labors, and so the study was modified to better understand this effect (Klaus, Klaus, and Kennell 1993). I ended up getting interested in the anthropology of birth, and found in the books of the anthropologist Wenda Trevathan the answer that I had long sought to the enigmatic picture on page 130. It has been so important to my work that I always quote this sentence from Wenda in my lectures and workshops, at the same time revolutionary and clarifying: "The roots of social support during labor and delivery are as ancient as the human species itself, and one of the reasons for the dissatisfaction with the way in which childbirth is practiced in many industrialized nations is the failure of the medical system to acknowledge and work with the evolved emotional needs of women at this time" (Trevathan, Smith, and McKenna 1999: 183).

The mists that surrounded the mystery picture on page 130 slowly began to dissolve. Step by step, I could understand more deeply that the contact, the gentle touch, the continuous presence, and the physically expressed affection were a part of the "deep unconscious" that women evolved during our adaptive process. My difficulty in surpassing culturally determined barriers was because of the fact that my condition as a man kept me from being able to act as I saw Dominique acting in Odent's book. Such closeness and contact would be prohibitive and scandalous if it were a man who was not her partner on the other side of that embrace. In the domain of the patriarchy, this kind of intimacy is forbidden. To break this invisible barrier and offer women the support that depended on accessing the more subtle layers of affectivity could happen only if I worked with women, substantially changing my structure of assistance. No more the omnipotence of doing everything, but rather the challenge of immobility and the humility of realizing that not everything was within my reach. I wanted to offer superior results, like those I read about at the Farm in Tennessee, where midwife Ina May Gaskin worked. Ina May says that there is a feminine aura that suffuses everything and everyone, which she calls "birth energy" (Gaskin, personal communication). The cesarean rate at the Farm was around 1.4%, and the neonatal mortality rates were similar to the rates achieved by the best obstetric services around the world, while both the maternal and neonatal morbidity rates were lower (Gaskin 1975). The mystery was solved: to improve my work it would be necessary to feminize it.

THE BEGINNING OF TEAMWORK

Our teamwork began in an unusual way. Cristina had never actually worked as a doula, nor did I have an exact idea about Cristina's spectrum of work. Our opening act was frustrating. A patient in her early forties came to my practice; she was interested in a normal birth and came to see me because the doctors in my city made it clear that at her age, a normal birth was contraindicated. She knew that she had little possibility of achieving her goal if she remained with those doctors; the odds were against her.

I talked with Cristina many times about what we might encounter during this birth. Slowly, I was acquiring confidence in her ideas and attitudes. But destiny didn't want our first patient to get what we were all hoping for. The fetal presentation was breech until the end of pregnancy, and all our attempts to turn the baby failed. (At that time, I had not learned how to do external version, which later I did learn from the traditional midwives of Mexico.) Because she was a *primigravida* (a woman pregnant for the first time), we opted for a cesarean. Cristina was present in the hospital during the prep and the surgery, and created a very strong and consistent attachment with the patient. I perceived that the work of doulas could be important even in the surgical ward because the calm, tranquil attitude of the patient had positive effects on the outcome of the surgery.

Little by little, as long as we were talking and exchanging ideas about our work, we began to establish a special way of organizing our assistance. Everything had to be created from scratch; nothing had been taught to me. This kind of labor support had never been discussed during my years of medical school and residency as part of any known medical approach. Even the word "doula" had never been said by any colleague obstetrician before my conversation with Cristina. We had to create a way of working that was completely different from what I had learned.

Our collaborative path unfolded as we faced each new birth, a challenge full of questions awaiting answers. Cristina gave yoga classes and group classes for pregnant couples about preparation for birth. She referred those of her clients who were eager for a humanized birth to me for prenatal care. Other clients took the reverse road: I referred them to Cristina to work with her during pregnancy. We were coming closer in our approaches and learning with each patient. We discussed every case, debating the failures, victories, doubts, and difficulties of each birth process, searching always for the most integrative view. So step by step, we built a model of assistance that combined technical obstetrical knowledge with holistic attention to the physical, emotional, psychological, and spiritual aspects of birth.

With time, we established some routines that emerged in a natural way as we learned from our patients. For a long time I had been noticing the iatrogenesis that resulted from a laboring woman simply being in a hospital. Clearly and consistently, one could observe the changes in the attitude and behavior of the "patients" when they entered that physical space. Contractions that had been rhythmic and strong simply disappeared when the mother entered the obstetric ward. There was something in this abrupt change of scene that produced profound psychological alterations in women whose bodies, exposed to a possible threat, reacted unconsciously to protect themselves, just as a deer's labor stops when the hunter draws near.

Ask any child why hospitals exist, and she will tell you without hesitation, "to treat sick people." That's why the German word for hospital is "Krankenhaus." When women are interned in maternity units, they transform into patients even when they have no pathology. The discourse of doctors constantly repeated that pregnancy was *not* a disease, but this discourse disappeared into an immense vacuum when I observed that their practices were diametrically opposed to what they were saying. The interventions they repeatedly applied could only be justified if one sees the women as sick. Under such conditions of "sickification," it is normal for women's bodies to react with tension and fear, opening the gates to adrenalin and its protective effects (Moberg 2003: 15).

Our cultural and social development as human beings occurred mostly during our long journey as hunters and gatherers, a period that encompasses more than 95% of our time on this planet. We lived in an environment of evolutionary transformation, and there, in the struggle to survive, we developed our most sophisticated systems of protection. The autonomous sympathetic nervous system is the result of millennia of sophisticated adaptation to changing environments, but it can become an obstacle to good labor progress. This fact is observable in the day-to-day operations of maternity units, and is the consequence of our inability to understand the phenomena that rule the deep physiology of birth. The massive migration of birth from home to hospital in the early decades of the 20th century left by the side of the road a good part of our evolutionary knowledge about birth, relegating to the emerging science of obstetrics the task of caring for women and their births. Unfortunately, besides some important progress in dealing with pathologies in birth, we saw the dismantling of women's previous systems of social and emotional support. Birth stopped being a social event, surrounded by social and religious rituals and symbols, and became a medical event, surrounded by medical and technological rituals and symbols in which, as Marsden Wagner says, "strangers manipulate strange machines that make strange sounds" (personal communication). Nevertheless, as Wenda Trevathan affirms, anyone with eyes to see will come to experience, in this separation from the affective nucleus of birth and in the denial of its immanent sexuality, the vivid sensation that something is wrong (Trevathan, Smith, and McKenna 1999: 183).

HOME LABOR

My medical training included some important, formative experiences. One of them was that I worked as a student (and also after graduation) in the services of *Pronto-Socorro* (clinics that provide emergency home assistance). On these occasions, I could note that people's homes held signs and clues related to the specific diseases they had. The elements present when I arrived to assist with an emergency (which varied from fractures to fights between couples) were extremely significant and rich, informing my diagnosis. The conversations with the family, the placing of the furniture, the fences, the well-kept (or unkempt) garden, the animus of the couple and children, the *psychosphere* of the house, were all elements constitutive of a whole that needed to be understood. Over the years, I made an effort to capture these elements as important clues in my search to understand the people who had asked for my help.

During this initial period of work with Cristina, I received a call from Ana, single and seven months pregnant with her first child. In a tense and apprehensive voice, she said she had been having contractions for some hours and was scared that her baby might come early. She needed a medical evaluation so that we could be sure it was not a premature birth. We agreed to meet at the hospital, but when I asked her where she lived, I realized that she was my neighbor, so I decided that it would be much smarter for me just to go to her house to check her. I grabbed a Doppler and some sterile gloves and headed out.

I talked for a long time with Ana. She explained her present difficulties—being single and without the support of a partner. The house, her room, the books on the shelves, the cold greeting I received from her mother, her bed, her introspection, and her fear—I would have known none of these elements had she gone to the hospital, decontextualized from her world of symbols and significances. The experience was remarkable, and I saw that full comprehension of a human being—one who suffers or (as in the case of a pregnant woman) one who is passing through a critical life stage—can be achieved only if her psychosphere and the environment she lives in are seen and considered as a integral part of the whole.

If we consider that the way we treat pregnant women individually or culturally determines the outcomes that we obtain in relation to birth, it becomes obvious that our *relationship* with the woman during pregnancy and labor—with its convergence of fears, anxieties, memories, and physical pain—will be key. According to Trevathan, it is highly likely that women have supported women during labor since the advent of bipedalism and the narrower pelvis it required (Trevathan 1987). The fact that we walk upright put us on the path that inevitably would lead us to the domains of symbol and language—semiotics—changing the course of our natural history. It also determined that childbirth assistance would be necessary, making birth a social and integrative event, in contrast to the births of the majority of mammals, who give birth in isolation.

Influenced by these important experiences and by the writings of Robbie Davis-Floyd, I began to abandon the hospital environment because I saw that it was a strong generator of tension. Cristina and I agreed that child-birth assistance should begin at the patient's home, so when a patient began to have her first consistent contractions, instead of meeting at the hospital, Cristina went to the woman's house to begin the exercises, the massages, the stretching, and all the other aspects of doula care. When the contractions reached a certain point of frequency and intensity, Cristina would call to give me a report. After confirming that labor was well established, we would all meet in the hospital where we would attend the mother until the baby was born. This model meant that many patients came to the hospital in advanced labor because the delay at home offered them the chance to escape early admission. The doula, even though she didn't do any medical or nursing activities, offered to the patient the tranquility she needed to labor at home. Cristina's presence in women's houses assured that the first part of the labor process would take place in a calm and familiar environment. When the women arrived to the maternity ward, they had already overcome many fears and achieved some centimeters of dilation.

Soon I decided that I would go to the houses of my patients, too. Instead of doing labor assistance in the tension-filled hospital environment, together with Cristina, I would allow them to stay in the warmth of their homes for as long as possible.

It quickly became clear that home labor assistance had incalculable advantages over the traditional model. The monitoring of contractions, fetal well-being, blood pressure, cervical dilation, and fetal descent could be done in a simple way with simple technology that any caregiver can bring. Helping the woman stay with her family, in her domain, positively reinforces her sense of safety and keeps her out of the vicious, adrenalin-loaded cycle of fear–tension–pain, as Grantly Dick-Read explained decades ago (Dick-Read 2004). Even the most gentle hospital care always carries the symbolic weight of being given in the hospital, where the patient is understood and treated as sick, and the technology—and thus the likelihood—of intervention is omnipresent. Many successful experiences taught me the multiple advantages of supporting the woman to stay in her home for as long as possible during labor.

ZEZA AND HOME BIRTH

Zeza, my wife, followed with curiosity the changes that my work with Cristina was producing. It is not inappropriate to note that a little bit of jealousy of the time I was spending with Cristina was part of what motivated her. Trained in nursing, she had decided to specialize in nurse-midwifery. Probably my deep interest in obstetrics and my all-absorbing passion for humanizing childbirth stimulated her to make this move, and Zeza had a special leaning toward midwifery. Her maternal way of acting, her sweetness, the love her patients feel for her, and her personal experience as the mother of two imbued her with the essential qualifications to care for women during this special time. She had not yet ventured to participate in births with me, but when my work with Cristina began to produce such good results, she thought it could be a great opportunity to recapture her nurse-midwifery leanings and her passion for birth assistance, and to put into practice what she had learned in her postgraduate midwifery program.

The work of the nurse-midwives in my region has a notable characteristic: nurse-midwives, postgraduates in obstetric nursing, are allowed to assist birth by law, but not by the hospitals or doctors, who limit them to working as obstetrician assistants. They perform the same work as obstetrical nurses in the United States—they work in the obstetric wards, they admit patients in labor and care for them, but they are forbidden to provide direct assistance in childbirth, such as checking dilation, administering drugs, catching babies, or giving prenatal care. Postgraduate training in midwifery generates in nurses the expectation and hope of assisting births and working with pregnant women, and the denial of this possibility produces frustration and resentment. Zeza was not an exception. Used to discussing obstetric cases with me every day for many years, she was saddened to see that her natural talent and desires were going to waste. She worked as a general nurse in the health centers of Porto Alegre, and despite receiving a good salary, she knew she could do much more with her midwifery training and skills.

But she felt tied to a model centered on the doctor as the authoritative figure in birth care. Her only short-term alternative would be to work as an independent midwife outside the hospital, attending home births. But which doctors would give her support and backup for this kind of work? Obstetricians in my city considered it dangerous, and they did not want the competition. How to face and fight the medical monopoly? More than that, how to overcome her own fear and lack of experience? Zeza probably would not find an obstetrician to give her this kind of support—but her husband obstetrician would!

Our collaborative work began in 1999 when a patient requested a home birth. At that time, home births were still a great challenge for me. In spite of having attended a few—described in my first book, *Memoirs of a Man Made of Glass* (Jones 2004)—the fear that home birth caused for me was still significant. The idea that the most important factor for the success of a normal birth was the ideological attitude of the caregiver (see the Conclusion to this volume) was already a part of me, but between rationality and fear, there was a considerable space still to cross. Nevertheless, my patient's firm insistence on a home birth helped us find the necessary courage. And so it was that Zeza and I went together to our first joint home birth.

Our patient lived in a middle-class apartment and was married to a young lawyer. Labor seemed to me to be surprisingly calm, as I had observed it usually was in the few other home births I had attended prior to that one. Home birth tasted different, with its aura of tranquility and familiarity. There was no fear and no hurry; pain was a part of the process and not its most salient feature. The contractions evolved smoothly, and the intervals between them were filled with smiles, caresses, low murmurs, and cinnamon tea.

Little Luis arrived to the world in Zeza's hands. He didn't cry. As soon as he was born, he was nested in his mother's lap, and there he remained until he began to breastfeed. Later, Zeza would tell me that "to be born at home is a whole other story." All that she had seen during her nursing training was insufficient to describe the magic of home birth. I recorded the birth on my first (huge) digital camera (which today would be considered a museum piece). This was the beginning of a custom I continue today—I use the birth photos we take to create a beautiful slide show set to music as a gift to the birthing couple. After every birth we attend, we come back to the patient's house, and all together, we talk over the events of the day before and watch the slide show. These are always very moving moments.

Zeza understood clearly that this moment was the awakening of a sleeping passion that had long been pulsing inside her. Her journey as an independent professional midwife had finally begun, and there was no turning back. From this moment on, Zeza became part of our team. We were now a team of three professionals: an obstetrician, a midwife, and a doula, offering support to pregnant women in hospitals and at home. This simple framework for birth care is intended to support women's needs from a fully humanistic perspective, centered in women and their needs. Its goal is to restore to birth the sacred feminine, stripped away from it by modern obstetrics. The core of this goal is *women helping women,* offering physical, emotional, psychological, and spiritual support to the ones who are passing through this important rite of passage, reclaiming a model that evolved over a hundred thousand years ago. My function is to guarantee that all is going as well as possible, to help Zeza with attention to the variables of maternal and fetal well-being, and primarily to take pictures. My presence as an obstetrician is especially useful in cases of hospital transfer and in the (rare) cases where there is real need for medical intervention. On these specific situations, I can keep the team together in the hospital and guarantee full continuity of care. This emphasis on continuity of care is one of the key features of this birth model that works.

THE DYNAMICS OF OUR MODEL

"The contractions are really strong. We've had four contractions in the last ten minutes. She is a little tired, but she is going to take a warm shower. I think you can come now." This is the standard conversation that I've gotten used to hearing over the last ten years. The doula calls me from the patient's house and gives me a brief report on her condition. Normally, she is the first to arrive, many times when labor is still prodromal (very early phase). In this phase, the excitement of the first contractions adds to the anxiety about what is to come. It's a complex moment, because many arrangements need to be made for the arrival of the baby, like sending the small kids to school or to the houses of friends, or calling somebody to come over and take care of them. Call the grandmother or another companion. Arrange the house and finalize the preparations. Discuss the details with the husband. The doula is responsible for bringing her own materials, such as the birth ball and the massage devices. Zeza and I bring the necessary equipment for the birth (see Table 10.2). When the pregnant couple ask me what kinds of things they should have on hand, I tell them that there are five essential things:

- Cinnamon tea
- Ginger crystals to chew on
- Confidence
- Patience
- Chocolate cake

The first two are natural stimulants of uterine contractions. Confidence is the only antidote to the natural fear that every human has of the unknown. Patience is the fundamental essence, the primary value for anyone involved

TABLE 10.2 Outcomes of births attended by
Ricardo Jones, 1999–2007

Type of Birth	N	%
Births attended	112	100
Vaginal births	94	84
Cesareans	18	16
Birth position		
Total vaginal births	94	100
Squatting or sitting	88	93.7
Lithotomy	04	04.2
Side-lying	02	02.1
Episiotomy		
Total vaginal births	94	100
Spontaneous births	89	94.7
Births with episiotomy	05	05.3
Birth location		
Total births	94	100
Home births	40	42.5
Hospital births	54	57.5
Planned home births		
Total births	44	100
Actual home births	40	90.1
Hospital transfers	04	09.9
Hospital Transfers		
Total transfers	12	100
Failure to progress	03	75
Maternal fever[a]	01	25
Attempted VBACs		
Total attempted VBACs	12	100
Normal births	11	91.7
Cesareans	01	08.3

[a] In all, 50% of the transfers resulted in normal vaginal
births.

with childbirth. "And the chocolate cake, what is it for?" asks the couple. "It's for the doctor!" I reply. In fact, I explain that the point is not to *have* a chocolate cake but to *make* a chocolate cake. The main idea is to offer the mother a repetitive physical activity during the early phase of labor (kneading the flour, rolling the dough, adding the ingredients, waiting for the rising, and so on) to help her neocortex rest and get out of the way. In these initial stages, the doula is frequently present, helping around the house, doing massage, and preparing the environment (when it has been decided that the birth will take place at home). Of course, there are exceptions: The doula is not always the first to arrive. Often, the whole team shows up at the same time, and we all begin working with the patient together.

At present, there are two basic types of low-risk patients who receive our team care. (Obviously, our high-risk patients always give birth in the hospital.) Both types begin with an understanding of the importance of woman-centered attendance and a respect for her desires and values; they also agree on evidence-based medicine. Nevertheless, they differ on place of birth. One group prefers the intimacy of their homes and the freedom to be with their loved ones; the other group prefers the hospital for several reasons, the most salient of which is fear that something might go wrong. Because our team understands the iatrogenic effects of the hospital environment, we decided that, whatever the patient's choice about place of birth, she will be attended for as long as possible in her home after labor begins. When the choice is a hospital birth, after a good dilation is achieved at home, the whole team moves to the maternity unit to assist the birth. Even in these situations, we go to the patient's house with all the necessary apparatus for a home birth because women sometimes change their minds during labor and decide to stay home. (This possibility is a discussion that we have with every couple during the pregnancy.) The reverse is also possible: someone who wants to have a home birth can decide to go to the hospital because she wants to (so far this has not happened, but it could), or we might have to transport. The main idea should always be the well-being and safety of the woman, while offering full agency to the couple in the decisions made.

The equipment that we use for home birth is based principally on what some American home birth midwives carry. These are the things that we find helpful in our own practice. It is important to realize that the equipment is related to the context: Dutch midwives who ride to births on their bicycles carrying only their midwifery bags will find it ridiculously long; American midwives who take minivans full of stuff to home births will find it too short; with our small car, we find it just right.

In recent years, we have had no emergency transfers of either mothers or babies, and we have only used oxygen twice to help two babies with transitory breathing problems.

Some time after I presented the results of my first 1,500 births in private practice at a conference, I decided to do an update analyzing the outcomes I attained in the later years of my practice as my paradigm shift became more integrated and complete. I evaluated my last 112 births, all of which

Home Birth Equipment

- Vehicle for transfer
- Cell phone or pager
- Blood pressure cuff
- Stethoscope
- Fetoscope (Pinard)
- Fetal doppler
- Sterile gauze
- Antiseptics: alcohol, iodine, peroxide, betadine, etc.
- Cotton soaked in alcohol and iodine gauze
- Flashlight
- Blood-collecting equipment
- KY gel
- Homeopathic medicines (birth kit)
- Oil for perineal massage
- Birth stool
- Oxygen tank with neonatal aspiration tube
- Oxygen mask for mother and baby
- Neonatal resuscitation kit (ambu bag, laryngoscope, tubes, etc.)
- Scissors, tweezers, needle-holders, suture thread
- Syringes and drugs (pitocin, methergine, etc.)
- Local anesthetics (xylocaine)
- IV equipment
- Bulb syringe or a DeLee catheter
- Hot packs to warm the baby
- Various hemostats and clamps
- Metric scale and tape measure
- Oral vitamin K
- Camera and video camera
- Music
- Incense
- Birth ball

had been conducted according to the PHOA and with the presence of the complete interdisciplinary team. The outcomes seem to be even more positive. As time passed, our ideology of support, continuity of care and the assistance centered in women's needs has deepened and strengthened. The main outcomes of these latest births, which took place between 1999 and 2006, are shown in Table 10.2.

It is evident that the small number of patients and their middle-class origins prevent more expansive interpretations of these data. Some years ago, we decided to stop working with private insurance companies because the payments from these companies—around $200 per birth— are incompatible with the kind of teamwork we use. This amount of money is only slightly more than our patients pay for the doula alone. Normally, the cost to the patient is around $2,000 for the whole team to make a prenatal home visit, attend the birth, and make at least three post-partum visits. (Prenatal care is paid for out of pocket to me directly or is paid for by the insurance companies as normal medical appointments.[1]) This amount of money is accessible only for the middle-class women of our city, but it is evident that there are extensive spaces for negotiation—I do work on a sliding scale according to ability to pay. My clients have the option of lump-sum or extended payments, and we often work pro bono with those who can't afford it. Given that our team normally only attends about twenty births per year, you can see that we don't make a lot of money from births.

Because we live in a very conservative area, any new idea about health care is viewed with automatic suspicion. The medical monopoly is strong and unquestionable. In a state with more than 10 million inhabitants, I am the only doctor who assists home births. The prejudice from the medical establishment and its attacks against the humanization of childbirth make it really difficult to assist more births. We need to be strict and careful: any problem—even the smallest—can cause discredit to the model (Wagner 1995, 2006: 99). Our "day jobs" help pay the bills. I work in my private office giving patient care, and Zeza works as a hospital nurse in obstetrics, pediatrics, surgery, and recovery room care. Now (after Cristina, our first doula, moved to São Paulo), we have several doulas who work with us at various times: a yoga teacher, a childbirth educator, and a government worker. It is possible that in the near future, my participation on the team will become superfluous because the midwife(ves) and the doulas will take care of birth autonomously, and my role will change to that of a consultant and backup doctor.

It is also evident that the women who look for this kind of birth assistance already tend to have an active and empowered attitude in relation to birth. Just a little effort is needed to convince them of the innumerable benefits of humanized birth from a physical and emotional point of view.

Even noting the limits of our small numbers, I believe that these outcomes can point to a better way for birth, and that personal initiatives are the trigger for great transformations.

THE BIG PICTURE: A STRATEGY FOR THE
HUMANIZATION OF BIRTH

Obviously, the changes I made in my practice could not happen without shock and confrontation. As I said before, the medical community around me could not accept behaviors that led away from the orthodox catechism. After all, the predominant medical model built its supremacy over childbirth assistance through doctors' use of technology, from forceps to cesarean extraction. So to criticize and question the unrestricted use of technology in birth would be seen as an attack on the core of the obstetric agenda. If doctors limited their use of technology to keep it from causing danger and disease, what good would be the professional, exhaustively trained in its use? To put the contemporary obstetric paradigm in the hot seat, as I was doing with my personal practice, brought discomfort to my medical colleagues, who could see me only as a threat to the hard-won power that obstetrics has gained over the last two centuries. The more I questioned, the more indignant I became as I began to believe that responsibility for the way we handled birth lay solely in the hands of the medical professionals. Yet over time, my unilateral assignment of blame to doctors gave way to a more nuanced understanding of the complexity of forces, visible and invisible, that influence the cultural and medical treatment of birth.

I began to see doctors and hospitals as more than individual players, caring only about their own benefit; in fact, they were pieces of a gigantic jigsaw puzzle. Birth is a social and human event, whose expression can be effected only through human beings. We are all immersed in the same cultural melting pot where beliefs, myths, values, and fears bubble up and mix around. Change in the ideologies that govern human birth can happen only through profound, instead of superficial, examination of our values. At present, the dominion of biomedicine over birth is an incontestable reality. Thus, it is essential that doctors be invited to participate in the creation of a new model of assistance. I believe that obstetricians have a great role to play in the transformation of the present paradigm, directing it toward a model centered on professional midwives (specialists in the normal physiology of birth) and no longer on doctors (specialists in the pathology of birth, the ones needed to rescue mothers and babies when physiology really does give way to pathology).

Birth activists consistently and insistently say, "The contemporary Western technocratic model devalues women, medicalizes birth, turns birth into a colder and more dangerous event, and is expensive and inefficient." And then they ask, "So what can we do? How can we give central stage back to women and, at the same time, offer them more safety when facing the problems in birth that do sometimes occur?" There are no easy answers. We cannot take a dictatorial approach to generating solutions because our humanization of birth movement developed in response, and in contrast, to the dictatorial attitudes of contemporary medicine. Our response needs to take a different direction: integrative, multifaceted, respectful, and profound.

After pondering these questions for more than two decades, I developed a set of global strategies for action, always keeping in mind that the humanization of birth can occur only if society as a whole is changed. Childbirth is a human event that carries an extensive cultural load of myths, beliefs, images, and ideas, and only when we acknowledge the roles of these powerful and invisible forces can we offer to birth the position that it deserves. To change birth is to change the way we understand the feminine. To value women and their cycles in a world ruled by patriarchy is to challenge the core of our most profound values. Any change of such proportions shakes the deepest structures of our way of living, and thus needs to be undertaken slowly and with caution.

This strategy for the humanization of birth provides space for taking action in different social segments and strata. The basic action points can be grouped in the following way:

- *Government action.* Central governments should be the greatest stimulators of wide-ranging, systemic change. For that, it is fundamental to create well-defined criteria for the implementation of policies of humanization so that we don't confuse the "humanization of birth" with "epidurals for all," "prophylactic c-sections" (Feldman and Friedman 1985) and other actions that don't favor the restitution of agency to women. Governmental action could begin with a slow and gradual process of decentralization of the obstetric units, stimulating the creation of unmedicalized, freestanding birth centers and a model for planned home birth with systems of rapid referral, national campaigns to support normal birth, and the necessary support for doctors and nurses who work in accordance with evidence-based protocols. Beyond that, humanization of health care in a global way should be stimulated and financed through structural modifications in hospital obstetric wards (the inclusion of birth pools would be a great step) and constant stimulation through continuing education for health professionals who work in public hospitals.
- *Educational action.* There must be a slow and gradual replacement of an iatrocentric (doctor-centered), etiocentric (pathology-centered) and hospital-centric paradigm by a postmodern model with better

outcomes—such as the midwifery model of care (see Introduction, this volume). We must not continue to encourage professionals who are highly trained and qualified to deal with pathologies to be sidelined into the assistance of normal and physiologic events like births. The midwifery model of care, in which midwives are the primary caregivers for normal births, is far more cost-effective and has far better outcomes than models in which obstetricians are in charge of all births, as shown by the differences in the rates of morbidity and mortality of developed countries in which midwives are the primary birth attendants (De Vries et al. 2001). Countries such as the Netherlands and Sweden, which use the midwifery model, have better outcomes across the board (see Chapter 1). It is the responsibility of the universities to discuss this reality and to invest in the training of professional midwives, to slowly change to a more rational and coherent model. It is equally important to create a humanistic curriculum in medical schools, nursing schools, and midwifery schools, emphasizing the relational and emotional aspects of the therapeutic process. Finally, it is fundamental to create strong links with evidence-based medicine, because such links will enable us to challenge the mythology of contemporary obstetrics, which charter rituals that empower professionals and institutions but disempower women and their babies, not offering the protection they promised, while enhancing risks in the process.

- *Action in the nongovernmental organization (NGO) sector.* For such initiatives to succeed, it is important to have effective bearers of this new message. For this, it will be necessary to strengthen NGOs that work for the humanization of birth, so that they can serve as a point of connection between the desires of women and governmental directives. I think of NGOs as points of intensification that enable people of like mind to come together to create social improvements stemming from their shared beliefs. Without these intensification points, the isolated signals emanating from individuals remain fragile and weak, unable to effect change. The strengthening and unification of these institutions is vital for the construction of a new woman-centered model (as illustrated by events in New Zealand; see Chapter 2).

- *Action in public education.* This is the most fundamental and complex part of my action plan. Social change happens inside individuals; the humanization of childbirth can happen only with women's participation. Top-down changes carry the tone of authoritarianism, and their outcomes thus can only be fleeting and inconstant. Profound and true changes follow the development of a new consciousness, and for this reason are slow and gradual. We cannot change values and myths (like the myth of technological transcendence) by decree: they can only be altered when a new social vision is able to fill in the gaps in our imaginary. Women are the most significant figures in this paradigm shift, and for this reason, dialogue among groups of feminists, mothers, consumers, birth and breastfeeding activists, and others is of vital importance to the success of these initiatives. The media can play a significant role in stimulating such dialogue, and members of such groups should develop close relationships with the media, encouraging and assisting with the creation of a public dialogue around the importance of changing childbirth.

- *Individual action.* Margaret Mead said, "Never doubt that a small group of thoughtful and committed people can change the world; indeed, it is the only thing that ever has." I would add that the great leaps in the development of civilization began in the lonely hearts of visionaries, whose enormous passion for an idea inspired others, transforming their dreams into reality. Large-scale government actions will depend directly on birth professionals, who work on the front line directly with the women. We can only change a paradigm that we know is wrong by working from both ends of the spectrum, from large-scale policies to individual initiatives. Only by combining high-quality, evidence-based technical care with emotional and social support—the best of both worlds—as Trevathan (1999) says, can we give women the best system ever created by humans in the realm of healing; one that includes constant presence and unconditional caring.

To criticize the paradigm that rules does not mean to get rid of modern medical resources that help us in truly pathological cases. But the mythology that permeates childbirth transforms the technical resources into a many-armed Shiva, an omnipotent being that occupies the place that religion used to have in our social imaginary (Clerc 2004). We need to transform technology from a mythological system offering magical solutions to our dilemmas to a set of tools serving mothers and babies. The humanization of birth does not represent a romantic return to the past, nor a devaluation of technology. Rather, it offers an ecological and sustainable pathway to the future.

ACKNOWLEDGMENTS

I want to thank

Zeza and Cristina, the ones truly responsible for my awakening as a birth activist
Lucas and Isabel Cristina, son and daughter, my best teachers
Maurice and Elba Jones, my parents

Marcus, Roger, and Eunice, my brothers and sister

Robbie Davis-Floyd, counselor, examplar, editor, and best friend, who played a huge role in transforming my thinking about birth, and thus in my practice

My friends and colleagues from ReHuNa (Brazil), HumPar (Portugal), IMBCO, Instituto Jean Bergès, and ANDO

All the writers, healers, activists, traditional *parteras*, doulas, midwives, humanistic doctors, anthropologists, and other experts in women's issues who have inspired my path, taught me how to honor the feminine, and helped me to keep my chin up, even in the darkest times

All my clients, who gave me the possibility to witness the miracle of life perpetuating

NOTE

1. Brazilian physicians do not carry insurance. They can be charged for malpractice, but the financial penalty is not enough to bankrupt them, and doctors are almost never sent to jail. This non-insurance-based system is advantageous to doctors in terms of mitigating their fear of bad outcomes; at the same time, it can create feelings of impunity.

REFERENCES

Agency for Healthcare Research and Quality. *Vaginal Birth after Cesarean (VBAC).* 2003. Summary, Evidence Report/Technology Assessment: Number 71. AHRQ Publication Number 03-E017. Rockville, MD: Agency for Healthcare Research and Quality. http://www.ahrq.gov/clinic/epcsums/vbacsum.htm.

ANS. 2008. *Destaque: Brasil tem uma das maiores taxas de cesariana na Saúde Suplementar.* Agência Nacional de Saúde Suplementar. http://www.ans.gov.br/portal/site/home2/destaque_22585_2.asp?secao=home.

Balaskas, J. 1989. *Parto Ativo—Guia Prático para o Parto Natural.* São Paulo: Editora Ground.

Balint, M. 1957. *The Doctor, His Patient, and the Illness.* New York: International Universities Press.

Bolande, R. P. 1969. *Ritualistic Surgery: Circumcision and Tonsillectomy. New England Journal of Medicine* 280:591–92.

Carroli G., and J. Belizan. 1999. "Episiotomy for Vaginal Birth." *Cochrane Database of Systematic Reviews,* Issue 2. Art. No.: CD000081. DOI: 10.1002/14651858. CD000081.

Clerc, O. 2004. *Modern Medicine: The New World Religion.* Fawnskin, CA: Personhood Press.

Coan, J., H. S. Schaefer, and R. J. Davidson. 2006. "Lending a Hand: Social Regulation of the Neural Response to Threat." *Psychological Science* 17:1032–39.

DATASUS/SINASC. 2005. Ministério da Saúde. http://tabnet.datasus.gov.br.

Davis, E. 1993. *Heart and Hands*. New York: Bantam Books.

Davis-Floyd, R. 1987. "Obstetric Training as a Rite of Passage." *Medical Anthropology Quarterly* 1.3:288–318.

———. 1992. *Birth as an American Rite of Passage*. Berkeley: University of California Press.

———. 1998. *From Doctor to Healer: The Transformative Journey*. New Brunswick, NJ: Rutgers University Press.

De Vries, R., C. Benoit, E. van Teijlingen, and S. Wrede (eds.). 2001. *Birth by Design: Pregnancy, Maternity Care and Midwifery in North America and Europe*. New York: Routledge.

Dick-Read, G. 2004. *Childbirth without Fear*. London: Pinter & Martin. Originally published 1959.

"Episiotomy." *Birth Messages* [http://www.birthpsychology.com/messages/contents.html]. http://www.birthpsychology.com/messages/episiotomy/episiotomy.html.

Feldman, G. B., and J. A. Freidman. 1985. "Prophylactic Cesarean Section at Term?" *New England Journal of Medicine* 312:1264–67.

Gaskin, I. M. 1975. *Spiritual Midwifery*. Summertown, TN: Book Publishing Company.

Goer, H. 1995. *Obstetric Myths versus Research Realities*. Westport, CT: Greenwood Publishing Group.

———. 1999. *The Thinking Woman's Guide to a Better Birth*. New York: Perigee Books.

Jones, R. 2004. *Memórias do Homem de Vidro—Reminiscências de um Obstetra Humanista* [Memoirs of a Man Made of Glass]. Porto Alegre, Brazil: Editora Idéias a Granel.

Jordan, B. 1993. *Birth in Four Cultures*. Long Grove, IL: Waveland Press.

Klaus, M., P. Klaus, and J. Kennell. 1993. *Mothering the Mother*. New York: Perseus Books.

Leboyer, F. 2004. *Nascer Sorrindo*. São Paulo: Editora Brasiliense.

Martin, E. 1987. *The Woman in the Body: A Cultural Analysis of Reproduction*. Boston: Beacon Press.

Moberg, K. U. 2003. *The Oxytocin Factor—Tapping the Hormone of Calm, Love and Healing*. Cambridge, MA: Da Capo Press.

Odent, M. 1984. *Nacimiento Renacido* [Birth Reborn]. Buenos Aires: Ed. Errepar S/A.

———. 1990. *Água e Sexualidade*. São Paulo: Editora Siciliano.

———. 2000. *A Cientificação do Amor*. São Paulo: Editora Terceira Margem.

Paciornik M. 1990. "Use of the Squatting Position for Birth." *Birth* 19.4:230–1.

———. 1997 *Aprenda a Nascer com os Índios* [Learn How to Birth with the Indians]. São Paulo: Editora Rosa dos Tempos.

RIPSA. 2007. *Indicadores e Dados Básicos para a Saúde—2007. Tema do ano: Nascimentos no Brasil. Sumário*. http://tabnet.datasus.gov.br/cgi/idb2007/tema.pdf.

Scaer, R., and D. Korte. 1992. *A Good Birth, a Safe Birth*. Boston: Harvard Common Press.

SINASC. 2005. *Porto Alegre*. http://lproweb.procempa.com.br/pmpa/prefpoa/sms/usu_doc/sinasc_2005.pdf.

Sosa, R., J. Kennell, M. Klaus, S. Robertson, and J. Urrutia. 1980. "The Effective of Supportive Companion on Perinatal Problems, Length of Labor, and Mother-Infant Interaction." *New England Journal of Medicine* 303:597–600.

Trevathan, W. R. 1987. *Human Birth: An Evolutionary Perspective.* Hawthorne, NY: Aldine de Gruyter.

———. 1999. "Evolutionary Obstetrics." In *Evolutionary Medicine,* edited by E. O. Smith and J. J. McKenna, 201. Oxford: Oxford University Press.

Trevathan, W. R., E. O. Smith, and J. J. McKenna. 1999. *Evolutionary Medicine.* Oxford: Oxford University Press.

Wagner, M. 1994. *Pursuing the Birth Machine: The Search for Appropriate Perinatal Technology.* Camperdown, Australia: ACE Graphics.

———. 1995. "Global Witch Hunt." *Lancet* 346.8981:1020–23.

———. 1999. "Episiotomy: A Form of Genital Mutilation." *Lancet* 353:1977–78.

———. 1999/2000. "Bad Habits—a Poor Basis for Medical Policy." *AIMS Journal* 11.4.

———. 2006. *Born in the USA: How a Broken Maternity System Must Be Fixed to Put Women and Children First.* Berkeley: University of California Press.

Woolley, R. J. 1995. "Benefits and Risks of Episiotomy: A Review of the English-Language Literature since 1980. *Obstetrical and Gynecological Survey* 50:806–20.

World Health Organization. 1985. "Appropriate Technology for Birth." *Lancet* 2. 8452:436–37.

Chapter 11

The CASA Hospital and Professional Midwifery School

An Education and Practice Model That Works

Lisa Mills and Robbie Davis-Floyd

La Misión de CASA [CASA's Mission]

Contribuir con calidad y calidez a elevar las condiciones de vida de la población más vulnerable, a traves de acciones en salud, educación, y cultura, promoviendo el desarrollo sustentable y el respeto a los derechos humanos, con una perspectiva de genero.

[To contribute with quality and warmth to elevate the life conditions of the most vulnerable people, through actions in health, education, and culture, promoting sustainable development and respect for human rights from a gendered perspective.]

Placard on the entry wall of the CASA School for Professional Midwives, Colonia Santa Julia, San Miguel de Allende, Mexico

INTRODUCTION[1]

The CASA maternity hospital and professional midwifery school are unique in Latin America, perhaps in the world. The *Centro para los Adolescentes de San Miguel de Allende* (Center for the Adolescents of San Miguel de Allende) (CASA), in the state of Guanajuato, central Mexico, has developed both birth and midwifery education models with concrete practicality and a judicious combination of science and caring. CASA is a nonprofit health and social service agency offering diverse services that focus on the needs of disadvantaged youth and women. It was established in 1981 by Nadine Goodman, an American-born social worker and public health specialist. It has received consistent funding from several international, primarily U.S.-based, foundations (Friedland 2000). The CASA program began by offering contraceptives and family planning services provided through peer counseling programs throughout the state of Guanajuato. From the start, Nadine's vision included choices for women across the reproductive spectrum: the choice when to have children, the choice of how they would be born, and choice about how they would be cared for when mothers had to work. Thus in 1994, in response to the lack of local reproductive and maternal health services offering such choices, CASA opened a maternity hospital with the intention that it would eventually be staffed primarily by midwives, whom Nadine saw as the only caregivers fully equipped to provide true choice in birth. In 1997 CASA opened Mexico's first professional midwifery school, *La Escuela de CASA de Parteras Profesionales* (the CASA School of Professional Midwives). The CASA campus now provides a range of reproductive health care services, as well as dental, pharmacy, and laboratory services. It operates a day care center to care for the children of working families in its region, a large public library, and a youth ecological awareness team, and it also has formed a theater group involving local adolescents, who perform dramas dealing with gender issues such as domestic violence. CASA has approximately 100 paid staff and 300 volunteers; its family planning and reproductive education services reach tens of thousands of people per year in San Miguel and surrounding regions (see www.casa.org.mx). CASA also has a live weekly radio program run by young people and midwives, and its programs are rebroadcast to a potential listening audience of more than 5 million through a network of nineteen government-funded Indigenous radio stations.

The CASA midwifery school trains professional midwives *(parteras profesionales)*, most of whom plan to live and work in rural communities that currently lack medical services and where most instances of maternal death occur. The CASA midwives are imbued with the woman-centered philosophy known internationally as the "midwifery model of care" (see Rothman 1982; Davis-Floyd 1998; Conclusion, this volume), and the CASA educational model ensures that their care will be not only woman-centered but also culturally appropriate. This model of care represents an alternative to the biomedical model practiced in Mexico, which is unnecessarily interventionist (Castro 1998; Castro, Heimburger, and Langer n.d.) and in rural areas and among the urban poor is often experienced as disrespectful and insensitive (Espinosa Damián 2004).

As part of their professional training, the CASA midwifery students leave San Miguel and go into rural areas to apprentice with traditional midwives *(parteras tradicionales)*[2] for periods of two or three weeks at a time, five times during their three-year training program. These *terrenos prácticos* are intended to equip CASA graduates with the cultural literacy required for practice in such communities, in synthesis and combination with the professional midwifery and medical literacy necessary to augment traditional knowledge. During these rotations, the student observes and learns from a *partera's* interactions with the community, her care for pregnant women, and her management of childbirth. The student also participates in these activities, as well as in the day-to-day activities of cooking and other household tasks. The CASA program does, therefore, follow Brigitte Jordan's recommendation for a reciprocal teaching model "in which [traditional birth attendants][3] would also instruct scientifically trained [maternal and child health] personnel in traditional practices" (Jordan 1986: 4).

CREATING THE CASA MIDWIFERY MODEL
OF CARE AND MAKING IT WORK

It is CASA's goal to

- *Contribute toward the formation of new, professional, autonomous midwives, thereby enabling more Mexican women and their families to have access to the midwifery model of care*
- *Produce new professional midwives who are steeped in and feel respect for the ways of their elders, our traditional midwives*
- *Work with our municipal, state, and federal governmental bodies to secure the right of every woman to have access to the midwifery model of care and to secure the right of the midwife to practice legally*
- *Advocate for the traditional midwives in Mexico and worldwide, securing the mechanisms that will enable them to continue to work*

Letter from NADINE GOODMAN, November 5, 2000

We have very good training, but we're never going to forget traditional midwifery. We are parteras, *and then we are professionals.*
CASA student

The First Step: Professional Training for Traditional Midwives

Nadine Goodman and her colleagues established the CASA School in the context of an historical relationship with *parteras tradicionales* in the San Miguel area that grew out of the peer counseling and family planning programs CASA developed during the 1980s, and resulted in the creation of training programs for traditional midwives. Subsequently, a cycle has been set in motion in which *parteras tradicionales* who received training as a result of their interaction with CASA participate in the education of the new generation of *parteras profesionales*, who upon graduation, may also train traditional or professional midwives in other parts of Mexico.

The first training was initiated by the traditional midwives themselves, who requested *pláticas* (informal lectures) about family planning, physiology, and anatomy. At the end of this informal course, which took place in 1990, the *parteras*, especially Antonia Cordova,[4] wanted to continue their education, focusing specifically on skills for managing childbirth. Antonia asked Nadine Goodman to find them a teacher, and eventually

Nadine located Patricia Kay, an American direct-entry midwife trained and licensed in New Mexico (see Davis-Floyd 2001 for Patricia's story), who taught a three-year training course (1991–1993) attuned to the *parteras'* needs, beginning by learning about their existing knowledge and proceeding from there. Three midwives—Antonia Cordova Morales, Leonor Cervantes, and Esther Lara Castillo—finished Patricia's course in 1993. Leonor and Esther went back to practice midwifery in their communities. Antonia returned to CASA to practice midwifery at the hospital, and initiated her own three-year course for *parteras tradicionales,* in which she passed on what she had learned from Patricia. Beginning in November 1994 and ending in April 1997, Antonia taught seven community midwives:

> I taught them what I had learned, what I had written down—what life had shown me and what Patricia had shown me—and what they themselves had shown me. We all learned: I learned from them, they learned from me. From there I got Belén and Manuela. There were other midwives in that group with very much wisdom, but they were from rural areas and, unfortunately, they couldn't come to work here in the hospital because they don't know how to read and write. But they have a lot of wisdom as midwives. (Quoted in Davis-Floyd 2001: 210–11)

After the course, Belén and Manuela joined Antonia at CASA. Antonia, Belén, and Manuela subsequently participated in the education of the professional midwifery students when the CASA school opened in 1997, with Antonia serving as the clinical director of the CASA School and director of midwifery services for the CASA Hospital.

Before beginning her training with Patricia, Antonia had attended seventy births as a traditional or, more precisely, "empirical" (see Note 2) midwife: she did not learn through a traditional apprenticeship but, rather, simply from attending births and then from the short course in the *Seguro Social* for traditional birth attendant (TBA) training—this course left her frustrated at the paucity of information about birth she was given.[5] When Robbie asked Antonia to describe the differences in her philosophy and practice before and after her time with Patricia, she said:

A: The difference, I think, is a big one . . . Before I studied with
     Patricia, I felt that I was respecting the women, but the respect—
     I gave it to them silently, I did not talk. I watched the woman suffer,
     that she screamed and cried, that she got mad and that she became
     desperate—what I did was to be silent, not saying anything. But
     now I have an appropriate word to say. . . . There are times when
     the women, almost the majority, say, "I can't do it." I tell them, "You
     can do it, you *can*. . . . Breathe, breathe in deeply, concentrate and
     focus your energy." I touch their perineum—"focus your energy
     here, and push there where you feel my fingers. . . ." I tell them a
     lot of times that their uterus is a rose, why? Because a rose will open

petal by petal, exactly the way the uterus opens. . . . And the women practically don't complain anymore, don't get desperate anymore. They are happy to wait for the rose to finish opening.

Q: *Robbie: How did you think of using this image?*

A: Antonia: When I was with Patricia, she had us do visualizations. And I liked that a lot. For me it was like a fairy tale, I closed my eyes and I heard her voice, but I was inside what she was saying, you see? (quoted in Davis-Floyd 2001: 209–10)

Through Antonia's participation in Patricia's course, the New Age met the traditional midwife, and they clicked.

At a more technical level, Antonia offered a fascinating reflection on her experience of midwifery before her professional training, describing the first birth she had attended, by accident, that of a neighbor:

There was a woman whose husband had abandoned her . . . on the seventeenth of May of 1985, her contractions started. . . . And I told her, "Let's go to the hospital." She was very stubborn, she said, "I won't leave my house. I die here, whatever, but I will have my baby here." So I put a plastic sheet down and a blanket, there it was the baby was born. . . . This woman passed out and she had a big hemorrhage. I had heard . . . from a *curandera* that a handful of chewed cumin seeds *(cominos)* stops a hemorrhage, so I gave her a handful of cumin seeds and told her to chew them. Then the woman started to react and I put cold compresses on her face . . . really without knowing. [Once the baby started to nurse, the hemorrhage stopped, and] fortunately the woman and the baby are alive. . . . Now when I think of it, sometimes it gives me goosebumps! To think, to relive everything that happened and I know that it was a very dangerous birth.

In this story we have an opportunity to look back, through the eyes of a midwife now professionally trained, at the first birth she ever attended, when she had no training at all. She tells this story with a dual consciousness, noting her naïve lack of awareness of the risks she faced but also appreciating her intuitive reactions and use of traditional knowledge. Speaking without self-denigration, she thereby also avoids denigrating other "midwives without training" (Lefeber 1994), demonstrating a keen awareness of the sensitivity of her political position in Mexican midwifery. Because she is Mexico's first traditional midwife to complete a professional educational program and enter hospital practice, she spans the boundaries between the traditional and the professional, and between the indigenous and cosmopolitan worlds. Even as she embodies and expresses their differences, she represents and remains responsible to all. Thus when asked about her midwifery identity, she still responds, "*Soy partera tradicional*"—with this statement of identity, she honors her traditional roots and affirms her respect for the skills and knowledge of all those *parteras tradicionales* who have not received professional training equivalent to hers.

In describing what she learned from Patricia, Antonia consistently stressed that, more than anything, Patricia had taught her not to stop at obtaining technical information but to deal with the woman's emotional and practical needs in a holistic way: "The midwife is like a big tree, because the midwife isn't just good for attending a birth: many people come to her for advice, for emotional counseling, for family planning advice, for health things, for everything, you see? . . . We are a big tree, and it depends on the tree, on the shade the tree gives, to do the women good" (quoted in Davis-Floyd 2001: 210).

The Second Step: Developing the CASA Midwifery Model

The expanded role that Antonia encapsulates in the metaphor of the midwife as a "big tree" became foundational for the approach to midwifery education that CASA ultimately adopted, which includes training midwives in both technical and holistic skills. Describing the CASA approach, Antonia noted that first of all, the midwives try to send first-time mothers home if they arrive in early labor because, from the time of admission to the CASA hospital, the mother and her relatives start counting the hours and get increasingly anxious if labor does not progress. If the woman who arrives in early labor is from a rural area far from the city, then they admit her but frequently remind her that the labor may take a long time.

> First we ask her all the questions: what time did she start? did she eat? did she sleep? has she been walking? is she tired? If she is very tired, well, then she should rest. We give her something to eat, not like in other hospitals that say "no more food, no more nothing." They eat what they want. Of course in heavy labor they don't really want to eat anymore, but yes, they can drink. Sometimes we listen to the fetal heart rate with the Pinard, but if the woman is very sensitive, and it bothers her to have us push into her belly with the Pinard horn, then we listen with the Doppler. But the Doppler often transmits a lot of noise: it gets confusing. So better with the Pinard. We don't shave, we don't do episiotomies, and we don't use the Kristeller (fundal pressure). Most women don't get IVs. They give birth upright most of the time—sitting, squatting, or on their hands and knees *(hincada)*—in that position, they don't complain about back pain any more. (Quoted in Davis-Floyd 2001: 211)

According to students, a CASA tradition is to hold the baby up at some point after the birth and ask the mother, "*Qué ves?*" (What do you see?), so that the mother can express her pride in saying, "My baby!" and all present can share in that happiness.

The CASA midwives attend breech births when necessary, but like traditional midwives, they prefer to perform external versions during the prenatal period. During an external version, the midwife encourages the baby to turn by talking to it, by getting the mother to lie with her head down and her hips elevated several times a day, and by applying cold compresses to the top of the uterus and hot compresses to the pelvic region where she wants the head to go, for, as Antonia says, "The head of the baby always seeks the warmest spot." And of course the midwife works by using delicate massage and fetal body manipulation, stopping if she encounters resistance to avoid potential dangers. She does not perform versions if she hears variations in the fetal heart rate because of the danger that the cord may be too short or may be wrapped around the neck.

Birth Outcomes at CASA

The CASA hospital charges means-tested user fees of 70 pesos for a prenatal consultation (approximately US$7); 1,500 pesos for a normal birth (US$150); and 4,500 pesos (US$450) for a cesarean. For those unable to pay at these rates, CASA offers a sliding scale and in addition conducts an annual campaign to raise funds to offer birth attendance completely free of charge to at least 200 women per year. There are six midwives on staff, one general practitioner, one obstetrician/gynecologist, and one pediatrician (Álvarez 2007, personal communication); the CASA team attends both low- and high-risk births. To give an idea of the midwife/physician birth ratio at CASA, statistics from births attended in the CASA hospital between May and October of 1999 show a total of 249 births, 207 attended by midwives and 12 by physicians. Thirty cesareans were performed, yielding a cesarean rate of 11.5% in 1999 (Goodman 2000). At present, physicians attend only about 5% of the CASA births (Goodman 2007, personal communication).

As of 2006, the CASA hospital team had attended approximately 7,000 births since the hospital opened, including approximately 800 home births; the team currently average around 40 births per month or 500 per year (Goodman 2007, personal communication).[6] Cesarean rates for the years 2000–2006 were as follows:

2000: 12.52%
2001: 13.44%
2002: 6.02%
2003: 9.72%
2004: 13.64%
2005: 15.77%
2006: 15.34%

Thus, CASA's average cesarean rate during these seven years was 13.25%, which falls precisely within WHO parameters. There were no maternal deaths (Walker 2006: 2). The average rate for low-birth-weight babies was 4.5%. Out of the 2,440 CASA-attended births that took place from 2002 through 2006, there were ten perinatal deaths (including stillbirths and postpartum deaths taking place within seven days of the birth), yielding for these five years a perinatal mortality rate (PMR) of approximately 5/1,000 (see Table 11.1). (As Table 11.1 shows, approximately the same PMR has held at CASA since its inception in 1995.) By way of comparison, the PMR for Guanajuato was 1,792 per 100,000 live births (Secretaría de Salud de Guanajuato 2006: 35), or 18/1,000. The CASA Hospital is only one of many in Guanajuato, all the rest of which are grounded in a biomedical model of care. In 2005 there were fifty-eight maternal deaths in the state; between 2002 and 2005, there were five maternal deaths in San Miguel (Secretaría de Salud de Guanajuato 2006) and none at CASA.

The CASA team achieves these good outcomes in spite of the fact that, for example, approximately 41% of the women attending CASA between 2001 and 2005 lived in rural areas of Guanajuato (Walker 2006: 1) and many arrived at CASA's door with no prior prenatal care, choosing that site because word had spread of its more compassionate care. The above figures indicate that CASA is doing an extremely good job of keeping mothers and babies alive and well, even under challenging circumstances.

The Third Step: Creating a Professional Midwifery School

Antonia's success in Patricia's program and in training Manuela and Belén, combined with the good outcomes these professional midwives achieved in a high-volume practice with a high-risk rural population, intensified Nadine's commitment to midwifery and inspired in her the desire to create the CASA school. Its first co-directors were Anne Davenport, an American nurse who had specialized in intensive care for neonates and later became a direct-entry midwife, and Gloria Metcalfe, Chilean *matrona* and former government director of Chilean midwifery; both were experienced in international maternal-child health projects. They developed a solid curriculum which, in 1997, was formally accredited by the Ministry of Education of the State of Guanajuato. The Ministry approved the CASA school as a technical, terminal-level career program in the specialty of professional midwifery.[7] So CASA, the first school of professional midwifery in Mexico, is a government-accredited vocational training program below the university level. Subsequent directors Rosa Hidalgo, Jennifer Goldberg, and Maricruz Coronado have expanded the curriculum and preserved the school's state accreditation. The first nine students entered the school in 1997; four of them—Carolina Alcocer Bolanos, Maricruz Coronado Saldierna, Maria Eugenia (Maru) Torres Ortíz, and Rosa Maria Arriaga Soria—graduated in August 2000. Maricruz, Maru, and Rosa remained in practice at CASA

TABLE 11.1 Perinatal deaths at the CASA hospital, 1994–2006

	1994	*1995*	*1996*	*1997*	*1998*	*1999*	*2000*	*2001*	*2002*	*2003*	*2004*	*2005*	*2006*
Perinatal deaths			0	1	4	3	3	0	2	1	1	3	3
Total births	0	263	591	626	579	539	551	439	498	535	535	520	352
% perinatal to total births									0.40	0.19	0.19	0.58	0.85

NOTE: The original text does not include percentage figures for 1994–2001.

for several years and are now in private practice. Maricruz also served twice as the educational director of the CASA school; she currently serves as director of CASA's entire comprehensive programs. Carolina served for two years as the Midwives Alliance of North America (MANA) representative to Mexico, and entered into independent practice in Guadalajara.

During their three years of professional midwifery training, CASA students receive a core education in areas such as biology, anatomy and physiology, pharmacology, and nutrition; they then specialize in an area such as obstetrics or neonatology. Because CASA contains both a hospital and a school, students are able to begin clinical work with pregnant women from the first day of their educational program. In fact, according to Goodman, the hospital was built in part because it would create a training site for midwifery students and in part because the cultural acceptability of the hospital setting would help to legitimate midwives in the public eye. In addition to its private hospital, CASA also has a home birth service for women who live in San Miguel,[8] so the students have opportunities to attend in-hospital births as well as out-of-hospital births in both rural and urban environments.

Even though CASA's midwifery students do gain clinical experience in the CASA hospital, the intent of the school is not to groom them for hospital practice but rather to enable them to live and practice in their home communities. The vast majority of the Mexican population completes only primary education (grades 1–6), especially in rural areas where most people do not have access to higher education. Facing up to this reality, CASA set its educational requirement at the ninth grade to avoid overly limiting the applicant pool, which CASA intends to include the daughters, nieces, and granddaughters of traditional midwives. Bolstering this decision is the fact that students with high school and university degrees are generally unwilling to remain in rural areas to practice. Some government officials and obstetric nurses have criticized the CASA model for this low educational requirement. In fact, many CASA students do have higher education, but certainly not all. Some insight into students' intellectual performance is provided by Alison Bastien, certified professional midwife (CPM), one of the teachers at the CASA School. Alison writes,

> I began teaching obstetrics for midwives at the CASA school in 2000. During my first couple of teaching years, the majority of the students had little or no secondary education, so their ability to write essays, to give short talks on selected topics to their classmates *(seminarios)*, even to report to one another on their *terreno práctico* experiences, were very rudimentary. Lots of embarrassed giggles, incomplete paragraphs, nobody knew how to look up information in our library—but they all learned.
>
> Within five years I found myself in the same classroom with similar groups of rural young women sharing their laptop to give their seminars

with PowerPoint presentations (even if the words were still spelled like third graders sometimes, by golly it was on PowerPoint; they were nervous, but they had their computer disc ready with graphics and all). They are accessing information, creating bibliographies, looking up international networks on natural birth and midwifery care all over Latin America. There really are fewer and fewer traditional midwives for them to apprentice within the *comunidades* every year. But we also have more models for them to learn with of a new breed, of these hybrids, if you will, slowly but surely. (May 2007, personal communication)

Further insight, this time into student's embodied learning experiences, is provided by Sandra Morningstar, CPM, an American direct-entry midwife who spends several months each year at CASA assisting in the students' clinical training. During a conversation with Patricia Kay and myself in 2002, Sandi noted that the students had recently attended a number of births in which the cervixes of the women became swollen, apparently because the students were telling them to push too soon; Sandi began to try to figure out why. While watching a student check dilation, Sandi noticed that right afterward, the student went into a corner, surreptitiously pulled out a measuring tape, and measured the width between her fingers, apparently to assure herself that the cervix was actually at 10 centimeters; reassured, she told the laboring woman to push. Sandi then checked the mother herself, and realized that her cervix was indeed at 10 centimeters, but that she was "not ready to push." And it hit Sandi that

we were teaching the students a number, but it's not really about a number— it is when the woman is complete and has the urge to push, which is about a baby's head (whatever circumference that is) filling up a woman's cervix, whatever circumference that is, and how low the baby is in the pelvis when all this starts to happen, which is different for every mother, every baby, and every changing moment. We teach a number when it is really a dynamic interplay of many factors including emotions, which let one relax or not.

The most important point for the CASA students I believe is simply that . . . they are trying soooo hard to do exactly what they are told. Hence the literalness: you are taught 10 cm is complete, so you are looking for 10 cm and not finding it, and so you can't see the obvious: the mother is bearing down, the baby is moving down and out, but the student midwife announces, "You are not complete, it is not time yet to have your baby." Or the opposite: the mother has no urge to push, the baby is high or big and nothing at all is happening, the student midwife measures 10 cm and announces that "you are complete and you can push your baby out." In the first mistake, no harm done, the baby comes out in spite of the declarations. In the second mistake, the mother wears out, the cervix swells, and a normal birth is threatened.

Sandi's insight caused much discussion and introspection among the students, and an expanded awareness of the "dynamic interplay" she describes. This vignette points up the importance of what is termed in the Introduction to this volume "reflective practice, in which practitioners continually reflect on what they are doing and make efforts at improvement on an ongoing basis." In their studies, clinical practice, *terrenos prácticos*, and presentations, the CASA students are continually urged to engage in such reflection.

It is expected that upon graduation, students will practice the professional, evidence-based midwifery they learned at CASA in combination with the traditional model of care that they have learned from their traditional teachers, and that they will provide the care their clients need, even if this means that they have to work beyond a standard schedule. Educators at the school also perceive the students' role in the community as social and political: "The idea is that they return to the communities, and they fight and work for their communities." The professional midwife, therefore, is expected to harness the community's skills and resources to ensure the health of its women and newborn babies—a powerful reason for keeping CASA's educational program at a technical level; again, those with higher degrees seldom return to serve their local communities.

The Fourth Step: Combining Traditional and Professional Midwifery

As Alison implies above, "these hybrids"—the CASA graduates and others with a similarly synthetic midwifery education[9]—may have to carry the future of Mexican midwifery. By the 1970s, traditional midwives, the primary birth practitioners in Mexico for centuries, were attending only 43% of Mexican births (Secretaría de Programación y Presupuesto 1979: 237)—a percentage that has declined precipitously since then. Between 1995 and 1996, traditional midwives attended less than 17% of births in Mexico (INEGI 1999), although they did continue to attend the majority of births in some rural areas.[10] As of 2004, there were 18,740 traditional midwives registered with the government, and it was believed that there were at least 9,000 unregistered. The majority of these women are over sixty-five years of age (Secretaría de Salud 1994); many are dying without training replacements. In general, young people in Mexico today seek a formal education and want to enter a profession. Biomedicine has not only taken over childbirth; it is also redefining its very nature. In vaginal deliveries, extreme interventions such as fundal pressure (Kristeller maneuver) and manual extraction of the placenta are common. The national cesarean rate in Mexico is over 40%, with much higher rates in the private sector (Belizán et al. 1999).[11] Traditional midwives are keenly aware of this situation and consider themselves to be the only viable alternative to a cesarean for many Mexican women.

CASA's founder Nadine Goodman has long been acutely aware that Mexican traditional midwives are vanishing. Powerless to prevent their disappearance, she feels passionately that CASA students should be a part of preserving and applying traditional midwifery knowledge. Although the students receive evidence-based biomedical training, and their goal is to be "professional" rather than "traditional" midwives, the apprenticeship program *(terrenos prácticos)*, and the inclusion of traditional midwives in the maternity hospital, does represent a new model of interaction between the "traditional" and "biomedical," and an attempt to create a new generation of midwives who incorporate both professional and traditional midwifery knowledge and skills in their practices, thereby creating a new, inclusive, and comprehensive midwifery knowledge system.

This incorporation has been facilitated by the development of relationships between midwives and apprentices, teachers and trainees, so that what is exchanged is not only technical knowledge but also knowledge of each other's life experiences and, ultimately, common humanity. Because the exchange is occurring in the context of ongoing relationships built over time between the organization and the community, a base for genuine dialogue exists and is being developed by the apprenticeship program.

The apprenticeships with traditional midwives are intended to educate the students in both the richness and the deficiencies of traditional midwifery knowledge, to develop the students' capacity to make decisions independent of medical authority that balance the medical and midwifery ways of knowing in relative ways, to trust their own judgment, and to create an amplified knowledge systems through judicious combination of the best elements of each.

In order to be effective in the communities, students need to know how to gain access to the community's resources: to know whom to call upon for assistance in an emergency, and who can assist with transporting someone to hospital. They are expected to be able to determine individuals' risk factors and to take action to reduce or avoid the risk. As one student noted, "The *partera* is involved for the duration of the birth; the doctor is not. Therefore, the students learn maturity and independence. They learn how to manage situations so that they don't fear them . . . when they return to their communities and there is no access to institutional services, they have the knowledge to provide a solution." Thus the CASA students' training is not limited by long lists of potential reasons for referral: they learn these reasons, but they also learn how to deal with situations when referral is not possible. They are taught to be autonomous midwives, relying on articulation with the medical system when possible, yet using the necessary knowledge and skills for dealing with what arises when they are in fact on their own.

Through the apprenticeship program, students recognize the *parteras'* skills and resources. One student reported: "I learned a lot. I learned how to manage herbs, I learned how to give massages, I learned something they call *mantear* (to toss in a blanket), which consists of putting a blanket underneath the woman in labor, when the baby is not situated properly, and moving the blanket to properly situate the baby. I learned how to manage the umbilical cord on the neck. I learned how to manage shoulder dystocia, and positions that facilitate the birth."

Subsequently, she integrated the *parteras'* knowledge into her practice. Pointing to an herb in her kitchen, she said, "For example, this herb that I have here was given to me by a *partera*. It helps to prevent miscarriage," and went on to point to other herbs that she uses currently. The student perceived that the *parteras* had resources that were valuable to her understanding and practice of managing birth: "The *partera tradicional* has a lot of wisdom and experience about everything . . . generally the *parteras* have a lot of natural resources in their houses to attend a birth. They have oxytocic herbs, they have herbs of all kinds, including some that we learn to use, so there are many herbs at the community level. Also, during pregnancy, and at the moment of birth, they have a bath of herbs in which they carry the woman after birth, a bath of herbs, of vapor from the herbs—it's exquisite."

The student recognized that her traditional teachers might be able to identify and manage risk factors even if they were unable to name them: "There are many *parteras* who have a lot of knowledge about, for example, what is preeclampsia, without knowing the names of the illnesses . . . they know the symptoms and the risks without knowing the names." Through this interaction, professional midwifery students develop an appreciation of "invisible" knowledge: traditional practices that cannot be articulated in biomedical language but which, nevertheless, can result in successful births. When this tacit knowledge coincided with biomedical knowledge— for example, when *parteras tradicionales* identified biomedically recognized complications—they and the students were able to share in a process of naming and exchange.

Students who participate in births in the community also learn to respect the wisdom of the expectant mother's body: "In the community, the women don't have anything. So I think that it is the best place to learn how to attend births—in the community. Because you respect [the woman's] body, the knowledge of the body, as does the *partera*. Both parties understand each other." Students shared in the experience of invisibility when they decided to trust in the birth process for reasons that could not readily be articulated. A student describes how she has taken this knowledge into her practice as a home birth midwife in San Miguel de Allende:

> I had a birth with a foreign woman. She had high blood pressure in the third trimester, a month before the birth, but it wasn't preeclampsia, her laboratory tests were normal. I trusted that she was completely healthy. The reality

was that we weren't anxious. If necessary, we could go to the local hospital, we were prepared, we had a car ready. But everything was fine, without complication, the birth was active, rapid, and after three hours the baby was born. She and I were a team, I explained the risks to her, together we made a decision, without the pressure of the medical team at the clinic. Because all the world wanted to take her to the hospital because she had high blood pressure. So, the relationship with the woman is very important, and also that the woman knows her own body. This is very difficult to explain to the doctors and to have them accept it, because these things are invisible. In the hospital, there are protocols, norms, and we can't dedicate ourselves completely to the woman.

In her own practice, therefore, the student came to understand the traditional practitioner's experience of a birth where the successful outcome cannot be explained in biomedical terms, and therefore becomes "invisible." She thought that one way to rectify this was to codify the traditional midwives' knowledge, to compile a midwifery textbook: "In the community there are many things that don't comply with the textbooks, for example the textbook says that you need to cut the cord after a certain time, but in the rural areas the midwives wait much longer. We need to write down these things, we need a textbook of *partería*." Interestingly enough, the most recent scientific evidence shows that waiting to cut the cord until it stops pulsing allows the maximum transfer of blood volume, nutrients, and oxygen to the newborn, preventing possible complications. The dedication to the woman that the students learn as a result of their experience in the community means that their choice of traditional or biomedical technologies depends on the woman's own choice:

> In my mind I'm using both: for example, many people have confidence in natural methods, in plants, and in this situation I would use my knowledge of traditional midwifery, because here the medical doctors don't use teas, plants, massages, all of these are from the traditional midwife. The traditional midwife can teach me things that a doctor can't. Therefore we try to use the two, together, and we have the security and confidence to use either. At other times, there are women who don't want anything natural, who want medicine. . . . If a woman wants one thing and we give her another, she is not going to believe in us, she won't have confidence in us. Now if the advantages and disadvantages of each approach are explained to her, she makes her decision, and depending on that decision, we are able to talk. Each knowledge [is relevant] because the two are useful for us because we are *parteras*, and we understand both, but we're not doctors nor traditional midwives. Sometimes it is confusing because we are at an intermediate position, and sometimes we are guided by the births themselves as to what to do.

What the CASA students learned during their apprenticeships with traditional midwives depended upon the skills, experience, and nature of the training received by the traditional midwife herself. Students recognized that the use of herbs differed according to the area in which the *partera* lived. They also became aware that the skills of the *partera* depended on the number of births she had attended, as well as the source of her training. One *partera profesional* observed that "a midwife who has thirty years of experience obviously has seen everything and knows the symptoms of, for example, preeclampsia. But a younger midwife with maybe five or ten years of experience lacks some knowledge. . . . When the knowledge is passed from generation to generation, these midwives have a lot of knowledge. But there are women who learned because their neighbor had no one to attend her, and in these cases, there is some lack of knowledge."

Sometimes the issue was lack of material resources to apply during labor, a consequence of which was a lack of intervention in the birth process; some students were unsure whether this was because the *partera* lacked the knowledge to intervene, or because her experience had led her to trust in the woman's own capacity to deliver without intervention. "[Births in the community] are very different because they never intervene, not for anything. I don't know if the *parteras* don't intervene because they don't know how, or because of their experience they know that they shouldn't disturb the body's natural process."

Students distinguished their experience with midwives whose skills had been acquired from their own mothers, grandmothers, and other *parteras tradicionales* from those who had been trained by the Seguro Social or medical doctors. A number of students were concerned about traditional midwives' use of oxytocin, which can be bought in any Mexican pharmacy—the traditional midwives who had undergone biomedical TBA trainings often used it indiscriminately and inappropriately. In some cases, the students' own earlier experience of traditional midwifery from their mothers or grandmothers (who never used drugs) heightened their reaction to the administration of oxytocin:

> The midwives that have been trained by the Department of Health use oxytocin and, in reality, this is not ideal because I believe that they don't know about the use of oxytocin during birth. I was with a midwife who had a lot of experience and used a measure of oxytocin and it really wasn't correctly used. Because of the use of oxytocin, the woman's cervix softened, and this generally does not happen. When they know how to use it well, the effect is different. It has its use in rural areas, it's possible that oxytocin can help a lot, but it's necessary to know *how* to use it.

The student's influence over the decision-making process—her own authority—is difficult to establish because authority is determined not only by the relationship between the midwife and the student but, as Jordan (1993) has suggested, by the acknowledgment of authority by the laboring woman, who recognizes the midwife, rather than the student, as knowledgeable. The student, too, recognizes the midwife's experience and knowledge: "It was very difficult because they are her [the midwife's] patients, not mine; therefore it's not easy for the woman to have confidence in another person, she has confidence in the midwife and not in you. And besides, the midwife is a much older woman, with a lot of experience, and I am a student. So, it cost me something, [to speak out about the use of oxytocin], but finally one of the midwives said to me 'you were right, it was a good thing that you acted when you did.'"

Obviously, the relationship and dialogue between *parteras tradicionales* and *parteras profesionales* has not been without conflict. The question of whose knowledge is "authoritative" continues to arise, particularly around the use of oxytocin. The issue is made more complex when those questioning the authority of traditional midwives' knowledge are students who have not yet completed their training and do not have their traditional teacher's years of practical experience. In this situation, students may not easily persuade others that their biomedically based knowledge is authoritative: "[The apprenticeships] open an opportunity, but there are certain conflicts. Certainly conflicts. Not with much frequency, but last year there was a case where one of the students brought a woman to CASA [the maternity hospital] and the [traditional] midwife had said no, it wasn't necessary, but yes, it was necessary. This midwife wanted one hundred per cent control, but that's not the case. The two [midwife and student] are equal. So this midwife doesn't instruct our students now; we have looked for others."

However, the CASA students and midwives recognized that errors and differences of opinion can occur with any health practitioner, not only between those with medical training and those without: "When you encounter errors [made by traditional midwives], it's the same if you encounter errors by a doctor. In the end I believe that the intention of people in the health sector is to help people who need it . . . there is no bad intention." Ultimately, the students and midwives believed it was possible to maintain relationships in spite of these conflicts, and did maintain them.

In addition to knowledge acquisition, this mutual learning process also resulted in a change of identity, a kind of personal transformation, for both the students and traditional midwives. "Empowerment" may be an overused word, but it seems apt here. Through their acquisition of biomedical knowledge from the students that they could share with others, *parteras tradicionales* gained status in their communities and respect from their families. The transfer of biomedical knowledge can result in a sense of diminishment as traditional practitioners come to see their practices as incorrect; it can also result in an increased sense of confidence as they acquire new knowledge and are able to articulate their existing knowledge in biomedical terms and transform it in evidence-based ways.

Biomedical learning, therefore, has neither completely positive nor negative consequences. It is difficult to avoid acquiring such knowledge without cost, because one can never stand from a vantage point completely outside one's knowledge system; the professional midwives and students continued to judge what was "right" and "wrong" according to the standards of their own system. However, although this issue seems unavoidable, in the case of the CASA students and their traditional midwife teachers, it may be ameliorated by the development of a relationship in which the skills and deficiencies of practitioners from both systems can be acknowledged, and in which the acquisition of new skills by both groups can be acknowledged and supported.

The CASA students' recognition of the ethical principles underlying both biomedical and traditional knowledge systems is a further step in resolving this dilemma. Students felt that Mexican women should have as great a right to a safe birth as a woman in the United States or Canada, and that the application of medical knowledge to save a mother's life is as ethical as the traditional midwives' practice of being *with* the birthing woman. Such a recognition allows for a dialogue based on a common ethical commitment, and presents a shift that allows for the sharing of power between professional and traditional practitioners.

One student's approach to midwifery was also influenced by her experience in a hospital in the neighboring province of San Luis Potosí, where she observed women who had been transported to the hospital when complications arose during births attended by traditional practitioners. She stated, "The traditional midwives, in some ways, have much knowledge, but there are also many myths that they work with, many myths." In conjunction with another medical practitioner, she developed a training program based on her observations of labor complications occurring during births attended by traditional practitioners (or family members, or not attended at all). The training program focused on actions the *parteras* and *parteros*[12] could take to manage and prevent these complications. For example, although it requires a specialist to *treat* a woman with preeclampsia, the CASA graduate taught techniques that traditional midwives could use to *change the profile* of a preeclamptic woman. She took the traditional midwives' own experiences into account: because many of her trainees had not attended a breech birth, she taught a technique for managing this circumstance. She also considered the practitioners' resources and circumstances: "We did not pretend that they had an operating theater available . . . but they can have clean clothes, they can have their instruments sterilized by putting them in liquid or in an oven, all this they can do in some way."

This CASA graduate felt that she was continuing the tradition of *partería mexicana* while integrating it with biomedical knowledge:

What I did during training was to facilitate a dialogue. I tried to teach a little of what I had learned, and they taught me a little of what they knew. Therefore, everyone gave me herbs and I quickly made a manual for their use. When the course ended, she gave each a copy of the manual she had made along with a book on the biomedical techniques taught during the course. Like other CASA students and midwives, she was concerned about the lack of recognition of traditional midwives' knowledge and its absence from official textbooks. She was able to reconcile the biomedical and traditional systems because both practices, she believed, embodied ethical principles: Here in Mexico I think that the importance of medical training should be recognized, because we need to recognize risks, because I think it's an ethical principle not to risk the life of another person and her baby . . . it's an ethical principle to have sufficient knowledge not to put a life at risk. But the practice of traditional midwifery is an ethical practice, the empathy, the warmth . . . this is also ethical behavior. Therefore, now we are trained as much by doctors as by traditional midwives, we have both formations, so I am able to give medical instruction like that I received at CASA, but without losing touch with traditional midwives. I believe that is very important.

Students who are the daughters, nieces, or granddaughters of traditional practitioners may have already learned some of their forebears' skills; in other cases, however, their mothers or grandmothers have been reluctant to pass on their skills for fear of legal liability, although they hope that their daughters' professional training will enable them to take responsibility for maternal health in their communities upon return from CASA. Although not all students with a direct experience of traditional midwifery had learned practical skills from their forebears, they appreciated the contribution that their mothers and grandmothers had made to the community, especially where no other medical services were available.

Students from rural communities—as well as CASA's *promotoras* and educators—were concerned about the maltreatment of poor and indigenous people and their lack of access to health services. Many have experienced the consequences of Mexico's underfunded rural hospitals and clinics for its pregnant women, witnessing psychological as well as physical maltreatment there. Young women from more affluent backgrounds have also sought their education at CASA, and have been transformed in their attitude toward more impoverished communities. One middle-class student reported that "the *partera* had very few resources, she lived in poverty, and I didn't like it when I arrived the first day. But each *partera* had such humility that actually I'm thinking of working in a community, I've changed my mind completely, and actually my intention is to serve regardless of what I earn. I believe that when you do something with love, everything follows."

One of the defining characteristics of dialogue is its reciprocity: both partners speak and listen. The CASA program has allowed for such a dialogue between traditional and professional midwives not only because it allows the traditional midwife to become the authoritative partner in her relationship with the student, but because through sharing her life and understanding her experiences, a relationship develops that allows the dialogue to be sustained through episodes of conflict. In the context of this relationship, students have learned how to apply traditional techniques, including massages, herbal teas, herbal baths, *manteada*, and other techniques for external version, and upright positions for birth that facilitate both normal and breech deliveries. What has been impressed upon the students most strongly, however, is the importance of working with the laboring woman in an egalitarian rather than an authoritarian fashion, respecting her body and desires, and developing an attitude of patience and empathy. This emphasis on respect for the laboring woman means that the professional midwife may choose either biomedical or traditional techniques, or a combination, according to the woman's own wishes and what will serve her best. In other words, the professional midwife can create an expansive and open, comprehensive knowledge system that accommodates multiple ways of knowing about birth.

In May 2000, Sandra Morningstar, with the help of the CASA staff, organized a "herstorical event" in San Miguel called *Cultura Viviente* (Living Culture)—"a gathering of hundreds of regional village midwives from Guanajuato to document their birthways, traditional ceremonies, and visions for the future" (personal communication). At this gathering, a new Asociación de Parteras de Guanajuato (APGAR) was formed, with Antonia Córdova Morales as its first president. In such ways, even as CASA proceeds with its professionalizing enterprise, its members continue to demonstrate support for, and philosophical and political solidarity with, traditional midwives.

The Fifth Step: Achieving Recognition and Pioneering New Paths

It took almost ten years and much hard work and political networking to ensure that the CASA graduates would obtain the federal professional seal (*cédula profesional*)[13] that recognizes them as independent health professionals qualified to practice in any state. In this quest CASA was opposed by those who want to equate "professional" only with a university education, as well as by various physicians and state government officials who disliked the idea of autonomous midwives. In a front-page article on CASA in the *Wall Street Journal*, reporter Jonathan Friedland (2000: 1) wrote:

> Carlos Tena, the secretary of health of Guanajuato state, where both the school and hospital are located, says that while he is all for giving existing midwives the training necessary to do their jobs better, he sees no point in

creating new ones. "I don't think Nadine's vision is workable," says Dr. Tena, a cardiologist. "And I will continue fighting with her as long as she demands that parteras be recognized as professionals. . . ." Roberto Uribe, a professor at the National Autonomous University of Mexico and an officer of the National Federation of Gynecologists and Obstetricians, says the idea of reviving the partera, even with clinical training, "is a tremendous step backward." "It doesn't matter if the parteras all die off," Dr. Uribe says. "The real issue is: How do you get rural women to the hospital on time?"

In fact, transport to the hospital in many rural areas is often simply not a viable option: many rural women cannot afford and/or do not have access to transportation. Professional midwives who can screen women for risk and (if necessary) bring them to the hospital in advance, who have the skills and equipment to handle sudden emergencies at home, and who live and work in the communities where women live and give birth—and where they can provide backup services to traditional midwives—constitute a far more viable alternative (Davis-Floyd 2003).

The national Instituto Mexicano del Seguro Social (IMSS) operates a branch program called IMSS-Oportunidades that provides medical services to rural people who do not have medical insurance with one of Mexico's social security institutes (which provide health care to those employed in the formal sector and their families). Individuals who are covered by the IMSS-Oportunidades program are more likely to be poor and indigenous. In 2003 an agreement was reached with IMSS to allow CASA graduates to practice in the rural clinics and hospitals associated with the Oportunidades program. By 2005 eight CASA graduates had undertaken their obligatory social service and residency training at IMSS-Oportunidades hospitals (Escandón Romero 2006).[14] This collaboration between CASA and IMSS was part of an IMSS strategy to increase rural women's access to obstetric care by qualified practitioners. IMSS evaluations of the CASA graduates have consistently rated their performance as good to very good (Escandón Romero 2006: 1).

A similar sort of agreement was finally achieved with the federal Ministry of Health in August 2006. In order for CASA graduates' qualifications to be recognized by Ministry of Health institutions, a federal organization, CIFRHS (Comisión Interinstitucional para la Formación de Recursos Humanos para la Salud [Interinstitutional Commission for Health Human Resources Training]) had to certify the school's curriculum. This certification was granted in August 2006. IMSS-Oportunidades supported CIFRHS's recommendation of CASA to the Ministry of Health, as did an evaluation by the National Public Health Institute (Instituto Nacional de Salud Pública). This evaluation, which compared CASA students' knowledge of safe birth practices with that of students from the National School of Obstetric Nursing and the Medical School of UNAM (the National

Autonomous University of Mexico), found that CASA students performed significantly better (Walker 2006: 1).[15]

Federal Ministry of Health recognition opens the possibility for CASA graduates to practice in the public health system. Because this system is decentralized to the state level, ultimately their work opportunities will be determined by the Ministry of Health in each particular state. Excellent relations have been established with the Secretaría de Salud of the state of San Luis Potosí, which has been hiring CASA graduates to work in its rural clinics and to establish training programs for traditional midwives. In 2005 the Secretaría de Salud from San Luis Potosí received a national prize from the federal health ministry for its excellent work in lowering maternal mortality rates in indigenous populations through the incorporation of professional midwives (graduates from CASA) into its interdisciplinary team. Although the graduates are now recognized as *parteras profesionales*— primary autonomous caregivers—this status has not permeated the system and is thus not recognized in their salaries; they are still paid as obstetric nurses.

The CASA students' education, both in a technical sense and in the sense of their development as individuals, does not end with their CASA training. The need to demonstrate that their training is legitimate continues beyond graduation. One graduate experienced a form of re-socialization when working for a government institution: "They were afraid of how I was going to work, so I had to teach them my method of working, I had to demonstrate that I wasn't running risks with the person I was attending, and I think that I had to learn a method a little more like a normal hospital . . . but I never forgot that I was a midwife."

The ultimate goal of the school is to graduate students from rural communities who will return to practice in those communities. But there is no guarantee that these women will be able to make a living if they do return home. Most traditional midwives are poor because they often are not paid for their services or are paid very little. Graduates of a rigorous three-year professional program are going to expect a more substantial and steady income. Goodman and her colleagues are keenly aware of this problem; they are also aware that the Secretaría de Salud (SSA) and the IMSS have built thousands of rural clinics that are drastically understaffed, and they hope to convince these agencies to offer permanent, government-funded posts to the CASA graduates. At these clinics, CASA graduates could serve as primary health care workers, interacting with traditional midwives, attending births, and providing well-woman and reproductive care under government auspices. Some graduates to date have succeeded in obtaining such posts, while others struggle to find their way. Future challenges include generating legal status for them in the State of Guanajuato and, perhaps, nationwide, which will necessitate the passage of new legislation.

As of May 2007, twenty-three students had graduated from CASA with twenty-six more on the way. Thirteen of the graduates were in private practice; six were working at CASA; one was working at a health center in San Luis Potosí; two were currently doing their social service, one in San Luis Potosí, one in Puebla; and one worked as a radiologist in Guanajuato. About these students, Alison Bastien (May 2007, personal communication) states,

> It is a huge personal commitment to be a midwife, in any epoch of human history. But the young women who choose to come and give over their lives for three years in our CASA school, and then another year of social service, for an uncertain future in part of their own sheer will and networking—it's awesome. Last summer we had a conference at CASA in which all of our graduates to date were invited back to give presentations on life after graduation. The entire auditorium was filled for the first time with us—*CASA people*— not visiting Americans, not local politicians, just midwives, and the current students rose to their feet, many in tears of inspiration, to give (for just one example) Nohemi from Guerrero a standing ovation after she talked about her work as a community organizer there.

Astonishing and promising is the fact that doctors running rural clinics for the government have recently been sent to stay with the CASA students in the dorm and take classes with them; in Goodman's words, socioculturally this equates to "the CEO of Enron staying at the janitor's house" and is a clear indication of recognition of the value of the CASA model.

For the first several years, the CASA midwives have worked as employees of the hospital. Several years ago, they formed a midwifery collective as independent practitioners, renting offices from the hospital for prenatal and postpartum care and attending births there. At present, this collective is composed of six midwives—Antonia Cordova Morales, the first CASA midwife, and younger colleagues Isabel, Nancy, Anabel, Fabiola, and Maru (Antonia's own daughter). Alison Bastien informs us that in a continued effort to make the CASA hospital more self-sustaining and to help the students gain decision-making skills and more confidence in additional aspects of woman and baby care, the midwifery collective recently let go of all the nurses so that the midwifery students can learn to perform all the caregiving that previously was in the nurses' territory. Alison notes,

> This is a tiny change, in the sense that there were never more than two nurses on shift at any given moment anyway, but I think it speaks volumes about what we want our midwives to be able to know and do. We will be celebrating the 25th anniversary of CASA this summer with a newly remodelled birthing area in the clinic, including two birthing bathtubs, birthing stools, and some other midwifery-friendly, mother-friendly modifications. CASA,

even though it is always having its share of problems, is always in a state of change, improvement, flux, adaptation. The project and its people are never stagnant. (May 2007, personal communication)

CONCLUSION: SUSTAINABILITY AND REPLICATION

Our reality in Mexico includes a lack of access and attention to obstetric emergencies and a lack of humanization in birth and respect for the woman. And much obstetric practice is not evidence-based and does unintentional harm to women. It is urgent that we work together in a movement to change this situation.

NADINE GOODMAN, "In Encouragement of the Active and Effective Participation of All Types of Midwives and Obstetric Nurses in Mexico," 2004

These words form part of a document Nadine wrote in an effort to generate ongoing communication and cooperation with Mexico's *enfermeras obstetras* (obstetric nurses), many of whom would like the ability to become nurse-midwives with the autonomy to attend births. Should they succeed, their large numbers could overwhelm the CASA direct-entry model, subsuming it in favor of nurse-midwifery education. Well aware of CASA's fragility in this and other political realms, Goodman has expended a great deal of time and effort to establish relationships with obstetrical nursing leaders, to bring them to CASA to see the model in action, to convince them of the value of this direct-entry model, to develop strong and harmonious working relationships, and to avoid possible political conflict. She supports the obstetrical nurses in their desire to become nurse-midwives, and at present, the obstetrical nursing leaders seem favorably disposed to supporting two kinds of midwifery education in Mexico.

As a result of grant-writing efforts by Goodman and her colleagues and the concrete results CASA has produced, over time CASA has received financial support from individuals and from groups such as the David and Lucile Packard Foundation, the John D. and Catherine T. MacArthur Foundation, the Turner Foundation, and the Moriah Fund. In all, to date CASA has raised more than $15 million to fund its activities. Its annual budget approaches $1.5 million; CASA's Development Office supports and manages its fundraising work. CASA has a paid staff of 100 and nearly 300 volunteers; their multiservice work reaches more than 60,000 people per year. CASA averages twelve international interns per year. Interns participate in all aspects of CASA's outreach programs.[16] Its peer counseling program has now been replicated in four other states, and graduates from its midwifery school attend to thousands of women in thirteen states throughout the Mexican republic.

At present, CASA's continued success depends on continued outside funding. Aware of the fragility of such dependence, CASA is making efforts to establish and build an endowment fund. CASA owns all of its multiple facilities free and clear: the hospital, the large school and day care center campus, its adolescent training center, and an income-producing apartment building. The hospital and school campus were designed and built by Goodman's husband, Alejandro Gonzalez, in traditional colonial style. The campus includes classrooms for the midwives and the day care children, spacious gardens and common areas, a large playground, and a dormitory with living area and kitchen where the midwifery students live and prepare their meals. To ensure access to the midwifery education program from individuals at all income levels, their education and dorm space are free to students who cannot pay.

Although its community has embraced and come to have a sense of participation in and ownership of CASA, at its most elemental level, this chapter tells the story of a particular woman's achievement of a comprehensive dream: to offer women choices in reproduction and effective access to the accomplishment of those choices. It's a *can-do* story. See a need for a family planning and reproductive education program? Create one. Need a better hospital? Build one. Need midwives to work in your hospital? Start a school to educate them. Need federal recognition for them? Lobby effectively and obtain it. Need more money? Write more grant proposals, and base them on the good work you've already done. Goodman has been called a "one-woman bulldozer"—she simply does not let apparently overwhelming obstacles stop her, a skill many of those who want to create birth models that work would do well to develop. In recognition of their work, Goodman and her husband received the Population Connections Leadership Award at a ceremony in New York City, April 27, 2006. Their story and the story of all those who do CASA's work is a powerful demonstration of the difference strong leaders can make.

Over time, the CASA midwifery school, and Goodman, have experienced a good deal of opposition from various government officials and physicians that helped Goodman hone her bulldozing skills. Although the state Ministry of Education has been supportive, the state Ministry of Health, which is run by physicians, has not. At one point in 1998, the health ministry threatened to shut down the CASA hospital by refusing to renew its license if the midwives were not removed. CASA and its many supporters gathered more than 10,000 signatures from people in San Miguel and the rural communities served by CASA workers, as well as 200 letters of support from CASA donors, and delivered them to then-governor Vicente Fox (Friedland 2000). Shortly thereafter, the hospital's license was renewed. Part of CASA's ability to garner such widespread, grassroots support stems from the multiple services it provides—as noted above, its family planning and reproductive education services reach over 60,000 people per year, far more than the 6,000 birthing women its midwives have attended. Its success to date is inscribed in concrete, plaster, and stone, and also in the bodies and lives of the many thousands its programs serve. Goodman is the first to admit that victory has not been achieved—CASA is still one tiny birth model that works in a vast region that needs many more—but it *has* opened a humanistic chink in the system, and its replication is ensured.

In 2008 CASA obtained agreements with the Health and Education departments in the Mexican state of Chiapas, to establish two new midwifery schools, with the objective of graduating hundreds of new *parteras profesionales* (see www.casa.org.mx). Discussions about establishing other schools are also underway with the Mexican states of San Luis Potosí, Guerrero, Michoacán, Durango, and Nayarit. Significant funding for these schools has been obtained from the Carso Institute for Health, with further funding pending from other institutions. The school in Chiapas, which will also serve students from Guatemala, is expected to open in January 2009. The CASA model, in other words, is achieving replication and its many supporters, including Goodman, hope to spread it throughout Central America and beyond.

ACKNOWLEDGMENTS

From Lisa: I want to thank the midwifery students and midwives at CASA for their time, their thoughts, their dedication, and their warmth in welcoming me to San Miguel de Allende.

From Robbie: I wish to express my appreciation to the Wenner-Gren Foundation for Anthropological Research for Grants #6015 and #6247, which supported the research on which this chapter is based, to Nadine Goodman for her careful review of the chapter and her work to obtain the statistics this chapter presents, and to *las parteras profesionales de CASA por su dedicación, y por haber compartido conmigo sus experiencias, sus motivos, y sus visiones para el futuro de la partería Mexicana.*

NOTES

1. This chapter is based on interviews and observations carried out by Lisa Mills and Robbie Davis-Floyd. Between February and April 2002, Lisa carried out sixteen interviews with professional midwives, teachers, and students at CASA, two interviews with IMSS officials in July 2004, two interviews with CASA midwives in July 2006, and a further telephone interview in March 2007. Robbie carried out interviews between 1998 and 2002 with CASA's founder Nadine Goodman, four consecutive directors of the CASA educational program (Anne Davenport, Gloria Metcalfe, Rosa Hidalgo, and Jennifer Goldberg—other directors not

interviewed during their tenures include Estela Motolo, Maricruz Coronado, and Fabiola Zarate); CASA's clinical director Antonia Cordova, two of CASA's first staff midwives, the four members of CASA's first graduating class, and nine other CASA students prior to their graduation. It is also informed on both our parts by ongoing conversations with our interviewees; attendance at a midwifery conference at CASA in 2002; on Robbie's part by continued visits to the CASA hospital and school, and ongoing communication with Nadine Goodman and with CASA staff midwives and students; and on Lisa's part by conversations with traditional midwives in the communities surrounding San Miguel and observation of the interaction between the two at the CASA maternity hospital and in the community. This chapter also draws on the findings published in "*La Partera Profesional:* Articulating Identity and Cultural Space for a New Kind of Midwife in Mexico" (Davis-Floyd 2001).

2. *Partera tradicional* and *comadrona* are usually translated as "traditional midwife" and *partera profesional* as "professional midwife," which is how we will use these terms here. The term "empirical midwife" is sometimes used to distinguish those who learned midwifery through attending women in childbirth or through short training courses from those who learned it through a long tradition of apprenticeship. However, most often the terms *partera tradicional* and *partera empírica* are used interchangeably. In this article, for the sake of simplicity, we will confine ourselves to *partera tradicional.*

3. For a discussion of the problematics encapsulated in the term "traditional birth attendant," see Pigg (1997), Davis-Floyd (2005), and Davis-Floyd, Cosminsky, and Pigg (2001):105–121.

4. The child of a family with nine brothers and sisters, Antonia Córdova Morales grew up taking care of the cows and working with her parents and siblings in the fields around her hometown of San Miguel. She received no formal schooling, and at the age of twelve she went to work as a maid. She married young and gave birth to six children, all of whom were born in her home with a traditional midwife in attendance. Although there were hospitals, she told me she was afraid to go to them because she knew how badly poor women were treated there, and because her mother had successfully birthed all her children at home, Antonia saw no reason not to do the same. She added that, since she became a midwife, in addition to all her other clients, she has attended every family member who has given birth (over twenty-five)—a fact of which she is very proud. Antonia became a midwife "by accident," when she was called to attend the birth of a neighbor, yet went on to internalize both the philosophy and the skills of professional midwifery.

5. Antonia's description of her government training course echoes descriptions of equally inadequate TBA training described by Jordan (1993) and, more recently, by various authors in the new collection *Midwives in Mexico: Continuity, Controversy, and Change* (Good Maust, Güémez Piñeda, and Davis-Floyd, n.d.).

6. Additional services provided by the CASA hospital staff by 2004 include attending 157,159 out-patient visits and administering 6,125 Pap smears to detect cervical cancer, 9,401 ultrasound examinations, 627 sterilization procedures, and 5,021 free HIV tests.

7. The CASA School of Professional Midwifery is accredited by the Guanajuato State Department of Education, Accord No. 176–97, 4 July 1997, Registration No.

11PETO143N. For more information, write to the CASA School of Professional Midwives, Santa Julia No. 15, Col. Santa Julia, San Miguel de Allende, GTO, Mexico 37700. See www.casa.org.mx.

8. In creating both the home birth service and the community apprenticeship program, CASA has been assisted by Sandra Morningstar, a certified professional midwife from Missouri, who moved to San Miguel in the mid-1990s to help make Nadine's vision a reality. Currently, Sandra works in the CASA hospital as a professional midwife for part of the year and helps with the clinical training of CASA students.

9. A few professional midwives unrelated to CASA (all of whom received training outside Mexico or apprenticed with those who did) who incorporate traditional techniques practice in Mexico City, Xalapa in the state of Vera Cruz, Cuernavaca and Tepoztlan in the state of Morelos, Oaxaca City, Chiapas, and a few other places (see Davis-Floyd 2001 for some of their stories). And a number of "postmodern" traditional midwives who incorporate scientific, evidence-based procedures in their practices work can be found, especially in the city of Cuernavaca, Morelos (see Davis-Floyd 2003). In 2007 these professionalizing traditional midwives started a new School of Traditional Midwifery (see www.partera.org for more information). And in Oaxaca City, an organization called *Nueve Lunas* (Nine Moons, for the nine months of pregnancy) has created a midwifery school called *Luna Llena* (Full Moon), in which both professional and traditional midwives serve as teachers (see www.nuevelunas.org.mx).

10. The 1997 *Encuesta Nacional de la Dinámica Demográfica* (INEGI 1999) showed that 16.41% of Mexican births were delivered in *otro lugar* (another place), which, for the most part, would be births at home attended by a *partera*. This number breaks down to 5.48% in places with 15,000 or more inhabitants, and to 31.17% in places with fewer than 15,000 people. (Our thanks to demographer Joe Potter at the University of Texas for this information.)

11. In 2001 the national cesarean rate in the public sector was 32.5% and in the private sector was 60%. (Secretaría de Salud 2001). In 2005 the overall national cesarean rate was 39.3% (OECD 2007).

12. *Parteros* are male midwives. They are rare in most of the country, but in some areas of San Luis Potosí, *parteros*, who learn their skills from their fathers and grandfathers, are more common than female midwives.

13. Upon completion of their social service, CASA graduates are eligible to apply for their nationally recognized professional licenses (*cédula profesional*) from the Department of Professions, Ministry of Public Education (File # 11–00043).

14. The graduates have carried out their year of social service at IMSS institutions in the following locations: San Felipe Ecatepec, Chiapas (2 graduates); Coalcomán, Michoacán (2); Zacopoaxtla, Puebla (2); Zacatlpán, San Luis Potosí (1); and Juitlpaán, Veracruz Sur (2).

15. The evaluation is outlined in a letter to Dr. Enrique Ruelas Barajas, Subsecretario de Innovación y Calidad Secretaría de Salud (Deputy Secretary of Innovation and Quality, Federal Ministry of Health), from Dilys Margaret Walker of the Centro de Investigaciones en Salud Poblacional, Dirección de Salud Reproductiva. Instituto Nacional de Salud Pública (Reproductive Health Directorate of the

Research Center for Population Health, National Institute of Public Health) dated August 14, 2006.

16. For more information, write casainterns@hotmail.com.

REFERENCES

Belizán José, Fernando Althabe, Fernando Barros, and Sophie Alexander. 1999. "Rates and Implications of Caesarean Sections in Latin America: Ecological Study." *British Medical Journal* 319:1397–1400.

Camey, Xochitl Castañeda, Cecilia García Barrios, Xóchitl Romero Guerrero, Rosa María Núñez-Urquiza, Dolores González Hernández, and Ana Langer Glass. 1996. "Traditional Birth Attendants in Mexico: Advantages and Inadequacies of Care for Normal Deliveries," *Social Science and Medicine* 43.2:199–207.

CASA. N.d. Pamphlet.

Castro, Arachu. 1998. *The Burden of Excess Cesarean Sections in Mexico: Its Impact on Infant Morbidity and Mortality.* Cambridge, MA: Harvard Center for Population and Development Studies. Unpublished document.

Castro, Arachu, Angela Heimburger, and Ana Langer. N.d. *Iatrogenic Epidemic: How Health Care Professionals Contribute to the High Proportion of Cesarean Sections in Mexico.* David Rockefeller Center for Latin American Studies: Working Papers on Latin America, Paper No. 02/03–2. Available at www.medanthro.net/docs/castro_mexicocity.pdf.

Castro, Roberto, Lourdes Campero, Bernardo Hernández, and Ana Langer. 2000. "A Study on Maternal Mortality in Mexico through a Qualitative Approach," *Journal of Women's Health and Gender-Based Medicine* 9.6, pp. 679–689.

Comité Promotor por una Maternidad sin Riesgos. 1997. *Cesáreas: Tendencias actuales, y perspectivas.* México: Secretaría de Salud.

Córdova Morales, Antonia. 1997. "El Futuro de la Partería en México." Ponencia presentada en el "Curso Internacional: Actualidades en la Atención Perinatal," Hospital Central Militar, Auditorio General, Ciudad de Mexico. 23 de enero. Copies can be obtained from Antonia Córdova Morales, CASA Hospital, Indalecio Allende No. 4, Colonia San Rafael, San Miguel de Allende, Guanajuato 37730, Mexico. (011–52–415–26181).

Davis-Floyd, Robbie. 1998. "The Ups, Downs, and Interlinkages of Nurse-and Direct-Entry Midwifery: Status, Practice, and Education." In *Getting an Education: Paths to Becoming a Midwife,* 4th ed., edited by Jan Tritten and Joel Southern, 67–118. Eugene, OR: Midwifery Today. Also available at www.davis-floyd.com.

———. 2001. "*La Partera Profesional:* Articulating Identity and Cultural Space for a New Kind of Midwife in Mexico." *Medical Anthropology* 20.2/3–4:185–244. Also available at www.davis-floyd.com.

———. 2003. "Home Birth Emergencies in the U.S. and Mexico: The Trouble with Transport." *Social Science and Medicine* 56.9:1913–31. Also available at www.davis-floyd.com.

———. 2005. "Daughter of Time: The Postmodern Midwife." *MIDIRS Midwifery Digest* 15.1:32–39.

Davis-Floyd, Robbie, Sheila Cosminsky, and Stacy L. Pigg, eds. 2001. "Daughters of Time: The Shifting Identities of Contemporary Midwives." Special triple issue. *Medical Anthropology* 20:2–4.

Escandón Romero, Celia. 2006. Letter to Roberto Lara Arreola, June 1 (Celia Escandón Romero, personal collection).

Espinosa Damián, Gisela. 2004. "Doscientas trece voces contra la muerte: mortalidad materna en zonas indígenas." In *La Mortalidad Materna en México: Cuatro Visiones Críticas*, edited by Martha Castañeda, Daniela Díaz, Gisela Espinoza, Graciela Freyermuth, Dora Sanchez-Hidalgo, and Cecilia de la Torre, 161–238. Mexico City: Fundar, Centro de Análisis e Investigación, A.C., and K'inal Antzetik, A.C. www.modemmujer.org/El_Estante/Web's/libromortalidadmaterna.htm#introduccion.

Fernandez de Castillo, Carlos. 1997. "Las Cesáreas en el Sector Privado." *In Cesareas: Tendencias actuales y perspectivas.* Mexico City: IMES, Comité Promotor por una Maternidad sin Riesgos en México.

Friedland, Jonathan. 2000. "An American in Mexico Champions Midwifery as a Worthy Profession," *Wall Street Journal*, February 15, A1, A12.

Goodman, Nadine. N.d. "Cómo podemos asegurar los derechos de salud reproductiva de todas las mujeres mexicanas?" Unpublished paper.

—————. 2000. "De Qué Se Trata La Partería?" Oral presentation to Grupo Interinstitucional de Recursos Humanos de Salud. March. www.casa@unisono.net.mx.

—————. 2004. "In Encouragement of the Active and Effective Participation of All Types of Midwives and Obstetric Nurses in Mexico." Unpublished manuscript.

Good Maust, Marcia, Miguel Güémez Piñeda, and Robbie Davis-Floyd, eds. N.d. *Midwives in Mexico: Continuity, Controversy, and Change.* Unpublished ms.

INEGI 1999. *1997 Encuesta Nacional de la Dinámica Demográfica.* Mexico City: Instituto Nacional de Geografía y Estadística. www.INEGI.gob.mx.

Jordan, Brigitte. 1986. *Technology Transfer in Obstetrics: Theory and Practice in Developing Countries*, Working Paper 126. Palo Alto, CA: Institute for Research on Learning (IRL).

—————. 1993. *Birth in Four Cultures*, 4th ed. rev. and updated by Robbie Davis-Floyd. Prospect Heights, IL: Waveland.

—————. 1997. "Authoritative Knowledge and its Construction." In *Childbirth and Authoritative Knowledge: Cross-Cultural Perspectives*, edited by Robbie E. Davis-Floyd and Carolyn F. Sargent, 233–63. Berkeley: University of California Press.

Langer, Ana. 1997. *Identifying Interventions to Prevent Maternal Mortality in Mexico.* Paper presented at the Technical Consultation on Safe Motherhood, October 18–23.

—————. 1997. *Over-Medicalization and Appropriate Technologies.* Paper presented at the Technical Consultation on Safe Motherhood, October. 18–23.

Lara Arreola, Roberto. 2006. Letter to Maricruz Coronado, August 31 (Maricruz Coronado, personal collection).

Lefeber, Yvonne. 1994. *Midwives without Training: Practices and Beliefs of Traditional Birth Attendants in Africa, Asia and Latin-America.* Assen, NL: Van Gorcum.

Mills, Lisa. 2005. "Naming the Invisible: Facilitating a Dialogue between Professional and Traditional Midwifery in Mexico." Paper presented at the International Confederation of Midwives Conference, Midwifery in the Americas/Partería en las Americas," Trinidad and Tobago, April.

Mohan, Gilles. 2002. "Beyond Participation: Strategies for Deeper Empowerment," in *Participation: The New Tyranny*, edited by Bill Cooke and Uma Kothari, 153–67. London and New York: Zed Books.

Organization for Economic Cooperation and Development (OECD). *2007 Health Dataset*. www.oecd.org/LongAbstract/0,3425,en_2649_33929_37441245_1_1_1_1,00.html.

Pigg, Stacy L. 1997. "Authority in Translation: Finding, Knowing, Naming, and Training 'Traditional Birth Attendants' in Nepal." In *Childbirth and Authoritative Knowledge: Cross-Cultural Perspectives*, edited by Robbie Davis-Floyd and Carolyn Sargent, 233–62. Berkeley: University of California Press.

Ponce Cortes, Blanca. 2006. Letter to Julio M. Cacho Salazar, Secretario Técnico de la CIFRHS, August 17 (Blanca Ponce Cortes, personal collection).

Rothman, Barbara Katz. 1982. *In Labor: Women and Power in the Birthplace*. New York: W.W. Norton.

Secretaría de Programación y Presupuesto. 1979. *Encuesta Mexicana de Fecundidad, Primer Informe Nacional*. Mexico City: Secretaría de Programación y Presupuesto.

Secretaría de Salubridad y Asistencia. 2001. *Boletín de Información Estadística Recursos y Servicios*, vol. I. Mexico City: Secretaría de Salubridad y Asistencia.

Secretaría de Salud [SSA: this agency was formerly known as the Secretaría de Salud y Asistencia, and the name is still abbreviated as SSA]. 1994. *La Partera Tradicional en la Atención Materno Infantil en México*. www.ssa.gob.mx.

Secretaría de Salud de Guanajuato. 2006. "Dirección del Área de Epidemiología: Mortalidad Materna y Perinatal." Slide Presentation.

Uribe Zúñiga, Patricia. 2006. Letter to Roberto Lara Arreola, Director General de Calidad y Educación en Salud, June 14 (Patricia Uribe Zúñiga, personal collection).

Walker, Dilys Margaret. 2006. Letter to Enrique Ruelas Berejas. August 14.

Chapter 12

Mercy in Action

Bringing Mother- and Baby-Friendly Birth Centers to the Philippines

Vicki Penwell

SYNOPSIS

I studied the first 7,565 women admitted for labor and delivery in two charity birth centers that I established in the Philippines through Mercy in Action, the faith-based, nonprofit organization our family founded (see www.mercyinaction.org). The births in this study occurred between February 8, 1996 (the day the first woman delivered in our newly established birth center), and December 31, 2003 (when we ended the study to begin compiling data for my master's thesis). All the women who were admitted for delivery are included in this reporting. (Women risked out prior to labor are not included in this study.) Midwives conducted all of the deliveries. These were certified professional midwives (CPMs)[1] or licensed midwives (LMs)[2] from the United States and the Philippines. In the vast majority of cases, student midwives under direct supervision helped "catch" the babies as they were born, and assisted in all aspects of maternity and newborn care. All students represented in this study were enrolled in Mercy in Action's program for midwifery and primary health care training, and dual enrolled as candidates for an accredited associate of science in midwifery degree from the National College of Midwifery (see www.midwiferycollege.org and Chapter 9). The birthing women were at higher than average risk of a poor pregnancy outcome because of demographic factors: most were poor, often malnourished, and living in crowded urban slum conditions. In all, 92% of the women and 34% of their spouses were unemployed, and the average income was the equivalent of less than US$2 per day. Only a little over half were married.

In spite of the poverty, 95% of these women had spontaneous vaginal births; 83% had blood loss less than 500 cc, with only 2% having blood loss greater than 1,000 cc. Eighty-five percent of the babies required no resuscitation effort; 67% of the labors were without fetal distress or meconium staining; and 90% of the babies were of normal birth weight. Transfers to a hospital after admission to the birth center occurred 7% of the time, with 3% of transports during first stage and 0.5% during second stage. Less than half of these transports resulted in cesarean section births. One and one-half percent of total deliveries transported occurred during the postpartum period, and 2% were referrals for the baby to be seen by a doctor. Neonatal mortality was 4.1/1,000, four times lower than the neonatal mortality rate of 18/1,000 for the Philippines as a whole. Maternal mortality was 53/100,000 births, compared with 200/100,000 births for the Philippines, also four times lower than the nation as a whole, and when adjusted for causes of death that were not directly related to the pregnancy or birth, that figure was halved, to 26/100,000 births (Penwell 2005a).

When I conducted the research for my master's thesis for the National College of Midwifery, my friend and mentor Elizabeth Gilmore suggested I write my null hypothesis stating that I expected our outcomes for these 7,565 births to be worse than the national average for the Philippines. My hypothesis read as follows:

> The null hypothesis is that all these women would have worse outcomes than a similar group of women, for the following reasons based on usual assumptions: because all deliveries were conducted by midwives and no deliveries were conducted by doctors; because the midwives conducting the deliveries were direct-entry-trained midwives at the Associate Degree level rather than nurse-midwives or physicians with advanced degrees; because the majority of patient care, including the "catching" of babies, also involved student midwives under supervision of Licensed Midwives or Certified Professional Midwives; because the deliveries were all conducted out of hospital; and because the staff had access to only simple technology—on site we did not have lab capability, ICU or NICU capability, or surgical capability. In addition to that, and maybe most important to this study being unique, the mothers were demographically high risk. (Penwell 2005b)

Elizabeth said that such results would be expected based on the fairly universally held belief that doctor-attended hospital births would be safer than midwife-attended births in an out-of-hospital setting, especially for high-risk women living in poverty. By the time I finished this research and my thesis, our number of deliveries had increased to more than 12,000 in the slums of the Philippines, all of them free of charge to women who would be considered the poorest of the poor. I knew that we were having good outcomes, so I balked at Elizabeth's suggestion, but now I am so glad I wrote my hypothesis the way she had suggested, because in proving this hypothesis wrong, a model that works has been revealed in an unlikely place.

WHAT WORKS AND WHAT DOESN'T

Based on my own research and my twenty-seven years of international midwifery experience, I firmly believe that the model that works (and will work anywhere in the world, under any conditions) is this: When birth is normal, nothing should be done to interfere; even seemingly small interruptions of the natural process can and often do cause pathology and a domino effect of complications. Conversely, if a labor becomes abnormal, everything possible should be done to correct the problem, quickly and efficiently, in the setting in which the birth is occurring. This means midwives must be trained and equipped to carry out many medical interventions that are often thought to be the domain of physicians only. All birthing women, regardless of ability to pay, should have a trained birth attendant close to where they live, and those midwives should be trained in advanced life-saving skills, as well as being taught to respect the normal physiological process of parturition. Women and babies should always be treated gently, kindly, and with utmost respect.

It is really so simple: reduce interventions in the normal physiological and social process of birth, be prepared to perform advanced emergency life-saving skills in the event of an emergency, and be nice. In my opinion, many midwives I have observed do too much fiddling during normal birth and are not trained or allowed to do enough in the event of a life-threatening obstetric emergency. Unfortunately, kindness and compassion are too often ignored during the delivery of maternity care in both developing and developed countries. The North American midwifery model of care, as described by Citizens for Midwifery (see www.cfmidwifery.org/mmoc/) has something important to offer the entire world.

In writing about a model that works, it is first necessary to describe the current model forced on most poor women worldwide. Hospitals and government-run birth centers that serve the poor are too often inadequately funded and understaffed, resulting in substandard care. In addition, the abuses that occur on a regular basis to women giving birth are not often discussed, although in recent years the World Health Organization (WHO) and the United Nations have begun to mention the problem of rude and culturally insensitive maternity care (see www.safemotherhood.org/smpriorities/index.html). From my years of traveling the globe as a midwife, observing births in many cultures on several continents and in dozens of countries, I am convinced that the problem is twofold:

1. Midwives are being trained largely by doctors, or at least influenced heavily by a medical model of intervention, so normal birth is being seriously compromised. This is especially true in developing nations, where you see midwives, even at home births, forcing mothers onto their backs for delivery, performing numerous vaginal exams, shoving the baby out

with fundal pressure, cutting episiotomies, and separating the newborn and mother at birth. Rough treatment and practices that rob dignity from the mother giving birth are the norm, rather than the exception, even within the practice of midwifery.

2. Midwives are not prepared with the necessary skills or resources for obstetric emergencies; the midwives I have witnessed working around the world often do not carry a full range of oxytocic drugs, IV fluid, suction or resuscitation equipment such as DeLees and ambu bags, or vacuum extractors for a second-stage obstructed labor or fetal distress. Nor have they been trained in manual removal of placentas or neonatal resuscitation. Furthermore, very often they have not been taught the principles of uterine massage and immediate breastfeeding to prevent postpartum hemorrhage, or basic hygiene and the importance of sterile technique after rupture of membranes, during cord cutting, and while suturing the perineum.

According to the WHO 2005 *World Health Report,* the world's greatest current health need is making motherhood safe and saving the lives of newborns. The WHO 2005 report goes even further by stating that the health care professional needed most to save the lives of the mothers and babies is the midwife—especially the midwife who is trained to work outside of hospitals.

Childbirth in much of the world is a study in contrasts. On the one hand, it is a time of joy and celebration of new life. Yet for far too many families worldwide, it becomes a nightmare that ends in death or permanent disability. Well over half a million women die each year attempting to give birth, with the vast majority of all maternal deaths occurring in Africa and Asia. For every one woman who dies during pregnancy or childbirth, 100 more women experience morbidity, often resulting in a lifelong disability. Newborns that die within the first few days of life account for 37% of all deaths among children under five years old.

The Philippines is a land of contrast as well. On the one hand, it is a beautiful tropical archipelago of more than 7,100 islands populated by warm, friendly people. Yet it is also a land of severe poverty and deprivation, where many families live in squatter huts without sanitation or clean water sources, and the minimum wage for a laborer is the equivalent of between US$1.00 and $2.00 per day. Philippine national statistics show that, on average, eleven mothers die of pregnancy and childbirth-related causes every day, and a newborn baby dies every twelve minutes.[3]

The World Health Organization understands the need for midwives. In order to save the lives of the mothers and babies now being lost, not only do midwives need to be involved, but they also need to be trained to work under a model that respects women and the process of normal birth *and* respects the fact that normal birth can suddenly and without warning turn into a life-threatening emergency. Midwives can and must be trained to protect the normalcy of birth while being ready for and equipped to jump into any possible emergency with skills and tools necessary to save lives. In *Priorities for Safe Motherhood,* WHO reinforced its stand that all maternity care should be delivered if possible in midwife-run facilities, provided close to the woman's home and with her cultural values identified and respected.[4]

I first read about the Safe Motherhood Initiative in the late 1980s, soon after WHO began to track the tragedy and the magnitude of maternal death. At the time I was running a small, nonprofit, freestanding birth center and home birth practice that I had established in Fairbanks, Alaska. In 1990 I went on a medical mission trip with my church to Thailand, Laos, and the Philippines, and what I experienced there shattered me. I saw firsthand the devastating effects of the lack of health care for women, or in many cases, the wrong things being done to women, with disastrous results. On this visit, and countless times since, I have witnessed women being treated roughly while giving birth; I have realized to my horror that it is the dirty little secret of maternity care in the developing world that much physical and emotional abuse of patients takes place at the hands of those sworn to protect them. I personally have witnessed doctors, nurses, and midwives punching, slapping, and viciously pinching women in the face, thighs, or buttocks during a normal delivery. There are often overly rough vaginal exams before and after birth that make otherwise stoic women cry out in shock and pain, and weep uncontrollably afterwards. I have witnessed verbal abuse of women and the common practice of blaming them when an outcome is bad. In one case a woman who presented with a fetal demise was told it was her fault because she was "so dirty and stupid." Sometimes sexual remarks are directed at women in the form of crude jokes. I have seen women lying in large open rooms, ten or twelve delivery tables all out in the open, where it is normal practice after the baby has been taken to the nursery to leave the woman lying spread-eagle for an hour or more, genitals exposed, while male cleaning staff mop the floors around her and dozens of people come in and out. I have seen fundal pressure exerted in second stage with such force that it cracked the birthing woman's ribs. I have witnessed utter disregard for hygiene and sterile technique, seeing many women put on delivery tables that were still bloody from the last patient, and leftover suture thread being reused on numerous women. Rubber gloves are rinsed out and used again and again for vaginal exams, including on women who had ruptured membranes.

Hospitals for those below the poverty line often make do with inadequate facilities. Bathrooms are communal and in short supply, showers are cold water only with dipper and bucket, and cleanliness is not a high priority because of the extreme pressure on the staff to manage a patient load as high as 120 births in a twenty-four-hour period. Open windows allow stray cats to come and go in the hospital, but no one chases them out, because they catch the mice and rats that are also commonly seen in the hospital wards. Open, unscreened windows also invite mosquitoes that carry malaria and dengue fever.

There is never an ambu bag or oxygen in the delivery room in the low-resource hospitals in the Philippines where I have volunteered or transported patients. Sometimes they have an infant resuscitation bag in the neonatal intensive care unit (NICU), but not in the delivery room, so resuscitation, if needed, is delayed. A few hospitals we transported to had only an adult-size resuscitation bag, and personnel had to pump it only partially to avoid exploding a newborn's tiny lungs. Fetal heart tones are rarely if ever monitored in labor, even if the mother is in second stage an hour or more, and most hospitals for the poor have only a stethoscope for auscultating the fetus. After being removed from their mothers, newborn babies are put three or four together in small bassinettes, naked, waiting to be bathed, where they are exposed to cross-infection and cold stress. Mothers are put two or three together in single beds to recover postpartum. Depending on the hospital, they are lucky if there is a mattress, much less a sheet, on this bed. Much of this is unavoidable because resources are few, but it all contributes to the lack of safety for the mothers and babies (on several occasions Mercy in Action has donated ambu bags, Dopplers, and other equipment to the labor and delivery wards of underequipped hospitals).

Early on in my years of volunteering in the Philippines, I was in a rural government hospital one night, and I saw a baby born not breathing, who was set aside as dead. Incredulous that no one was doing anything, I pushed over to where the "stillborn" lay, and began to do mouth to mouth resuscitation and chest compressions. After just twenty seconds of cardiopulmonary resuscitation (CPR) the baby came around and cried. The nurses were astonished. The doctor looked up from suturing the mother and said, "Oh, it's alive!"

Family members are sent outside the hospital to buy IV fluids, drugs, and even blood for a transfusion, while the patient can only hope they will be brought back in time. Often the relatives have to borrow from unscrupulous money lenders who prey on the poor to be able to afford the medications needed. One night I went all over the city of Manila trying to buy blood for a woman who had delivered and hemorrhaged. When I finally found the type needed, I literally carried it back and passed it through the door of the surgical suite. Other times I have donated my own blood, as have many of our midwives, because even if we have a different blood type from our patient, they will give her a free unit of her blood type in exchange for our donation.

I have witnessed similar circumstances in numerous hospitals of the Philippines and during my travels to Laos, Thailand, Ecuador, Mexico, Guatemala and Nepal. Midwives I have trained have reported to me that they have seen the same situations I have just described in India, China, and countries of Africa as well. Last year, I set up an opportunity for one of our midwife graduates, Christy Martin, who was a registered nurse as well as a CPM, to work in a hospital in Tanzania. This is an excerpt from an e-mail she sent me after her first shift:

> I was completely unprepared for what I saw. I went in to working *[sic]* there with the attitude to serve and be helpful, not be a white woman know-it-all. Oh Vic, it was brutal. That's the word that best describes the whole experience. The horrible fundal pressure (done with great intensity like chest compressions, just downward), pinching the woman's legs when she would try to close them, trying to insert a very non-sterile catheter, the midwife sticking her fingers in the woman's rectum to try to speed delivery and then sticking those same fingers into the woman's vagina, cutting a big mediolateral episiotomy, digging into the woman's vagina and into the uterus after the placenta was out to remove anything that might be left in there though the placenta was complete. Oh my heart broke! (Martin 2006, unpublished private correspondence)

This is the care many resource-poor women are receiving, and it is not a model that is working, as evidenced by the horrific maternal and newborn mortality rates being recorded in Asia, Africa, and some countries in Latin America. The maternity system in most developing nations is badly flawed, a result of not enough funding, inadequate facilities and supplies, corruption that diverts funds meant for health care, overworked and burned-out medical staff and midwives, the influence of Western medical care that seems to be taken from the 1940s and 1950s, and a general culture of disregard for women and the disadvantaged.

In the Philippines, over half of all births in the nation still occur at home, but in many cases, the home births being conducted are also lacking in safe, evidence-based practice. In the areas of the Philippines where I have worked, on Mindanao, Cebu, Luzon, and Mindoro Islands, traditional birth attendants also use fundal pressure to speed birth, often beginning early in labor before full dilation has occurred. Basics of cleanliness are ignored, and newborn babies are often left unattended on the floor until after the placenta has delivered, resulting in cold stress that can lead to death. Even at home, the baby is often separated from the mother for hours while it is bathed and dressed. The woman is not necessarily encouraged to breastfeed until her milk has come in on the third day. By that time, bottle feeding may already be established. Neither traditional birth attendants (TBAs) nor licensed midwives in the Philippines are trained in neonatal resuscitation for the newborn. Only rarely do they carry the proper combination of oxytocic drugs to control a serious hemorrhage.

CREATING MERCY IN ACTION

In light of this great tragedy involving pregnant women and infants, and in light of the global shortage of trained midwives as reported by WHO, I felt strongly that I could no longer concentrate solely on maternity care in America. In 1991, along with my husband, Scott, and family members, colleagues, and friends, we conceived the idea of establishing teaching birth centers offering no-cost care in low-resource areas in the Philippines. In addition to the Philippines, we simultaneously established a prenatal clinic in Mexico and helped other doctors, nurses, and midwives establish outreaches to pregnant women in various countries.

At the same time, I began a life of travel to teach maternity care to groups that were sending primary health care workers on missions to the third world, such as Youth with Mission, Heart for the World, and numerous churches around the United States. We founded Mercy in Action, Inc., as a charitable, nonprofit organization that establishes, funds, and operates birth centers and medical missions, and trains other midwives to do the same all over the world.

One of the first steps was to research how to set up a nonprofit corporation, known as a 501(c)(3), with the U.S. government. I checked out books from the library and consulted with a friend who was an attorney. In the end, I just followed the advice from the books and used the sample forms to begin the process, which took about a year to complete. We identified a board of three—a minister, a Certified Public Accountant, and myself— and used an advisory board of medical and legal friends. From that point on, I began to solicit donations from family and friends for the purpose of helping women in childbirth in low-resource countries. Some of my early donors, many of whom have remained staunch supporters to this day, are my former midwifery clients from my first thirteen years in private home birth practice in Alaska. Upon hearing my stories, they embraced the moral responsibility to help other women in less fortunate circumstances to have good and safe births, and readily joined the cause with their financial support. Our fundraising has always been grassroots and based on relationships. We have no mailing lists or glossy brochures, no television ads or mass marketing. We depend on God to provide by nudging people to share what they have with the less fortunate.

I try to accept requests to speak in churches, schools, or service organizations whenever asked, as I am passionate to share the needs of women around the world with people who for the most part are unaware. I have always felt that if people only knew the terrible plight of women and children in the world, they would care and respond in some way. Occasionally, a donation or ongoing pledge for support will come to us through my speaking and teaching, but I am just as happy if the group decides to start their own project. Last year I was honored with a Making a Difference for Women award from the Soroptimist club, and with that came a $1,000 donation to Mercy in Action. I take every opportunity to speak about Safe Motherhood, to raise awareness and funds on behalf of the mothers we serve, and others like them.

The model we developed was to operate birth centers in the Philippines in which midwifery students could get their training while their tuition funds the operation of the center, providing a symbiotic situation wherein midwifery care can be given at no charge to the pregnant women. Private donations, occasional awards or grants, donations of supplies, and judicious budgeting have enabled us to do this work. It is important that maternity care be free if we are to reduce maternal and neonatal mortality. Because birth is a normal process and usually requires no medical intervention, poor families will gamble on not needing a birth attendant (and not going for prenatal care) if they are unable to afford the fees associated with that care. However, because complications can occur suddenly, a trained birth attendant needs to be at each delivery. Maternity care is the one area of health care that should be subsidized so that all women can have equal access.

Salaries have been paid to staff in different ways. The director and clerical staff are given a set salary by the board of directors of Mercy in Action, based on need and operating budget. Staff midwives from the Philippines are given a monthly salary based on a scale slightly above the average wages for a midwife, and they are provided with housing as well. Volunteer foreign midwives serving as missionaries in the Philippines raise monetary support and are paid monthly in the form of a salary from their churches. As founder and director, it is my full-time job to raise funds for the needs of the mission, and when money is designated for me personally, this money is deposited into the general fund. The board of directors set an annual salary, or stipend, for my own family's living needs. This has fluctuated over the years, from below the poverty line at times to somewhere around a reasonable salary for a midwife in the United States with a small private practice. During particularly lean times when donations are down, as happens occasionally when there is general nervousness about the economy, I have voluntarily asked the board to reduce my salary. Always it has been our goal to first pay for the health care projects we are funding overseas. My husband has for many years worked another job on top of his administrative duties with Mercy in Action, so that we could raise our children and help them with college. At this point, our children are all grown, and we live full-time in the Philippines, where neither of us, as foreigners, can work for wages. We are currently scaling back our training of North American midwives in order to concentrate on training TBAs and national midwives in the Philippines and other Asian countries, so we are more dependent on donations to continue this work than ever before.

Over the years during which we have trained midwife students, we have been committed to keeping our tuition costs low while still providing an excellent learning environment. Unlike most colleges that raise their tuition each year, the midwifery tuition we have charged over the years has not significantly increased. According to the *Trends in College Pricing Report 2006* (see www.collegeboard.com), college tuitions have gone up 35% in the past five years. Mercy in Action tuition has increased only 12% in twelve years. In 1995, when we began the projects in the Philippines, our tuition was US$12,500. In 2007 the charge was US$14,000, and there has been no increase in the past five years, even though our costs have risen, both for overhead and for fees we pay on the student's behalf to the National College of Midwifery. This tuition pays for a two-year-equivalent study program, culminating in qualifying to take the North American Registry of Midwives (NARM) exam to earn the certified professional midwife (CPM) credential (see Chapter 15) and be awarded an accredited associate of science degree in midwifery from the National College of Midwifery (see Chapter 9).

Once we knew where the funding would come from—private donations, church donations, and midwifery student tuition—it was a matter of finding a suitable place to build the first birth center of our own in the Philippines. In 1992 I had taken over the running of a birth center in Manila from a Canadian missionary family that was going home on furlough for one year (Penwell 1994a). Before that, I had been involved in a small church project in a northern province of Luzon. The clinic project was temporary but it gave me a good idea of what was needed to gather and educate pregnant women from a poor area. Running Gentle Hands Ministry (and doing all the fund-raising for one year to keep it going) gave me hands-on experience not only in high-risk births, of which we had many, but also in the day-to-day operation of a birth center in the Philippines. That experience taught me that the need was great for affordable maternity care in the Philippines, and that kind, charitable midwifery care was welcomed and appreciated.

When we contemplated that first birth center, the question on all our minds was where to begin. The need was great everywhere. I felt a strong inclination to begin in Davao City, on the southernmost island of Mindanao. I knew no one on that island, and in fact many people, both Filipinos and Westerners, were frightened of Mindanao because of the troubles there were, and still are, with Muslim terrorists and insurgents on that island. But the prompting in my spirit was strong, so I contacted a friend in Australia who knew missionaries in Davao, and, when asked to do so, they showed us the poorest slum area in Davao and introduced us around. We located a building to rent (a much wiser option for non-citizens) and began. Unlike setting up a hospital, the furnishings and equipment needed for a birth center are relatively simple: not much more than a few beds, a kitchen area, and a large meeting room for classes. The birth equipment needed is no different from a home birth kit, with the exception of trading a portable oxygen tank for a large, stand-up oxygen tank. Because of the high-risk nature of our practice, and according to guidelines written up by the International Confederation of Midwives and WHO, we also stocked our birth center with advanced life-saving equipment: a vacuum extractor for prolonged labor or fetal distress; IV fluids; needles and tubing for fluid replacement, delivery of IV antibiotics, and hemorrhage control; and a refrigerator set aside for anti-hemorrhage drugs and vaccines.

To date, we have established eight birth centers in the Philippines on four of the largest, most populated islands (Luzon, Cebu, Mindanao, and Mindoro). Three of these birth centers are currently being funded and overseen by me through our organization, Mercy in Action. Three more are currently being run by former midwifery students who trained in those centers and later returned, and two have closed. With every birth center we founded in the Philippines, we started by recruiting national licensed midwives to work for us on the project. These nationally trained and licensed midwives have been the backbone of every birth center, and have been present at every birth, bridging the gap between the foreign volunteer midwives and the patients. Our success in the Philippines was facilitated by the fact that English is an official national language, so it was easy for us to communicate. The initial stages of our work were also facilitated by the fact that the law governing the practice of midwifery in the Philippines exempts midwives who do not charge for their services, as is the case with us, so as humanitarian workers within the country, we did not have to be licensed. However, in recent years, this exemption has been called into question. Now, we make sure that an experienced, nationally licensed midwife or doctor is in charge of each clinic, and Westerners play a more behind-the-scenes role.

On February 8, 1996, a thirty-four-year-old Filipina woman named Bebe came with her husband to our first fledgling birth center in Davao City on Mindanao Island and delivered a baby boy, the first of many thousands more babies we would eventually deliver at no charge to the parents. In 1998 we began another birth center in Cebu City on Cebu Island. In 2003 we began a small birth center in Kalinga Province among tribal women, and in 2004 we began a birth center in a large urban slum of Manila, both of these on Luzon Island. This year (2008), our newest effort is a pilot project to combine our Mother-Friendly/Baby-Friendly birth center model with an existing primary health care clinic in a rural area of Mindoro Island. Midwives will conduct all normal deliveries, and the clinic doctor will be consulted for complicated cases. This will combine the best of midwifery care with the safety of good medical backup, because we are over two hours away from a hospital here in Mindoro. Besides having delivered more than 12,000 babies (as of December 2006), midwives in our birth centers have trained hundreds of midwifery and primary health care students to date, and the work described here continues.

HOW THE MODEL WORKS

The mission of the midwives of Mercy in Action is to reduce maternal and infant risk, and to protect and defend the dignity of women, by demonstrating Christ's love, compassion, and mercy in action. Let's consider what this means to a woman giving birth in the Philippines.

What follows is a description of how a woman in labor is treated at a Mercy in Action Birth Center. Prenatal days are quite festive, with free, nutritious food served to the pregnant patient and any family members she has brought with her. Often, there is music and singing. Later, interactive health teaching is done in her language. Using the book *Facts For Life* published by UNICEF (see www.ffl.org), we explain the information every woman and family has a right to know about safe motherhood, child spacing, breastfeeding, child development, hygiene, immunizations, and HIV/ AIDS prevention, among other topics. One by one, the patients are then called into a private area for an individual prenatal exam, which includes blood pressure check, weight, the measuring of fundal height, auscultating the baby's heart rate, Leopold's maneuvers for determining fetal position, and determination of due date. In addition, dietary counseling is done, and if we have the resources, the patient is given a bottle of vitamins free of charge. All women are given a simple lab test for anemia, and this hematocrit test is done several times during pregnancy. When appropriate, according to Mercy in Action policies and procedures, the patient may be sent for an ultrasound, further and more detailed lab workup, or referral to a physician for assessment.

Vaccinations are also a part of our midwifery and primary health care services. Tetanus vaccinations are given to all pregnant women in developing countries to protect against neonatal tetanus; we give two shots per pregnancy, at approximately six and eight months of gestation. At times, we have also given childhood immunizations. In the Philippines these vaccinations begin at birth with a BCG *(Bacille Calmette Guerin)* vaccination against tuberculosis. Later, we give immunizations to protect our babies from polio, measles, diphtheria, tetanus, and whooping cough—all diseases that kill many babies and young children in developing countries.

When a woman arrives in labor, she is greeted warmly and shown to a bed made up with clean sheets over a waterproof mattress. Her bed is kept private by a system of curtains that completely enclose her into a private cubicle. A team of two or three midwives, at least one of whom is Filipina, assesses her. If determined to be in active labor without risk factors that would necessitate a hospital birth, she is checked in and given an informed consent form to sign. Her family members are welcome to stay and are offered water, coffee, or other refreshment. The woman is allowed to wear her own dress, walk around the outside courtyard, interact freely with her partner and loved ones, and is offered water or juice on a regular basis. She can eat if she wishes. A clean bathroom with toilet, shower, and sink is made available to her, and she is also instructed to urinate often. All procedures are explained to her, as well as instructions on how to maximize contractions and how to minimize pain. Vital signs are monitored often, but vaginal internal exams are kept to a strict minimum, ideally only a few during an entire labor. In pushing stage, the woman is offered her choice of positions, with upright being the preferred position for birth. The atmosphere during the delivery is kept calm and quiet, and the mother is supported and gently encouraged. As long as the baby is born in good condition, he or she is given to the mother to hold immediately after birth, thereby lessening trauma and stress to both mother and baby. The baby is put to the breast immediately, reducing the risk of excessive blood loss and ensuring bonding and successful breastfeeding, both known to be important to infant survival. Third and fourth stages are monitored closely for signs of hemorrhage or shock, and treated accordingly using any or all of the following: oxytocic drugs, IV fluids, oxygen, fundal massage or bimanual compression, and urinary catheterization.

At all times, cleanliness is paramount. One of the best ways we can prevent the spread of HIV/AIDS, sepsis, and other diseases is with careful attention to how we handle blood and body fluids during and after birth, and how clean we keep our hands and our surroundings. Clean, fresh gloves are worn for all appropriate situations. Instruments used for the births are sterilized in an autoclave. Sinks are available for frequent hand washing, and midwives are required to keep their fingernails short and free of polish. Careful attention is given to sterile technique whenever it is called for, such as during suturing or following rupture of membranes. Floors, bathroom fixtures, and vinyl mattress covers are washed with soap and a chlorine solution between patients.

Mercy in Action midwives practice according to Mother-Friendly/ Baby-Friendly practices as outlined in the Mother-Friendly Childbirth Initiative created by the U.S.-based Coalition for Improving Maternity Services (CIMS) (see www.motherfriendly.org), and the WHO-UNICEF Ten Steps of the Baby-Friendly Hospital Initiative (see www.unicef.org/ programme/breastfeeding/baby.html). I find that by adhering to the tenets of Mother-Friendly/Baby-Friendly care, we are giving the best care possible both from a medical and psychosocial standpoint.

Mercy in Action midwives practice within a culture of shared knowledge, which includes sharing knowledge with student midwives and interns and with the patients and their families. We teach the women constantly through each prenatal visit, helping each mother to feel empowered by understanding her own vital signs, what is normal in position and growth charting of the baby, as well as how she can improve her chance for a good outcome through healthy nutrition. Our motto is that we should know nothing about the patient that she does not know about herself. Student midwives are included in everything, and have a wonderful opportunity to learn by observing and doing. There is a richness to the way we learn from each other, and from the patients themselves. I have always said that my real teachers are the mothers and babies, and we want our students to realize and appreciate this fact.

Care given is based on kindness, gentleness, and compassion. It must be noted here that Mercy in Action is a faith-based Christian ministry established on service and mercy, and all who work with Mercy in Action are consciously following the teachings of Jesus to care for the "least of these" as if they were in fact Christ himself (Matthew 25: 34–40). Routine maternity care includes prayer, and this prayer takes the form of staff praying in general for all patients who will come at the beginning of each prenatal day, prayer for a safe delivery at each birth, and a prayer of thanksgiving for each newborn baby. Each woman is asked if she would like a prayer said for her, and if she declines a verbal prayer, the midwives respect this; however, most patients do ask to be prayed for either during their prenatal exam or during labor.

Most often the person presiding over the actual "catching" of the baby is a student under direct supervision of a certified professional midwife or a licensed midwife. The certified professional midwives in my study were all graduates of the National College of Midwifery (see Chapter 9). Licensed midwives from the Philippines were graduates of a two-year, direct-entry midwifery college within that country. Because the training system in the Philippines does not allow for much hands-on clinical experience, if the Filipino licensed midwives hired by Mercy in Action have limited experience, they are paid by our organization for an additional year of hands-on training before they conduct deliveries without supervision. When student midwives are properly educated and trained, their involvement in actual patient care appears to be a benefit and not a liability. Our training of midwives from the Philippines and a variety of other countries helps us to achieve several important aspects of this model.

First, we are not just helping the women we deliver, but we also are training the next generation of midwives. According to WHO, the developing world needs at least 300,000 persons qualified to attend births in order to reach the Millennium Development Goal of a two-thirds reduction in maternal mortality by 2015.[5] It has come to my attention recently that some midwives from the United States have speculated aloud that perhaps it is not in the best interest of Third-World women to have students "practicing" on them. Hopefully, the excellent outcomes in this study, as well as the high level of personal satisfaction with their birth experiences expressed by the families, will put that concern to rest. Evidently, those who have voiced this concern have no idea of the actual quality of patient care being given and the good outcomes achieved. Having student midwives present is seen as a plus by the women we serve: there are always several pairs of hands and loving hearts to help them navigate the difficult waters of birth. In addition, it is relevant here to note that all centers of higher learning involved in the training of medical and/or nursing students use students in patient care in adjoining hospitals. If a life-threatening complication occurs, the senior midwife steps right in and guides the student or takes over altogether.

Second, also not unlike medical or nursing schools, the student tuition helps fund the teaching facility and underwrite the free care given to indigent patients. This is certainly the case with Mercy in Action: families are not charged for midwifery services or for a facility fee at the Mercy in Action birth centers. Yet because the student tuition supplements private donations to fund the facility, the excellent care continues to be available to all, regardless of ability to pay (families are given a chance to make a donation to cover any medications used during the birth). This is a model that could be used worldwide to alleviate the burden of cost of health care for the poor, while continuing to train much needed midwives to serve among them.

Women and their families continually express gratitude to the midwives of Mercy in Action by verbal words of thanks, thank-you letters and cards, frequent smiles, gifts, and even the common practice of naming their baby after one or more of the midwives involved in their care. I have often noted the beautiful smiles on the faces of our mothers and compare this to the stoic facial expression often seen in the hospital maternity wards. Years ago I took a simple poll of 200 women who had delivered with us, and asked them the main reason they had chosen to give birth in our birth center. I thought the obvious answer would be that the care was free. However, less than 1% said that they came because it was free. The majority, over 66%, said they came because the midwives were kind. This shows me that the model that works is a model that considers the often overlooked aspect of kindness in offering maternity care.

DETAILS ON THE FIRST 7,565 MERCY IN ACTION BIRTHS

What makes my study so unique is the fact that we did keep such detailed statistics on such a large population of women, from the moment we started the first birth center and including each and every woman who checked in for labor for the next ninety-five months (see Table 12.1 and Table 12.2).

TABLE 12.1 Characteristics of care provided to women delivering in Mercy in Action birth centers in Davao and Cebu, 1996–1999

Characteristics of Care Provided	% of Women Receiving Care (n = 7,565 women)
Birth Attendants	
Deliveries conducted by midwives	100
Prenatal Care	
Trimester prenatal care began	
First trimester (1 to 3 months)	6
Second trimester (4 to 6 months)	57
Third trimester (7 to 9 months)	37
Number of prenatal exams	
1 to 5 exams	36
6 to 9 exams	41
> 10 exams	17
Women receiving no prenatal care	6
Deliveries	
Spontaneous vaginal birth	95
Position for birth	
Birth stool (supported squat)	28
Squatting	1
Hands and knees	1
Semi-sitting	18
Dorsal	50
Side-lying	2
Mobility 1st stage	
Walked around	86
Stayed in bed	13
Movement restricted for medical reason	1
Mobility 2nd stage	
Moved around, changed positions	33
Stayed in one position	66
Lacerations of the birth canal	
No laceration of birth canal	49
First-degree laceration	31
Second-degree laceration	18
Third-degree laceration	1
Fourth-degree laceration	0.1
Episiotomy	0.4
Nulliparas	
No laceration of birth canal	24
First-degree laceration	35
Second-degree laceration	38
Third-degree laceration	2

TABLE 12.1 *(continued)*

Characteristics of Care Provided	% of Women Receiving Care (n = 7,565 women)
Fourth-degree laceration	0.2
Episiotomy	0.3
Multiparas	
No laceration of birth canal	61
First-degree laceration	29
Second-degree laceration	9
Third-degree laceration	0.3
Fourth-degree laceration	0.08
Episiotomy	0.4
Compound presentation (arm alongside head)	5
Persistent posterior presentation	4
Face presentation	0.02
Breech	0.5
Babies	
Birth weight	
< 2,500 grams (5 lbs, 8 oz)	10
2,501–3,460 grams (5 lbs, 9 oz–7 lbs, 10 oz)	79
3,461–4,000 grams (7 lbs, 11 oz–8 lbs, 13 oz)	11
> 4,000 grams (8 lbs, 14 oz)	.06
Smallest birth weight 892 grams (1 lb, 15 oz)	
Largest birth weight 4,930 grams (10 lbs, 14 oz)	
One minute APGAR of 7 or greater	92
Breastfeeding	
Breastfeeding at birth	99.8
Bottle or NG tube	0.2

The demographic statistics show that most of the pregnant women are unemployed (92%). Over a third (34%) of their spouses or partners are unemployed as well. For the men who held jobs, the average daily salary was US$2. Only a little over half of the women were legally married (54%), though being pregnant and alone was rare (6%). A common situation was for women to live with a man (40%), though that did not always afford security, as some men moved frequently between live-in situations, sometimes even keeping two families at the same time in different parts of town. It is not known how often domestic violence occurred among our patients, as the question was not asked on official forms, but we do know that it was present in a considerable number of cases. Teenagers accounted for 14% of our population, while only 7% were over thirty-six years old.

TABLE 12.2 Complications and interventions of women delivering in Mercy in Action birth centers in Davao and Cebu, 1996–1999

Complications or Interventions	% of Women or Babies Experiencing Complication or Intervention (n = 7,565 women)
Neonatal Complications	
Meconium-stained amniotic fluid	33
Light	13
Moderate	12
Thick	8
Fetal distress during labor	25
APGAR < 7 at one minute	8
Infants requiring stimulation	17
Infants requiring full resuscitation	3
Low birth weight	10
Newborns requiring transfer to hospital	2
Neonatal mortality	0.5
Maternal Complications	
Postpartum hemorrhage > 500 cc	17
Postpartum hemorrhage > 1,000 cc	2
Hypertension > 140/90	5
Delivery requiring assistance (vacuum extractor)	2
Delivery requiring manual assistance	3
Shoulder dystocia	3
Maternal mortality	0.05
Interventions/Drugs	
Postpartum use of oxytocin	33
Postpartum use of methergine	9
Suctioning of baby with DeLee mucous trap	33
IV fluids in labor or postpartum	15
Oxygen to newborn	12
Vacuum extractor assisted delivery	2
Maternal catheterization	2
Infant resuscitation-PPV or CPR	3
Manual removal of placenta	2
Episiotomy	0.4

The youngest mother was thirteen years old; the oldest fifty-two years old. Multiparas accounted for 70% of the population, with 4% being grand-multiparas. The highest parity recorded was twelve. The average number of children in the Philippines is five per family, with some stopping at two and others having eight to ten children or more.

More than half (57%) of the women first came seeking prenatal care in their second trimester. Thirty-seven percent began prenatal care in their third trimester, considered to be dangerously late; 6% of the women had sought no prenatal care at all, just showing up at our door in labor. Reflecting their late start in availing themselves of prenatal care, 42% of the women received fewer than six exams before birth. Delivery positions were suggested but not enforced, except in 1% of the cases for medical reasons, such as when the woman was asked to lie on her left side to reduce blood pressure. The vast majority (86%) of the women chose to walk during labor. Forty-eight percent chose an upright position for delivery, and 52% chose to lie down or assume a semi-reclining position. Twenty-eight percent of the births occurred on a simple birth stool, usually with the husband supporting from behind.

Most women (79%) went into labor on their own and needed no augmentation, but in 21% of the cases, non-drug methods of induction or augmentation were used, such as nipple stimulation, castor oil, or stripping the membranes. This was deemed necessary especially if the water had broken or the woman was post-date. Minor or no lacerations of the birth canal occurred in 80% of the deliveries. Second-degree tears involving the perineal muscle and requiring stitches occurred 18% of the time, with more serious lacerations or episiotomy occurring in less than 2% of the cases. Women who had given birth previously had minor or no lacerations of the birth canal 90% of the time. Sixty-eight percent of the deliveries involved some perineal support or counter pressure to the emerging head, with 32% being what we call "hands off," allowing the baby to emerge without hands touching the baby or perineum. This reflected differing philosophies among midwives, and did not seem to affect the overall rate of tearing. [Editors' note: At this time, the randomized, controlled study by Leah Albers (2007) at the University of Mexico on reducing genital tract trauma is still not published, but it does confirm that supporting hands on the perineum and hot compresses neither harm nor protect genital areas from splitting or separating.] Some sort of manual assistance with the birth, such as forcefully stretching the vaginal opening, was used 3% of the time in difficult deliveries. A vacuum extractor suction device was used 2% of the time, for fetal distress or prolonged second stage (all the midwives and students are trained in its use, according to a joint recommendation by World Health Organization and the International Confederation of Midwives that midwives working in developing countries have advanced life-saving skills). Episiotomy was rare at 0.4% and was done for fetal distress only.

By far the largest number of babies arrived head down, with 99.5% in a vertex position. Four percent were born persistent posterior, and there were two face presentations during this study. Breech birth occurred at our center 0.5% during the study, for a total of thirty-five breech deliveries.

High-risk breech deliveries according to the breech scoring chart described by Rahima Baldwin and Valerie El Halta were referred to the hospital before labor, if there was time.

Pregnancies known to be premature, post-mature or complicated by hypertension were also referred out unless the labor was too far advanced. The majority of the babies (90%) were between 2,501 grams (5 pounds, 9 ounces) and 4,000 grams (8 pounds, 13 ounces). Ten percent were considered low birth weight at 2,500 grams (5 1/2 pounds) or under. The smallest baby was 892 grams (just under 2 pounds), and the largest was 4,930 grams (10 pounds, 14 ounces).

Practically all (99.8%) of the babies were breastfed at birth. At the parents' request, 97% of the babies received Ilotycin eye ointment, and 73% received vitamin K. Neonatal complications included meconium-stained amniotic fluid, with moderate to thick staining being present 20% of the time. Fetal distress occurred 25% of the time to varying degrees, but only 8% of the newborns had an Apgar score of less than 7 at one minute following birth. Twenty percent of the babies required some stimulation or blow-by oxygen, while only 3% required positive pressure ventilation (PPV) or CPR. Two percent of the newborns were transferred for hospital care at some time following birth. These mothers or babies who transferred to a hospital were followed up with a midwife visit and were included in the study.

Maternal complications included hemorrhage, shoulder dystocia, and placenta problems. Although many texts now define hemorrhage as blood loss over 1,000 cc, because the women in this study were malnourished and often anemic, I chose to use the more conservative definition of hemorrhage as blood loss of 500 cc or greater. By that definition, 17% of the mothers suffered a hemorrhage; however, only 2% had hemorrhages defined by blood loss greater than 1,000 cc. Intravenous fluids were given in 15% of the cases, oxytocin in 33%, and methergine in another 9%. Because of the high number of cases in which the placenta partially separated with accompanying bleeding, the placenta was assisted to deliver with gentle controlled cord traction in half of all cases (54%), and manual removal of the placenta was required in 0.2% of all deliveries. Maternal catheterization was required 2% of the time. Shoulder dystocia happened in 3% of the cases.

Transfers to a hospital after admission to the birth center because of maternal factors occurred in 5% of the cases. The intrapartum transport rate was only 3.5%, and less than half of these transports resulted in cesarean section births, for a cesarean rate under 2% (these were women who had already been screened as suitable for an out-of-hospital birth by the Mercy in Action midwife team, according to our own internal protocols). When a woman or baby was transported to a hospital, a midwife accompanied her and turned over pertinent data to the attending physician. Rarely were Mercy in Action midwives allowed in the delivery room once we arrived at the hospital, but it was our practice to visit the woman later in the hospital or at home if at all possible, and record the outcome and any interventions on her chart. These data were included in the study.

Neonatal mortality was 0.5%, but it might have been higher because not all parents brought their babies for follow-up exams through six weeks. The deaths recorded did not occur while in our facility, with the exception of stillbirths, but rather the babies died some hours or days later in the hospital where we had transported them, or after being discharged back home. Many complicating factors surrounded neonatal deaths because of the poverty of the parents and the lack of access to medical care for many. Even after transporting a baby who was having respiratory problems to the hospital, the parents were often not able to afford a respirator, or an incubator may not have been available for a premature baby. Some babies died weeks after birth from unhealthy conditions in their homes. Because autopsies are not done in the Philippines when a baby dies, it is impossible to ascertain the true cause of death. Sepsis and birth defects were the most commonly named causes on death certificates.

Maternal mortality, defined as a death within forty-two days of giving birth, happened four times, for a statistic of 0.05% of births. In all cases, the mother had checked out of the birth center, and only later was it reported back to the midwives that she had died. In one of the four cases, a woman arrived as a "drop in" (our name for a patient we had never seen for pre-natal care) in advanced labor, obviously very ill. She refused transport to a hospital, went home the next day, and died two days later of tuberculosis, a common ailment in the Philippines, with which, according to her family, she had been diagnosed previously. The second reported maternal death was a woman who had checked out healthy but went to a local "healer" and received a massage rubdown with a gasoline and kerosene mixture, only to die days later in the hospital of full-body chemical burns. Neither of these cases had anything to do with where the woman gave birth or the quality of maternity care. In the remaining two cases, it was reported to us that a postpartum patient had died weeks later, one from supposed infection and one of unknown etiology.

The problem of possible underreporting in our statistics is the same for the Philippines as a whole. Experts tracking maternal and neonatal death postulate that the published rate of neonatal and maternal mortality is definitely underreported all across the developing world. Even in the United States, the rates of maternal mortality are said to be grossly under-reported (see Kim 2000). The Centers for Disease Control and Prevention warned in 1998 that "the actual number of maternal deaths in the United States is estimated to be 1.3 to three times that reported in vital statistics records" (CDC 1998). The World Health Organization warns that "cross country comparisons should be treated with considerable circumspection because different strategies have been used to derive the estimates for different countries, making it difficult to draw comparisons (Abou-Zahr and Wardlaw 2004).

All in all, this study suggests that demographically high-risk women (anemic, malnourished, physically abused, unmarried, and impoverished) can still have good birth outcomes using a model of Mother-Friendly/Baby-Friendly care run by midwives in an out-of-hospital setting in a poor and underdeveloped country such as the Philippines.

TRIALS AND TRIUMPHS

The birth centers described here offer a model that provides excellent midwifery care, as well as love, comfort, and support to women and their families during pregnancy, birth, and the postpartum period. Few types of maternal/child health services available are as appreciated by the Filipino people as these Mercy in Action freestanding charity birth centers. Here people are welcomed and loved, regardless of their circumstances. Here they find the values of home birth they are used to, but in a cleaner, more spacious setting than their own homes. In the birth center they find the skilled midwives, emergency medicines, and equipment that make birth safe, without sacrificing the comfort, kindness, and personal care they crave.

Still, not all of the birth centers we started since our inception are in operation today. Over the years, we have faced turnovers, staffing shortages, disagreements over management styles, and conflict over whether or not students should be part of the team. We have been awarded Model Clinic status and also been issued a cease and desist order, both coming from the Department of Health of the Philippines. In one recent instance, we faced unavoidable and overwhelming opposition to one of our birth centers. The cease and desist order closed a busy and successful birth center we ran in Manila, and only later did we learn it was because we were seen as competition to doctors who sat on our licensing board and owned their own for-profit birth centers in the area. These situations of government corruption are disheartening, to say the least, when you are in a country faced with so much need.

Some opposition we were able to overcome by complying with new regulations, like the new law a few years back requiring licensing for all birth centers. We got a copy of the regulations, and went out and purchased all the things they required (for instance, the stirrups for the end of our birthing bed that we were required to have but have never used). Other times, we would call meetings with the doctors at the local hospital and ask to be included in peer review. This went a long way toward defusing any animosity over transports we brought to them. At times over the years, opposition took the form of workers in the mission having clashing viewpoints about how to do things, or about how students fit in the organization. There was a constant tension between the needs of the birthing women, the needs of the student midwives, and the needs of the supervising midwives. When things were running according to plan, these needs were symbiotic; but the world is not perfect, and even the best-intentioned humanitarians are flawed human beings, so conflict arose at times. The one thing I found most disheartening was when other American midwives, who had themselves been trained by us in the apprenticeship model, did not seem to value the young students on our team the same way I did. Because of this issue, Mercy in Action turned over two different birth centers we had founded and invested in for years, in order to allow the clinics to continue to operate for the communities' sake without interpersonal friction. In one case, the birth center eventually closed down, but another was later established in its place by a former student, who hired the same staff of Filipina midwives. In the other case, the new directors eventually started their own midwifery training school, which is successful to this day. What I value most is that poor women would be helped and served by trained and compassionate midwives, whether or not we agreed on exactly how to go about providing that service.

Young North American midwives who have stepped into leadership roles in these birth centers have found it both a joyous experience of a lifetime, and a stress beyond anything they could have imagined. A few have even had to seek counseling for posttraumatic stress disorder following their time on staff with Mercy in Action in the Philippines. To understand the high burnout factor, consider that these clinics were often delivering 80 to 100 babies each month, and seeing approximately forty women per day for prenatal care. All that on top of regular home visits, follow-up with labs and hospitals, and teaching of students. Midwives and students were often witness to heartbreaking scenes of wife or child abuse, abject poverty, corruption, and alarming injustice issues. Part of the stress was in feeling powerless to change these situations. It is also important to note that although our outcomes are excellent in terms of overall mortality, it is overwhelming for a midwife to experience even one mother or infant death. Even when we save lives, the constant battle against injustice, the constant fight for life, is soul wearying: the average volunteer midwife stays only two years. Westerners coming over tend to have little experience in dealing with death and thus no conceptual grid for coping with the reality. The following is an excerpt from one young midwife's journal entry shared here with permission from the writer, Amy Osborne, about her time with Mercy in Action.

The things of this time will haunt me for the rest of my life, and for that I am grateful. I am only 24 years old and I have felt the weight of the world on my shoulders. I have fought to save the life of a newborn and lost. I have held a dead infant in my arms and sobbed over the loss of her life. I have put my fingers inside a lifeless little hand and prayed that she would grasp it— knowing that she never would. I will never forget the feel of her silky hair as I cut off a lock for her parents, or the sound of her mother's anguished cries as we handed her a tiny bundle, dressed in Winnie-the-Pooh. I have slid down a wall, pulled my knees to my chest, and wished that I was dead. I have fought to save the life of a newborn and won. I have forced air into tiny lungs— seeing her skin turn pink, and her limbs flex. I have rejoiced at seeing her lower lip quiver as she gathers her strength to scream in protest. I have wrapped her up and given her to her mother who reached out for her child, crying with relief. I have fallen to my knees in gratitude, knowing that this life could have easily been taken. (Osborne 1998)

We have found that even when North American midwives are not able to handle, on a long-term basis, the painful things they see and the intense working conditions, they are changed for the better. The young woman who wrote this journal entry in 1998 eventually went on to Afghanistan to train midwives with the organization Samaritans Purse, and later served as a midwife in Darfur with Doctors without Borders. She is now in medical school with plans to become an obstetrician, determined to return to the Third World with even more skills to help the less fortunate. This basic altruism that comes from awareness of the acute needs of the world is a common denominator among graduates of the Mercy in Action midwifery training.

In staffing these birth centers, we have now increasingly turned over responsibility for leading to Filipina midwives, and for staffing help, we depend on short-term volunteers and interns, both Filipino and foreign. We have this past year begun another new model, working with a Filipino doctor to make available maternity services within his existing rural health clinics.

CONCLUSIONS

Through all of our victories and defeats, I do believe we have found a model that works. This type of provision of maternity care is innovative, cost-effective, and evidence-based. The environment, the facility, the providers, and their level of education all appear to be beneficial on many levels. Maternal and neonatal mortality rates are significantly lower than in the country as a whole; families appear happy and well pleased with their birth experience; and this type of natural birth philosophy, combined with advanced life-saving skills on the part of the midwives, reduces mortality and morbidity that come from both too much or not enough intervention. In addition, this model of care encourages early and successful breastfeeding, which has been shown to be an important factor in reduction of under-five-year-old death rates in the developing world.

As the whole world strives to achieve the United Nations Millennium Goals (www.un.org/millenniumgoals/) by the year 2015, let it be noted here in conclusion that five of the eight goals are being directly addressed by the work of Mercy in Action midwives: to eradicate extreme poverty and hunger, to promote gender equality and empower women, to reduce child mortality, to improve maternal health, and to combat HIV/AIDS and other disease through prevention and immunizations. These are lofty goals, but ones that are attainable using birth models that work.

NOTES

1. Certified professional midwife, (CPM) is a designation granted by North American Registry of Midwives (NARM): www.narm.org

2. Licensed midwives from both the Philippines and the United States. Vicki Penwell holds a license from the state of New Mexico and the certified professional midwife designation from the North American Registry of Midwives. For other examples of her work, see Penwell 1991, 1994 a, 1994b, 1995, 1998, 2001a, 2001b, 2004, 2005a, and 2005b.

3. See www.unicef.org/pon96/leag1wom.htm, www.who.int/countries/phl/en/, www.childinfo.org/files/Countdown2015_Philippines.pdf, www.unicef.org/philippines/children/.

4. See www.safemotherhood.org/.

5. See https://gn.rti.org/news/index.cfm?fuseaction=detail&id=92.

REFERENCES

Abou-Zahr, Carla, and Tessa Wardlaw. 2004. *Maternal Mortality in 2000: Estimates Developed by WHO, UNICEF, UNFPA.* Geneva: World Health Organization. http://www.who.int/reproductive-health/publications/maternal_mortality_2000/mme.pdf. Accessed November 18, 2008.

Albers, Leah. 2007. Address at the American College of Nurse Midwives on Reducing Genital Tract Trauma at Birth. May 29, 2007.

CDC. 1998. "Maternal Mortality—United States, 1982–1996." *Morbidity and Mortality Weekly Report* 47.34:705–07. http://www.cdc.gov/mmwr/preview/mmwrhtml/00054602.htm.

Johnson, Kenneth C., and Daviss, Betty-Anne. 2005. "Outcomes of Planned Home Births with Certified Professional Midwives: Large Prospective Study in North America. *British Medical Journal* 330.7505:1416. Available at www.bmj.com/cgi/content/full/330/7505/1416.

Kirn, Timothy F. 2000. "Maternal Mortality Rates Grossly Underestimated," *Ob/Gyn News,* January 11.

Penwell, Vicki. 1991. "Midwifery Education: A Global Perspective." *Midwifery Today* 20.

———. 1994a. "Gentle Hands across Manila." *Midwifery Today* 30:36–38. Reprinted in *MIDIRS* journal.

———. 1994b. "Cross-Cultural Childbirth Education." *International Journal of Childbirth* 9.2.

———. 1995. *Down Mercy Road.* Self-published.

———. 1998. "Midwifery Education: A Global Perspective." In *Paths to Becoming a Midwife,* edited by Jan Tritten and Joel Southern. Eugene OR: Midwifery Today.

———. 2001a. "Mercy in Action: Training Missionary Midwives to Serve the Poor." *Midwifery Today* 60:58–59.

———. 2001b. "Philippines: In the Night Lorega." *Midwifery Today* 58:61

———. 2004. "Mercy in Action Philippine Birth Center Statistics." *Midwifery Today* 70:56–57.

———. 2005a. "Mercy in Action: Philippine Birth Center Statistics." Abstract for M.S.M. thesis, National College of Midwifery, Taos, NM.

———. 2005b. "Mercy in Action: Philippine Birth Center Statistics." M.S.M. thesis, National College of Midwifery, Taos.

Ronsmans, C., S. Holtz, and C. Stanton. 2006. "Socioeconomic Differentials in Cesarean Rates in Developing Countries: A Retrospective Analysis. *Lancet* 368.9546:1516–23.

World Health Organization. 2005. *World Health Report.* www.who.int/whr/2005/en/.

PART FOUR

Making Models Work

Chapter 13

Circles of Community

The CenteringPregnancy® Group Prenatal Care Model

Sharon Schindler Rising and Rima Jolivet

INTRODUCTION

CenteringPregnancy® Program Description

CenteringPregnancy®, a copyrighted program design, is a multifaceted model that integrates the three major components of prenatal care—health assessment, education, and support—into a unified program within a group setting. Eight to twelve women with similar gestational ages meet as a group with an obstetrical provider—midwife, physician, advanced practice nurse—and a co-facilitator for ten sessions throughout pregnancy and the early postpartum period. Together, they practice self-care skills, participate in facilitated discussions, and develop a support network with other group members. Standard physical health assessment is completed by the practitioner within the group space. Through this unique model of care, women are empowered to choose health-promoting behaviors. Health outcomes, specifically increased birth weight and gestational age for mothers who deliver preterm, and increased satisfaction expressed by both the women and their providers, support the effectiveness of this model for the delivery of prenatal care.

Groups provide a dynamic atmosphere for learning and sharing that is impossible to create in a one-to-one encounter. Hearing other women share concerns that mirror their own helps women in CenteringPregnancy® groups to normalize the experiences of pregnancy. Groups are also empowering because they provide support to the members and increase individual motivation to learn and change. Professionals report that groups provide them with renewed satisfaction in delivering quality care. The model has been widely implemented across the United States, in private practices, and public health clinics, among women of different ages and different ethnic and cultural backgrounds, and with women whose pregnancies unfold under special circumstances, such as infection with HIV or incarceration. CenteringPregancy® programs are under way in Australia and Canada, and there is active model development in England.

Sue Monk Kidd's words illuminate the power of women sharing with other women: "Sometimes another woman's story becomes a mirror that shows me a self I haven't seen before. When I listen to her tell it, her experience quickens and clarifies my own. Her questions rouse mine. Her conflicts illumine my conflicts. Her resolutions call forth my hope. Her strengths summon my strengths. All of this can happen even when our stories and our lives are very different" (1995: 172–73).

That power is what fuels the CenteringPregnancy® group prenatal care model. Pregnant women in group care reflect, learn, and share ideas and self-disclosures with other pregnant women. In so doing, they experience an affirmation of self that nourishes them as they participate in CenteringPregnancy® groups. Their confidence in their ability to manage their own pregnancies grows as they learn to measure their own weight and blood pressure. Their sense of agency and personal responsibility grows as they learn to interpret these measurements and record them in their own medical charts. Women learn about childbearing by tapping into their own knowledge and the collective wisdom of the group during discussions that are facilitated by midwives and other childbirth professionals. The solidarity and community that grow out of group sharing becomes a base of support for women as they cultivate their growing bellies and their growing confidence in their ability to be mothers.

The group provides a circle of safety for the expression of questions, troubles, and anxieties. The circle is also a place for sharing of joys, hopes, and dreams. As trust grows among the members, so does the quality and depth of intimacy and caring. It is natural for this sense of community to extend beyond the framework of the pregnancy and to persist after all the babies in the group are born, "because when you get to know everybody, you get to care about everybody," as one woman in an early CenteringPregnancy® group commented.[1]

THE NEED FOR REFORM IN PRENATAL CARE

Health care providers continue to search for ways to optimize the delivery of prenatal care. There is a recognized need to improve the process to provide the best possible outcomes for mothers and babies. It is problematic that in this era of evidence-based practice, the structure and the content of prenatal care continue to be defined largely by tradition. Almost two decades after the publication of the seminal U.S. Public Health Service Task Force report, *Caring for Our Future*, which highlighted the lack of evidence to support most of the prenatal care as it is delivered in America, there is still not an adequate body of evidence on which to base reform. Equally problematic is the uncertainty about how the various components of prenatal care translate into birth outcomes.

In the United States, much of the recent focus on outcomes has been directed toward the persistent problems of low birth weight and preterm birth, neither of which is fully understood. Increasing credence is being given to those complex components of care that influence the health and well-being of the mother. It is particularly challenging to address the complex psychosocial needs of the mother and her family, as well as the basic concerns for safe physical outcomes for the mother and infant, within the usual parameters of prenatal care. The CenteringPregnancy® model of prenatal care is designed to meet this challenge.

Underlying Philosophy of Centering

The conceptual foundation for CenteringPregnancy® is composed of several underlying philosophical elements. These influences meld like key ingredients in a savory Crock-Pot to yield the secret recipe's singular aroma and flavor.

The stock, which provides the basis for the Centering program, draws on the frameworks of feminism, particularly Andrist's (1997) feminist model for health care, Kennedy's (2000) relationship-centered midwifery model of care, and the theories of social support and self-efficacy derived from the behavioral and social science literature.

The main ingredients are found in CenteringPregnancy®'s Essential Elements (Rising, Kennedy, and Klima 2004):

- Health assessment occurs within the group space.
- Women are involved in self-care activities.
- A facilitative leadership style is used.
- Each session has an overall plan.
- Attention is given to the core content; emphasis may vary.
- There is stability of group leadership.
- Group conduct honors the contribution of each member.
- The group is conducted in a circle.
- Group composition is stable but not rigid.
- Group size is optimal to promote the process.
- Involvement of family support people is optional.
- Opportunity for socializing within the group is provided.
- There is ongoing evaluation of outcomes.

In completing the creative kitchen metaphor, there is ample room in the CenteringPregnancy® model for using flexibility and improvisation, for adapting the details to reflect the needs of the model's consumers, for personalizing the recipe with signature variations from contributors to the pot, or for changing aspects of the presentation to appeal to the palate of each new group.

The CenteringPregnancy® Essential Elements reflect and fulfill the Institute of Medicine's Ten Rules to Redesign and Improve Care, from their seminal 2001 report entitled *Crossing the Quality Chasm* (Rising, Kennedy, and Klima 2004):

- Care is based on continuous healing relationships.
- Care is customized according to patient needs and values.
- The patient is the source of control.
- Knowledge is shared, and information flows freely.
- Decision making is evidence-based.
- Safety is a system priority.
- Transparency is necessary.
- Needs are anticipated.
- Waste is continuously decreased.
- Cooperation among clinicians is a priority.

GROUP SHARING

In the spirit of group sharing that is at the core of CenteringPregnancy®, several Centering practitioners from different settings, including program founder Sharon Schindler Rising, share their experiences with the model in first-person narrative form below. The members of this circle of Centering providers share from their experiences implementing the model in private practices and public health clinics, among women of different ages and different ethnic and cultural backgrounds, and with women whose pregnancies unfold under special circumstances, such as infection with HIV or incarceration.

The Birth of CenteringPregnancy®

SHARON SCHINDLER RISING

It was 1993, and I was in my twenty-sixth year of providing prenatal care. I was working as a midwife in multiple settings in Connecticut, including a private office, a hospital clinic, and a community health care center, and caring for many, many pregnant women—all of whom shared common issues as they moved through the childbearing process. I began thinking there must be a better way to do prenatal care, a way that would benefit both the women and me.

Several years earlier, before moving to Connecticut, I had established the Childbearing-Childrearing Center at the University of Minnesota in Minneapolis. There, pregnant couples who were due during the same month joined together early in the third trimester and continued meeting regularly through the first three months postpartum. This became a time of preparation for the birth experience and parenting for the couples, and provided an opportunity for them to build community. My husband and I were in one of these groups during our first pregnancy, so I personally experienced the power of group support and appreciated the confidence that sharing gave me as I began my own journey of parenting.

Because of these earlier experiences, it was natural for me to turn to groups as my frustration grew with the care I was able to provide at these three locations in Connecticut. But the question was, what kind of groups? Prenatal classes abounded, and participants often formed a type of support system for each other. However, fewer women were interested in formal childbirth classes, partly because their lives were busier and they were getting more of their education through media and books. Also, formal childbirth classes were not financially feasible for all women. The answer seemed to be to combine the assessment component of traditional prenatal care with time for education and support.

I initially focused on the hospital clinic site, which managed approximately thirty births per month, most assisted by Yale Hospital ob/gyn residents. Most women there were healthy, young, of low income, and approximately equally divided ethnically among Caucasian, African American, and Hispanic. I gathered the medical director, the clinic nurses, the women's health supervisor, and the social worker and suggested that we group eight to twelve women of similar gestation, starting at about sixteen weeks, for all of their prenatal care. The care would be provided by a nurse practitioner or a nurse-midwife along with a nurse—a provider dyad that would follow the women for ten sessions throughout pregnancy. If women developed medical problems, they would be referred to the medical staff for evaluation.

A curriculum was developed using self-assessment sheets that each woman could use to get in touch with her thoughts and needs on a variety of topics related to pregnancy and childbearing. These were used to springboard a facilitated discussion. As the provider in the group, I had to learn to really listen to women. In that process, I found that I was learning much more than I was "teaching." Women participated in self-care activities, assessing their own blood pressure and weight and entering these data on the chart. The chart itself became demystified as terminology was explained, and each woman was able to claim her own data. It was amazing to me to see how empowering this was for the women and how, when given a chance to really speak, they were able to claim their considerable knowledge.

A lack of appropriate space in which to conduct groups is sometimes a challenge with the CenteringPregnancy® approach, as is difficulty with the process of recruitment. Fortunately, I had a conference room available in the hospital. Because it was also used for other activities, we needed to set up and take down the room for each use, which was not ideal. However, the clinic staff was very enthusiastic about the program and readily helped with recruitment of the women. Also, because I was the primary provider of prenatal care at the clinic, I was able to do much of the promotion. We found we easily could involve half of our women in groups by starting one group a month. Women loved it!

The nurses working with the program also loved it. As one said, "This is what nursing should be!" and another commented that "in Centering, a connection is made between the women and the staff that is empowering to all." The initial pilot program included thirteen groups, of which three were teen groups. At the final evaluation, 98% of the women said they enjoyed being with other women to receive their care (Rising 1998). This figure is consistent with findings from across the country: 96%–97% of all women, whether primigravidas or multiparas, say they prefer getting their care in this model. And midwives comment, "I was ready to get out of midwifery but this has totally re-energized me, by getting me back to why I became a midwife."

With that first site, my enthusiasm for the model really grew, and I was soon able to begin the program at both of my other locations. Eventually, I started facilitating translated groups for our Spanish-speaking women. All of these groups were successful, and the word got out. As interest grew, I started speaking to groups about Centering. My first national presentation on CenteringPregnancy® took place in 1995. Since then, the number of training workshops has continued to increase steadily. The power of groups is contagious.

CenteringPregnancy® in Private Practice

Women to Women, Yarmouth, Maine

SUSAN FEKETY AND BETHANY HAYS

Women to Women is a progressive group practice located in a renovated Victorian house in a suburb of Portland, Maine. Women to Women encourages client autonomy, awareness of the emotional content of illness, and the use of complementary and alternative medicine. Our clients are affluent; most pay out-of-pocket or have private insurance, 75% are college educated, and consistent with Maine's overall demographics, virtually all are white. The practice drew a fair number of women who had previous traumatic labor and birth experiences, who mistrusted conventional medicine, who were sexual abuse survivors, or who were in recovery from substance abuse.

We (an obstetrician and a certified nurse midwife [CNM]) offered CenteringPregnancy® from 1998 to 2001. Both of us were ready to try something that supported women to reclaim the prenatal and birth process in an innovative way, and which offered us a refreshed perspective on our work. Aging, flirting with fatigue and burnout, we found the notion of simultaneously leveraging our clinical time and reframing women's prenatal care experience by facilitating group support completely tantalizing. We asked ourselves, "Why didn't *we* think of this? It makes so much sense!" "Because we were too tired from being on call!" we exclaimed as we rode home from the first CenteringPregnancy® workshop in 1998.

Our CenteringPregnancy® groups were offered in the living/waiting room of the practice after the office day was over. CenteringPregnancy® was the standard option at the practice—all women were assigned to a group and were expected to attend. No one was risked out of group care, and though it was possible to opt out, few did. Our clients loved the idea of knowing their visit schedule in advance and having an opportunity to meet other women and involve their partners in their care. Women who worked outside the home really liked the evening hours.

One of the unanticipated benefits of the Centering model in this practice was its ability to welcome and support the partners in the group. Men discussed their experience of the role transition to fatherhood and strategies for balancing fatherhood with a consuming professional career. They arranged to help one another with home renovations. For the clinicians, access to partners in the group setting offered an opportunity to address the realities of providing labor support directly, and to facilitate an open discussion about the differences between "support" and "control." Once, a pregnant woman was unable to attend the group, but her husband came anyway because he enjoyed the meetings so much.

Strong friendships developed among the women, some of which have lasted for years, with ongoing socialization, shared child care, and play dates. One woman who had been in an early Centering group was diagnosed with breast cancer when her baby was two, and she immediately sought emotional support from other members of her group. Another group has developed a website where baby photos and family updates continue to be shared.

We did an informal comparative analysis of our statistics for the women who went through Centering, parity matched to a group of women in the practice who had not experienced groups. Although ours was already a low-intervention practice, we observed fewer cesarean sections and instrumental deliveries, fewer labor inductions and augmentation with pitocin, shorter first stages of labor, less use of regional methods of pain control, and more medication-free labors with the Centering group. Mean birth weight among women in Centering was slightly higher, but the difference was not significant.

Although we have moved and no longer offer maternity care, we remain staunch advocates of the CenteringPregnancy® model and of patient-centered groups in general. We saw that the emphasis on horizontal relationships, conscious speaking and listening, and the building of community were powerful tools for change for women, and a delightful and refreshing approach to care for us. Both of us are demonstrably better listeners now than we were prior to Centering. We learned early on that our tendency to "go didactic" or take control of the group had to be resisted because the best groups were those in which the issues that arose were permitted to evolve on their own.

Unquestionably, Centering offered a hedge against burnout because it was simply pleasurable, fun, and human. Women who had been through the program with us actively sought it during subsequent pregnancies—and helped stimulate another local midwifery private practice to offer the model when Women to Women morphed into a new organization that didn't offer prenatal care. They're still up and running.

CenteringPregnancy® in Private and Academic Practices in Cambridge, Massachusetts

GAIL PHILLIPS

I was immediately attracted to the CenteringPregnancy® model of group prenatal care when I heard a presentation about it at the 1995 American College of Nurse-Midwives' annual convention because

- I had a great interest in the concept of group health care.
- I thought the model fit beautifully into the midwifery model of care.
- I had some past professional experience of the power of groups.
- I wanted to incorporate more of the rich community resources available into our prenatal care.
- I realized my own limitations both as a midwife and as an individual to meet the specific needs of every woman on a one-to-one basis.
- I knew the limitations of what could be accomplished in a thirty-minute visit.

After a few years of being excited about this model, I was finally able to bring it to fruition in Women Care, our unique, private midwifery practice. Our population, located in Cambridge, Massachusetts, was composed of older, highly educated professional women. They were empowered and curious, and questioned many things during their prenatal care, yet they also wanted the support and guidance of a capable, loving midwife. They were both a pleasure and a challenge. My assistant was the office manager/ medical assistant. She had worked at our midwifery practice for almost twenty years and was near burnout, but had gone to the training with the rest of the staff and was enthusiastic about our new adventure.

The very first session foreshadowed the overall success of this model in our practice. The topic of prenatal testing evoked a heated discussion that reflected the sharing of different convictions and value systems. This group was not shy about expressing their beliefs. They were confident, open, and well informed during the discussion, and at times my group facilitation skills were not even needed. The discussion just flowed, reinforcing my own belief in the power of the group model. The process helped the group participants create their own unbiased, informed consent. The discussion included the benefits, risks, and alternatives to testing. Participants expressed their fears, clarified their values, and in the end, more decided not to test.

With Centering, the relationship with my clients and their partners seemed more intimate than in traditional care. I was able to "see them" more clearly in a group, and because I was better able to understand and appreciate them, I felt more able to meet their individual needs. Their intellectual energies were channeled more easily in a group setting. People were able to share their expertise with each other, exchanging information and resources, such as Internet sites and technical information. The open charts stimulated amusing questions and discussions, especially about ultrasound exams because of the scientific background of many of the group members.

It seemed very natural to include partners, and it certainly contributed to the richness of the discussions. The bonding and the support within the group grew progressively, culminating with the reunion. Every woman in the group cried as each couple told their birth story and recounted the particular challenges they had faced. How often does a couple get the opportunity to share their birth story, uninterrupted, to others who listen with understanding and compassion, and without judgment?

Interestingly, my assistant's stress level dropped dramatically. She particularly identified with the stress management component that I incorporated into the groups. She became more energized, and her productivity increased at work. She began to nurture herself and ultimately lost over 100 pounds.

The group attendance rate was near 100%, the evaluations were all positive, and everyone in the group rated their satisfaction 10/10. The cesarean rate was 11%, everyone was still breastfeeding at the reunion, and 50% of the births were "natural" [Editor's note: an astounding figure for the United States, given its usual high intervention rates].

Perspectives on CenteringPregnancy® for Teens

San Francisco General Hospital, San Francisco, California

DEENA MALLAREDDY

In 2004 I helped San Francisco General Hospital start a Teen CenteringPregnancy® program. I had been the Teen Clinic coordinator for a few years before we decided to build on the successes of our adult Centering program and offer the model to our teen patients.

I believe the biggest advantage of Centering for teens is peer support. Teens have a developmental need for peer-based interactions, and reach out to each other for information about their body, sex, and identity issues. Group interaction is fluid and normalizing. Group members share the same bellies and pregnancy clothes and the same concerns about parenting, stretch marks, and day care. Centering provides a place to feel validated and be accepted by other pregnant teens. They express themselves in so many different ways—by the CDs they bring to share, the way they decorate their name tags, and the clothes they wear. They respond enthusiastically to interactive games such as charades or Red Rover, and to activities that may be based on TV shows such as *Jeopardy*. These young women have to grow up quickly. Inevitably, many fall out of contact with non-pregnant friends. They assume lives that revolve around self-care and parenting activities as opposed to social events. The friendships forged in Centering can make up for the lack of support and understanding from past social networks and society at large.

I have also seen the advantages of consistent, quality time with adult providers in group. Teens seem to love the two dependable and fun hours they have with the same people over and over again. Many pregnant teens lead chaotic lives, and have very few engaging and mutually respectful relationships with adults. I have been told that group was the first place they felt they could trust adults with their "stuff," and have heard teens disclose substance use and hold complex discussions about peer pressure and risk taking in groups. One teen practiced role plays in the group and was able to ask her mom to cut down on smoking around her. She eventually quit smoking herself.

Teens who are defensive around authority figures or mistrust the system are less suspicious when they own their groups and discuss topics they pick. They are encouraged to empower themselves at a critical time in their self-esteem and identity formation.

Teens are notorious "no shows." They will skip their appointments if they feel overwhelmed by labyrinthine health care systems. In San Francisco, the Teen Centering program is in the same building as the community teen advocacy agency, as well as the continuation high school for pregnant and parenting teens. Teens can go straight to Centering from school without going outside. This unique arrangement allows them to continue with their pregnancies while preserving their routine along the route of their daily lives. In Teen Centering, there appears to be higher attendance, earlier entry into prenatal care, and less loss to follow-up.

Teen Centering holds a special place in my heart. These young ladies start so tender and fragile, but they really grow into their own. They are curious at the first session, but somewhat tentative. By the last session, they hold their heads higher, demonstrating a budding sense of confidence that I rarely saw in regular Teen Clinic. If it gives *me* such hope, I can only imagine what it must give them.

Centering under Special Circumstances

HIV-Positive Pregnant Women, Miami, Florida

THERESA GESSE

My budding enthusiasm for group care increased after I attended a CenteringPregnancy® workshop. I was convinced that this would be a model that would work with vulnerable populations. I decided that HIV-positive pregnant women, who are often isolated in their dilemma without a support person to share feelings and fears, would be the particular population on which I would focus.

The University of Miami and its medical center provide services for pregnant women with HIV in their immunology clinics, but these clinics are overcrowded, and it is often difficult for women to obtain sufficient attention there. In addition to prenatal care, the providers must also cover a host of topics related to living with HIV. I believed that CenteringPregnancy® would generate a support system as well as encourage an exchange of coping strategies for these pregnant women. A certified nurse midwife (CNM) from the Immunology Clinic, a nurse, and a social worker who attended the workshop shared my beliefs and enthusiastically agreed to be part of our Centering team. The final team member was an attending physician, board certified in maternal-fetal medicine.

In our practice, the lowest-risk members of this high-risk population are identified by the CNM in consultation with the team physician. She explains the program to eligible individuals and offers them the choice to join a group for their prenatal care. A woman in Centering care who subsequently develops problems that place her in a high-risk category is either co-managed by the maternal-fetal medicine specialist while she stays in the group, or if the problems are severe, followed individually in the Immunology Clinic. We have modified the standard CenteringPregnancy® materials and self-assessment sheets to include some added content about HIV.

During the groups, a nurse-midwife, a registered nurse, and a social worker are present for each session and participate in the many discussions related to pregnancy, labor, birth, postpartum blues, contraception, changing feelings, and parenting. The social worker is always available to meet in a private setting if necessary, but often the questions raised by one person are of value to everyone. The attending physician serves as a consultant for problems and special needs that arise for the women in the group.

By the final session (when we give each group a "baby shower"), the interaction among the women is always remarkable. There are exchanges of phone numbers and instructions such as, "Now you call me if you need anything," or "Call if you don't have anyone to stay with your other children when you start labor," or "Call if you just need to talk and I will do the same, because I still get down and depressed sometimes."

The bonding is significant and obvious. The team and observers have concluded that this model works well with this population. There is increased self-esteem, a sense of responsibility, trust, and a feeling that there are other women out there in the same situation who are no longer living in isolation because of these groups.

Most of all, the women learn a lot, not only about their HIV status, but about themselves, their pregnancy, and their future. They feel better about themselves and regain a sense of self-worth. The team recognizes that the women in groups are developing friendships and a sense of belonging.

An Incarceration Center, Louisville, Kentucky

JACQUELYN REID AND MIMI MCKAY

In the summer of 2002, a psychiatric mental health nursing colleague asked me to visit a group of pregnant women with whom she was working at a correctional facility. She said they had "lots of questions she couldn't answer." The questions the women raised were those that would commonly be addressed in a childbirth education class. The discussion was lively, and I was moved by the plight of these women: imprisoned and pregnant, with no access to childbirth education classes. Another issue that drew my attention was their discussion of relinquishing their babies. I left the group wondering how I could help.

A review of the literature on incarcerated pregnant women revealed a number of alarming facts. First, 85% of women inmates are behind bars for nonviolent offenses. Second, the number of women behind bars increased tenfold between 1986 and 1996. It also distressed me to learn that incarcerated pregnant women often receive little or no education about prenatal care and nutrition, and that their pregnancies are frequently categorized as high-risk as a result of substance abuse, smoking, or infectious diseases. In addition, they receive inadequate family support during pregnancy and childbirth and often have histories of physical and sexual abuse. Another practice the majority of pregnant inmates in the United States face routinely is shackling during childbirth. This makes it is easy to understand why incarcerated pregnant women and their offspring have a higher morbidity and mortality rate than those who are not imprisoned. After this eye-opening review, I felt compelled to try to influence the care of this group of women.

I attended a CenteringPregnancy® workshop and realized that many of the components of Centering could easily be adapted for incarcerated women. After returning from the course, I discussed CenteringPregnancy® with my colleagues. They were enthusiastic about the program and wanted it implemented immediately. Upon receiving approval to conduct research about our proposed intervention and a grant from the March of Dimes to fund our startup, the program was introduced at the prison in the fall of 2003. Since then, seven groups of women have completed the Centering-Pregnancy® program.

The content for the women in the correctional facility is identical to that in regular CenteringPregnancy®, up until the infant care sequence. Because incarcerated women must relinquish their infants immediately to a family member or a state-approved foster care program, we have a discussion that deals with the emotions associated with separating from one's infant.

At the first and last meeting of each group, the women complete several questionnaires that test knowledge about pregnancy, locus of control, self-esteem, and psychosocial attributes. In addition, at the last session of each group, the women evaluate the program. These tools have allowed us to evaluate the influence this unique program of education and group support has on women's experience of pregnancy in a correctional facility.

The age range of incarcerated women who have participated in CenteringPregnancy® to date is between twenty and thirty-four years of age. About 75% are Caucasian, 23% African American, and 1% Native American. Ninety percent smoke. Their evaluation of the CenteringPregnancy® groups has been very positive. Our questionnaire results demonstrate increased knowledge about a broad range of educational topics, and increased internal locus of control among women who have attended CenteringPregnancy® groups. These women also reported increased social support during the group and demonstrated a modest increase in self-esteem scores from group beginning to end. Women have cited the support they received from the group leaders and each other as the greatest strength of the program. They also appreciate the group process "where no one lectures us, but helps us to learn."

Here are some things that pregnant incarcerated women said they like best about CenteringPregnancy®:

- "Meeting all the pregnant ladies, and now we meet outside class and speak to one another and talk about our babies."

- "Being a part of a group of women like myself and learning from an experienced midwife."
- "That you do learn more and you're made to feel good about others. I think highly of the program."

Spanish-Speaking Women, Goshen, Indiana

BETH ELMORE

CenteringPregnancy® groups offer a number of advantages to Spanish-speaking women and to their prenatal care providers. The most obvious is that these women benefit from the comprehensive education that is offered in groups, but because of the language barrier is often missed or misunderstood in traditional settings. Providers have the advantage of being able to educate several women at once. Equally important, a Centering group offers immigrant women a community of other women. Groups allow care providers the pleasure of joining that community themselves, of coming to know something of the context of immigrant women's lives, not marginally or academically, but directly and personally. Ultimately, the act of providing health care in the context of community may change everything about the way care is provided and the way it is received.

In sharing my experience with Spanish-language Centering groups, it is important to establish that my Spanish is only passable, not nearly adequate to facilitate a group discussion, so I have done Centering groups for six years with a translator. In Centering groups, the group leader and the translator need to work as a team, together observing and responding to group dynamics to facilitate the multidirectional flow of communication and energy. I have been fortunate to work with several translators who have been not only bilingual but bicultural as well, and who have therefore been able to convey cultural context, when needed, along with words.

The CenteringPregnancy® model changes the dynamic of prenatal care by substantially reducing the power differential between the care provider and the women. Centering groups open a context in which care providers and women from disparate cultures can begin to set aside their differences and assumptions in order to learn from each other.

One example of our reaching successfully across the cultural gap was a group discussion regarding breastfeeding. American health professionals who are strong supporters of breastfeeding generally believe that giving supplemental bottles to breastfed babies often inhibits successful breastfeeding. Many of us, therefore, have been frustrated when our Mexican and Latin American clients insist that breastfed babies need supplemental bottles for various reasons. A Centering group discussion gave me a context for understanding this issue. When asked about their plans for feeding their babies, almost all women in the group had responded that they planned to give both breast milk and formula. I asked why a woman might want to give supplementary bottles. One woman said, "You need formula for times when your milk is not good for the baby." I asked, "When would that be?" The women around the group answered variously: "When you're sick," "If you're taking medicine that's bad for the baby," and "When you're angry or upset."

This last idea was news to me, so I asked more about it. All the women agreed that an angry or upset mother's milk is bad for her baby and will cause anger or upset in the baby. To avoid this, the mother pumps and discards her milk during and soon after the time she's upset, and gives the baby a bottle. As soon as she feels better, the milk is fine again, and she resumes breastfeeding.

It took me several days to realize fully what they had told me. These are women for whom breast milk is not a food commodity that merely provides calories and nutrients for a baby. Rather, it is the product of a relationship, and everything that affects the participants in that relationship affects the milk.

In this way, mothers in my groups are slowly broadening my awareness of the myriad ways in which the world can usefully be understood. At the same time, my factual, scientific explanation of the events of the menstrual cycle and the anatomy of the male and female reproductive systems may be allowing them to choose effective methods of contraception and use them correctly. My pictures and demonstrations of the mechanisms of labor may be helping them understand why sitting on a huge ball is a good thing to do in labor.

For some time, my nurse and I wondered whether our group women didn't like the American food we were bringing for snacks—although it seemed that fruit, cheese, and quick breads should have a universal appeal. Our translator suggested that it might seem rude for a woman to help herself to the food even though it was set out and available. She thought we should serve the women, taking the food around the circle and inviting each woman to try some. Passing around plates, cups, and food is now part of each group just before the discussion begins.

In many ways, the CenteringPregnancy® model, itself, has power to create the openness that we need to see things in a different light and make necessary adaptations. As in other situations involving language barriers, things are undoubtedly "lost in translation." However, things are gained as well. In any case, whatever allows people to connect personally despite differences in race, culture, and language is a hopeful thing and perhaps the only way to heal our fractured, post-9/11 world. What better place to start than at the point at which we welcome children into the world?

CENTERINGPREGNANCY®: A BIRTH MODEL THAT WORKS

The CenteringPregnancy® model meets all of the criteria identified by the editors in the Introduction to this volume to characterize "birth models that work." Centering group care is women centered and community based. Moreover, it is community building. Centering groups provide a mechanism for continuity that moves beyond continuity of health care into the wider scope of "continuity of caring" for women and families who form strong bonds during their group experiences together. The Centering model is one that provides added support for all women, but it may particularly benefit those high-risk women for whom the barriers to care are especially high within traditional care models. This group includes, but is not limited to, women from cultural and ethnic minorities, teens, low-income women, those with high-risk pregnancies, and those who are incarcerated. The Centering model values the time of the women in group care, who can count on group sessions that start on time and end on time (allowing them to plan for child care needs and time off from work at the beginning of their pregnancy), and whose content is tailored to their needs and interests.

CenteringPregnancy® provides a supportive framework for providers of prenatal care as well. The Centering model encourages multidisciplinary cooperation and creative collaboration among providers of care. It reduces provider burnout and fosters professional growth. It provides a supportive educational environment for students, and one in which ongoing evaluation promotes continuous quality improvement. Groups conducted in a variety of languages offer women from all backgrounds opportunities to fully participate in their care and give providers an important glimpse into diverse cultural beliefs.

From an institutional or system perspective, the Centering model results in statistically sound outcomes, improving the quality of care for all participants and particularly for those who are most vulnerable. A matched cohort study of CenteringPregnancy® published in *Obstetrics and Gynecology* (Ickovics et al. 2003) demonstrated that among women in the study with preterm births, those who received their prenatal care in a Centering group gave birth on average two weeks later to babies that weighed on average one pound more than their counterparts who received traditional prenatal care.

The Centering model encourages optimal use of system facilities and resources, and promotes staff development and satisfaction. In addition, because comprehensive prenatal care is what happens in the group, Centering programs are fully reimbursable, making the model sustainable and financially viable. Centering groups also serve as a marketing tool for institutions, attracting media attention and increasing clientele. CenteringPregnancy® changes the paradigm of prenatal care from a traditionally linear, top-down model, with a narrow emphasis on physical outcomes, to one that reflects the qualities of an inclusive circle: group centered, democratic, egalitarian, and with a broad, holistic approach that emphasizes health empowerment and well-being.

COMING FULL CIRCLE:
THE CENTERINGPREGNANCY® MODEL IN 2008

More than a decade has passed since the model was first piloted in a hospital clinic in Connecticut. Since that time, over 300 sites, both private and public, in almost all states have active CenteringPregnancy® programs, and international sites are found in Australia, Canada, Germany, Sweden, and the United Kingdom. Research and evaluation studies in academic settings and practice sites are multiplying.

The results of the Yale/Emory five-year randomized controlled trial, a study that includes over 1,047 women and examines a range of outcomes in Centering group care compared to traditional prenatal care, has been published in *Obstetrics and Gynecology* (Ickovics et al. 2007). The birth outcome data demonstrate a 33% reduction in preterm birth for women randomized to group, two-thirds of the total sample. And the African American women in group, 80% of the sample, had a 41% reduction in preterm birth. In addition, women in group demonstrated increased knowledge of labor and birth, increased satisfaction with care, better psychosocial functioning, and increased breastfeeding rates. This study, under the direction of Dr. Jeannette Ickovics, Yale University, is the first of several major Centering research projects and was funded by the National Institutes of Mental Health. It is being followed by another randomized study involving multiple community health centers in New York City. Another randomized study through the University of California–San Francisco, funded by a tri-service military grant, involving two military pilot sites on Navy and Air Force bases showed high satisfaction among the women in the group and increased support for family readiness. Researchers at the University of Illinois at Chicago are studying the process that characterizes Centering groups and also have developed a new empowerment tool that will help to evaluate the extent to which groups contribute to the building of self-confidence in the women who participate in them. The University of Kentucky Dental School has developed CenteringPregnancy® Smiles with a strong dental component. Data from the first year show improved oral health and decreased preterm births and low birth weight.

March of Dimes chapters across the United States are funding Centering workshops and providing seed money for startup. One of the early programs funded is still going strong at Montefiore in the Bronx, New York. The Healthy Start and Healthy Mothers/Babies programs also have provided financial support for Centering activities. Programs in several states are benefiting from funding from these organizations. A variety of local, state, and national foundations are supporting other projects.

Strong Centering consortiums have developed in the Bay Area of San Francisco, funded by the Aetna Foundation, and in Texas, funded by the March of Dimes. Other consortiums are emerging in Illinois, Massachusetts, Louisiana, Tennessee, New York, North and South Carolina, and Georgia, to name a few. Programs in other areas are gathering strength as one site helps to spark others. Residency programs in obstetrics/gynecology and family practice are providing opportunities for medical trainees to lead groups, and midwifery students are being trained to provide prenatal care within the model. Many sites have been doing Centering groups long enough to notice that women are coming back for a next pregnancy and asking when their new group will start.

The Centering Pregnancy and Parenting Association (CPPA) incorporated in 2001 in order to support the spread of the Centering model; it recently changed its name to Centering Healthcare Institute (CHI) to reflect the broader mission of Centering throughout the life cycle. In March 2006, CPPA sponsored its first national conference on group health care, The Power of Connection: Group Health Care for the 21st Century, which focused on changing the paradigm of care throughout the lifespan. Over 200 people from thirty-one states, Canada, and Australia, and representing a diverse group of health care providers, administrators, and researchers, attended the first conference. The conference featured balanced content, some of it geared to health care reform and some focused on the heart of group leadership and personal connection. This was a typical comment: "Amazing, fun, empowering conference. I go back [home] renewed, refreshed and better prepared for ALL the groups in which I participate! You have prepared me to make a difference!"

We are also training for CenteringParenting®groups that provide well-woman and well-baby dyad care during the first year of life and beyond. There are several sites using the model, both in family medicine and in pediatrics/well-woman care; a small randomized controlled trial (RCT) involving the pediatrics department and women's center staff at Yale–New Haven Hospital in Connecticut will look specifically at the issues involved when specialists work together. It makes sense for prenatal groups to continue to meet whenever possible through this intense time of adjustment; many sites are finding that it is the women who are insisting on continuing their group into the first postpartum year. There are many issues that women and families face with the advent of a new child, and there is much to learn about caring for and interacting with a baby. All of this provides very rich content for learning and discussion.

Within the field of maternal and child health, we are striving to provide evidence-based care in our health care delivery models. Although we are all searching for ways to reduce preterm birth and low birth weight, it is also important that we choose to examine additional outcomes that reflect issues pertaining to quality of life. Outcomes such as satisfaction with care, self-esteem and empowerment, maternal-infant attachment, rates of breast feeding initiation and duration, assertiveness within relationships, safe sexual practices, pre- and postpartum depression reduction, goal setting and self-efficacy, stress reduction, adequate contraception, and child spacing all are appropriate outcomes to evaluate. Pregnancy is a time for a woman to grow herself as a mother. We need to continue to identify measures that will help us to understand how we can support mothers to do this successfully.

The prenatal period encompasses a major life event for women and their families. It heralds the birth of a new family constellation, which brings with it the awesome responsibility of parenting. It presents a unique opportunity for health professionals to be truly present to the needs and values of the families they serve, at a time when these families are ripe for learning and in real need of support. By fully realizing this opportunity and harnessing the power of the group, what is facilitated is the development of those very skills and resources needed to ensure the healthiest possible outcomes, over the short and the long term, for all who participate. It is, without a doubt, a privilege for us to be with women during this time of vulnerability and accelerated growth. Because we recognize this honor, let us continually strive to be present in the best possible manner. Claire Westdahl, nurse-midwife and CenteringPregnancy® group leader, put it best: "In truth, I continue to be awed by the power of the group. We are having such a good time, and such laughs. I am learning that it doesn't matter what we *don't* talk about, because we are talking about what *matters* to the group."

ACKNOWLEDGMENTS

The authors wish to thank Susan Fekety, CNM,MSN; Bethany Hays, MD; Gail Phillips, CNM, MS; Deena Mallareddy, CNM, MSN; Theresa Gesse, CNM, PhD; Jacqueline Chinnock Reid, CNM, EdD; Mimi McKay, ARNP, EdD; and Beth Elmore, CNM, MSN for their contributions. We sadly acknowledge the death of Theresa Gesse in 2008.

For more information: www.centeringhealthcare.org.

NOTE

1. Comments included were made by women in Centering groups on evaluations collected at the end of the group series.

REFERENCES

Andrist, Linda. 1997. "A Feminist Model for Women's Health Care." *Nursing Inquiry* 4:268–74.
Ickovics, Jeannette, Trace Kershaw, Claire Westdahl, Sharon Schindler Rising, Carrie Klima, Heather Reynolds, and Urania Magriples. 2003. "Group Prenatal Care Improves Preterm Birth Weight: Results from a Matched Cohort Study at Public Clinics." *Obstetrics and Gynecology* 102:1051–7.
Ickovics, Jeannette, Trace Kershaw, Claire Westdahl, Urania Magriples, Zohar Massey, Heather Reynolds, and Sharon Schindler Rising. 2007. "Group Prenatal Care and Perinatal Outcomes: A Randomized Controlled Trial," pt. 1. *Obstetrics and Gynecology* 110.2:330–39.
Kennedy, Holly. 2000. "A Model of Exemplary Midwifery Practice: Results of a Delphi Study. *Journal of Midwifery and Women's Health* 45:4–19.
Kidd, Sue Monk. 1995. *The Dance of the Dissident Daughter*. San Francisco: HarperCollins.
Massey, Zohar, Sharon Schindler Rising, and Jeannette Ickovics. 2006. "Centering-Pregnancy Group Prenatal Care: Promoting Relationship-Centered Care." *Journal of Obstetric, Gynecologic, and Neonatal Nursing* 35.2:286–94.
Rising, Sharon Schindler. 1998. "Centering Pregnancy: An Interdisciplinary Model of Empowerment." *Journal of Nurse-Midwifery* 43.1:46–54.
Rising, Sharon Schindler, Holly Kennedy, and Carrie Klima. 2004. "Redesigning Prenatal Care through CenteringPregnancy®." *Journal of Midwifery and Women's Health* 49.5:398–404.

Chapter 14

Humanizing Childbirth to Reduce Maternal and Neonatal Mortality

A National Effort in Brazil

Daphne Rattner, Isa Paula Hamouche Abreu, Maria José de Oliveira
Araújo, and Adson Roberto França Santos

SCENARIO # 1: ITABUNA

*A town by the south shore of Bahia, Itabuna became famous in Brazil because of
the books written by Jorge Amado about the life of people living in this cacao growth
region with names like Gabriela, Clove, and Cinnamon. Until January 2006,
women used to have babies in Itabuna's hospital just as they did in most hospitals
in the country: as soon as they arrived in labor, they were admitted (even in very
early labor), their pubic hair was shaved, they were given enemas, they were made to
lie down with a drip of oxytocin, and they were not allowed any food or drink—and
although there were so many norms, no protocols were available for the professionals.
Other common, non-evidence-based practices included routine amniotomy, routine
episiotomy, no personal companion during labor and delivery, and no use of the
partogram (an evidence-based tool for tracking the progress of women in labor).*[1]
Cesarean sections were fairly common—in January 2006 the rate was 50.8%.

In July 2006, about six months after participating in one of our seminars,
Dr. José Leopoldo dos Santos, director of the Hospital Manoel Novaes, a
proud presenter at a state seminar, described the current care offered to
delivering women: no early admission, amniotomy only according to the
partogram, no routine or liberal use of oxytocin, defined protocols, no
restriction of fluids during labor (and soon women will also be allowed to
eat), freedom of movement during labor, empathic support from doulas—
now women are allowed a companion of their choice by their side—as well
as other changes. Now medical interns and residents in this hospital are
being taught to care for childbirth following these guidelines, a reform
that has introduced to them the importance of adopting practices based
on scientific evidence. In that month of July, the cesarean rate dropped to
37.4%—not yet ideal, but a significant improvement. But not all is rosy in

this story: the medical professionals are having a hard time—and giving their director a hard time—accepting the presence of the woman's companion, which, though it is her prerogative by force of Law No. 10,108 of April 7, 2005, does not come easily.

This successful story is one of many, and it introduces the focus of this chapter: a program created by officials of the Ministry of Health to humanize childbirth in Brazil through the adoption of a snowball strategy. It started with a few hospitals in 2004 (one in each state) and, by involving them in a process of multiplication, by the end of 2006, almost 500 hospitals and more than 2,000 health professionals had participated in the process.

In this chapter, we also describe how the Ministry of Health is working to integrate traditional midwives into the public health care system. All the authors of this chapter work or worked for the Brazilian Ministry of Health. Daphne Rattner, a public health physician and epidemiologist, is responsible for government strategies to reduce unnecessary cesareans, among other assignments. Prior to her admission to the Ministry of Health, she was the national coordinator of the Brazilian Network for the Humanization of Childbirth—ReHuNa, a nongovernmental organization (NGO) that influenced this public policy. Isa Abreu, a public health physician, was responsible for training traditional midwives from 2000 to May 2007, among other assignments. Maria José Araújo, also a physician, was the coordinator of the Women's Health Program of the Ministry of Health from 2003 to May 2007. Adson França Santos, the national coordinator of the Pact for the Reduction of Maternal and Neonatal Mortality and currently the director of the Department of Programmatic and Strategic Actions of the Ministry of Health, is an obstetrician/gynecologist and a member of the Brazilian Federation of the Societies of Obstetrics and Gynecology. All helped shape the strategy and develop the classes, and all have served as seminar instructors.

MEET THE CONTEXT

With a territory of 3,300,000 square miles (8.5 million square kilometers) spreading from the equatorial zone in its north down under the Tropic of Capricorn at its south,[2] Brazil is the largest country of South America, composed of twenty-six states and a Federal District distributed in five major regions: North, Northeast, Southeast, South, and Central-West, with 5,565 municipalities.

Brazil was the third name our country received: when the Portuguese discovered it in 1500, they thought it was an island, so they called it Island of the True Cross (Ilha de Vera Cruz). When they realized it was much larger than an island, it became the Land of the Sacred Cross (Terra de

Santa Cruz), and finally, it was named after a precious tree of red wood (pau brasil), used to dye textiles. Now this tree has almost disappeared as a result of predatory exploitation,[3] but the country has grown, carrying its name, and has become one of the major economic powers of the world.

In 2004 Brazil's population was estimated to be 181 million, with higher demographic density in the Southeast and South. Great geographic, climatic, population, and cultural diversity distinguish the regions. The Northern region encompasses the Amazon Basin—an area of rain forests and rivers very different from the rest of the country. The Amazon's natural riches are a counterpoint to the difficulty of communication and transportation: its population is dispersed across a large territory and lacks access to goods and services such as health care. The most common method of travel is by boat. Most native Brazilian tribes live in this and the Central-West region, although various tribes are scattered all over Brazil. There are no major economic activities in this region, and many people live on what nature offers, collecting fruit, fishing, or hunting.

The economics of the Central-West are based on agribusiness (cattle, soy) and tourism. The Southeast has experienced centralized economic development for many years. São Paulo is the most industrialized of all Brazilian states, where most of the automobile and metallurgic industries built their plants, along with textile and graphic industries, and others. Many immigrants, mostly from European countries but also from Japan, settled in the Southeast (and in the South) at the end of the 19th century and at the beginning of the 20th century, bringing their culture and traditions, and bolstering economic development. The Northeast is where the highest levels of absolute poverty may be found, and where income distribution is more concentrated. Health indicators are worse among women, in general, and among African descendants, both women and men. The South, Northeast. and Central-West economics are based on agriculture and cattle, and Brazil is a major exporter of soybeans, sugarcane, coffee, and meat.

Caring for People's Health

According to the highest law of the country, our Constitution (the most recent version of which was approved in 1988), every citizen has the right to health and to the use of health care services according to her/his needs. The right to health means that the State should guarantee to all inhabitants the conditions in which to live with dignity, as well as universal and egalitarian access to services that promote, protect, and recover health in all its aspects. In order to achieve these principles of universality and equity, the Brazilian Healthcare System (SUS) is structured and organized into a very complex network of services. The main strategy has been to create a public structure organized around participation in all levels of the system: there are national, state, municipal, and regional health councils, on which different sectors of society are represented and where most of the policies, problems of implementation, development of programs, and specific health issues are collectively discussed. Even though its resources and services have not yet reached adequate standards compared to those of developed countries, efforts to extend health coverage and improve health quality are under way. These efforts have resulted from broad-based, popular health movements led by left-wing health professionals promoting health care as a right guaranteed by the Constitution.

The federal level defines the policies and guidelines, the municipal level is responsible for at least primary health care, and the state level technically and logistically supports the organization of the health services in the state, including specialized care not offered by the municipality. Therefore, in the public health care system, prenatal care is offered at the municipal level, while childbirth might be cared for either at the municipal or the state level. Although responsibility for health care is within the public health care system, most of the hospitals are privately owned: the SUS buys their services, delivery care included.

Around 36 million inhabitants are clients of the supplementary sector through HMOs and private insurance providers, and their internal policies started being monitored by the federal government only in the last few years. Cesarean section rates in this sector average 80%.

Brazil has been called "The Land of Contrasts" by some and *Belíndia* by the famous anthropologist Claude Lévi-Strauss, because here (as in other Latin American countries) you may find the contrasting realities of a highly developed Belgium and a very underdeveloped India in the same country—and sometimes in the same locations—coexisting in parallel.

Childbirth care in Brazil as a whole has been heavily marked by medicalization: many unnecessary and potentially iatrogenic interventions, abusive use of cesarean sections, isolation of the childbearing woman, lack of privacy and respect for the woman's autonomy, and lack of involvement of the family in the process. In many locations, the lack of a formal referral system for childbirth has meant that childbearing women have had to seek hospital beds on their own, knocking at many hospital doors before being accepted and thereby delaying care for any complications.

The information displayed in Table 14.1 demonstrates our diversity of care as revealed by numbers. Most of the deliveries are attended in hospitals. Resources, including physicians and specialized care, are concentrated in the Southeast region and are associated with the higher rates of hospitalized births and interventions that are characteristic of the technocratic model (Davis-Floyd 2004), including its higher

TABLE 14.1 Selected indicators of resources, health status, and type of maternity care for Brazil by region

Index	Year	Brazil	N	NE	SE	S	CW
Resources							
Physicians/1,000 inhabitants	2006	1.7	0.8	1.0	2.3	1.8	1.7
Nurses/1,000 inhabitants	2006	0.6	0.5	0.5	0.6	0.6	0.6
Hospital beds/1,000 inhabitants	2007	2.73	2.18	2.52	2.84	3.00	2.32
Public hosp. beds/1,000 inhabitants	2007	0.93	1.22	1.22	0.81	0.61	1.06
Health Indices							
Natality/1,000 inhabitants	2005	17.9	22.2	20.1	16.1	15.5	18.2
Infant mortality rate/1,000 live births	2005	21.2	25.5	31.6	14.2	13.8	17.8
Early neonatal mortality rate/1,000 live births	2005	10.9	12.9	16.6	7.2	7.0	8.8
Maternal mortality/100,00 live births	2005	74.7[a]	...	...	40.7	55.1	54.5
Low birth weight (%)	2005	8.2	7.0	7.5	9.1	8.6	7.6
Type of Maternity Care							
Hospitalized births (%)	2005	97	91	95	99	99	99
Cesarean section births (%)	2005	43.2	32.4	32.0	51.6	50.0	49.3
Cesarean section births in the public healthcare system (%)	2007	31.8	28.3	28.5	35.2	33.7	34.6
Live births ≥ 7 prenatal care visits (%)	2005	53	29	37	67	66	58
Population covered by private health insurance (%)	2007	20.6	7.4	9.1	32.5	19.0	13.0

SOURCES: Ministry of Health databases: www.datasus.gov.br; www.ans.gov.br.
[a] The correction factor of 1.4 was applied, based on Laurenti et al. (Ministério da Saúde 2006b)

cesarean section rate (cesarean rates in Table 14.1 include both the public and private health care sectors). The Northern region (which includes the Brazilian Amazon) displays the lowest rate of hospitalized births. Because of the difficulties of transportation and access to health care, this is where traditional or indigenous midwives are the caregivers to women in childbirth: many towns only have physicians or nurses for short periods of time, if ever. The Southeast and the South have lower natality, but also lower infant and early neonatal mortality rates; in addition, these regions have better information systems—for instance, their information on maternal mortality is available.

Our extremes, then, are the Southeast, with a Western kind of development, and the North, with the remaining traditional, indigenous population and culture; the other regions are in between, in the following order: South, Central-West, and Northeast.

As a result, both the technocratic model and the more humanistic traditional model coexist, with the technocratic model prevailing in the Southeast, South, and part of the Central-West, and the traditional model occurring more in the North and the Northeast (and part of the Central-West). Unnecessary interventions common to the technocratic model occur all over the country, although there are towns in the North region where traditional midwives attend almost 100% of all childbirths.

Home birth prevailed in Brazil until the 1970s, with midwives as the predominant caregivers in childbirth. Starting in the 1940s, but more pronouncedly in the 1970s, childbirth care moved into hospitals and hence became a medical issue. The availability of equipment and new technologies increased, and they were immediately introduced in professional practices, strengthening a hospital-centered and interventionist model of childbirth care. One of the consequences of this trend was the increase in cesarean rates, which reached unacceptable levels in many Brazilian states as early as the 1980s. We described this model of childbirth care above, taking Itabuna as a prototype.

The Brazilian Ministry of Health has been adopting official policies to reduce cesarean section rates in the public sector since 1998, either by defining limits on hospital rates for reimbursement (1998) or by sharing the responsibility with the state governments (2000), for example by establishing the Pact to Reduce Cesarean Section Rates. By signing this pact, the states became responsible for the cesarean section rates in their territories. However, the impact of these measures was limited to the first two years, and soon the rates began to rise again, as shown in Figure 14.1. As higher cesarean rates are found in the private and supplementary sectors, this reduction in the public sector presents a major challenge: often the same professionals work in the public and private sectors, and adopt the same professional habits in both.

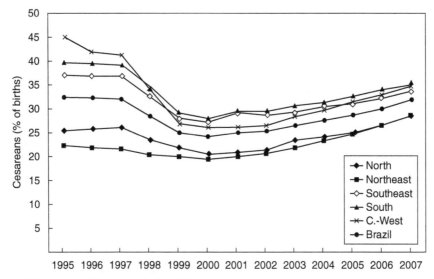

Figure 14.1. Cesareans in Brazil by region.

Cesarean sections in Brazil have risen to the extent that our country has long been an international anecdotal example of questionable practices and a topic of interest for national and international scholars. When asked the reasons for performing so many surgical interventions, many obstetricians would excuse themselves by stating they were only responding to women's demand.

Recent studies have shown that such allegations are inconsistent. For instance, Potter et al. (2001) showed that of 1,136 women interviewed throughout Brazil who gave birth by cesarean, 70%–80% would have preferred vaginal births; there were no significant differences in preferences between public and private patients. Barbosa et al. (2003) interviewed 909 women in Rio de Janeiro, and the majority (75.5%) preferred vaginal birth; only 17% asked for a cesarean, and of those, 75% made this request during labor. Qualitative studies also contributed to a better understanding of other reasons: Dalsgaard (2000) studied cesarean section associated with female sterilization; Hotimsky et al. (2002) revealed the complaints, fears, and expectations of pregnant women, revealing a marked preference for vaginal birth; and the results of the study by Behague, Victora, and Barros (2002) showed that many lower- to middle-class women sought cesarean sections to avoid what they considered poor-quality care and medical neglect resulting from social prejudice.

According to Faundes and Cecatti (1991), a variety of factors influence Brazil's high cesarean rates, all underlined by sociocultural, institutional, and legal issues. Just as a reminder, there are two different scenarios in Brazil: cesarean rates reach 100% in some hospitals in the supplementary and private sectors, but average 30% in the public health care system.

Brazil's so-called cesarean culture was generally thought to derive in part from the fact that some of those who can afford to negotiate demands for cesareans are opinion makers such as famous actresses and sportswomen who, under the influence of their physicians, have helped shape a positive notion of cesarean as a procedure full of value and glamour that takes away the pain of delivery. In this view, Brazil's high cesarean rates stem from (1) women's desires to emulate such figures; (2) the "modern" status associated with cesareans, which makes vaginal birth appear to be "primitive"—a touchy subject because of the extreme class distinctions in Brazil between the poor and indigenous and the more modern middle and upper classes; and (3) Brazilian women's reputed desire to be "nice and tight" for their husbands, which they assumed vaginal birth would ruin. But in fact, the studies mentioned above showed no foundation for such a culture, and when specifically questioned about the third point, most women stated they never considered it at all.

The institutional component of the cesarean-as-routine derives from the way health care services are organized: physicians simply find it more convenient and cost-effective to perform cesareans rather than waiting around for vaginal birth. Brazilian obstetricians are trained solely in the technocratic model of birth: they believe that birth is pathological. and that cesareans, over which they have control, are safer. Thus, they tend to invent reasons for convincing women to schedule cesareans in advance and for performing unnecessary cesareans once labor has begun. And even when obstetricians are paid the same for a cesarean or a vaginal delivery, performing cesareans enables them to get out of the hospital and return to their offices, where they can make more money attending private patients. Ideology and economics conveniently merge to create our high rates of cesarean section.

Regarding the legal realm, Faundes and Cecatti (1991) mention the fact that for many years, the public health care system would not reimburse analgesia nor surgeries for female sterilizations. A way to bypass this limitation was to artificially recommend cesarean sections: in the case of sterilization, the family would give an extra fee to the physician "under the table."

Thus, it became clear to us in the Ministry of Health that reducing unnecessary cesarean sections would require complex and comprehensive measures, including a massive reeducation of maternity care practitioners. This was our motivation for the organization of the series of nationwide seminars on Humanized Obstetric and Neonatal Care Based on Scientific Evidence that are the subject of this chapter.

CHANGING CHILDBIRTH: THE SEMINARS

On March 8, 2004, during the commemoration of Women's International Day, the Brazilian government accepted a great challenge: the institution of the National Pact for the Reduction of Maternal and Neonatal Mortalities by all levels of government—federal, state, and municipal—and civil society. Representatives were present from state and municipal levels of government, popular movements, women activist groups, and scientific and professional associations. The pact defined strategic actions to improve the quality of care for women, adolescents, and children, and placed the effort to reduce maternal and neonatal mortalities on the state agenda because the majority of these deaths are avoidable.[4] The goal of the pact was to reduce both types of mortality by 15% by the end of 2006 and to reduce them to internationally acceptable levels in the next two decades, because it is assumed that avoidable deaths are a violation of women's and children's human right to survival.

During the past decades in which childbirth became more and more medicalized, a number of "culture heroes" of the movement to humanize birth began specific efforts in their areas to create better birth models. These pioneers include obstetrician Moysés Paciornik, who studied childbirth among the Kaingang tribes of Paraná state and is well-known for his early film *Birth in the Squatting Position* (produced in Curitiba and launched in 1979); his son Cláudio, who continues his work; and obstetrician Hugo Sabatino, a professor of obstetrics who started the Group of Alternative Practices in the State University of Campinas, state of São Paulo, introducing in the academy the possibility of learning and practicing in a humanistic way. In October 1993, Dr. Sabatino invited a group of professionals dissatisfied with the current status quo for a three-day meeting, during which the Brazilian Network for the Humanization of Childbirth— ReHuNa (Rede pela Humanização do Parto e Nascimento)—was born.

Central among these pioneers was Dr. Galba de Araújo, chief of obstetrics and gynecology at the Maternidade Escola Assis Chateaubriand Hospital in Fortaleza, the primary regional hospital for the state of Ceará in the Northeast region of Brazil. Dr. Araújo took his responsibility to the rural women of the state seriously, most of whom were attended by traditional midwives. Visits to rural towns and many conversations with traditional midwives taught him that their major needs were clean places for women to give birth (most rural houses had dirt floors) and transport to the hospital when necessary. He oversaw the creation of small birth centers in a number of these towns, made sure they were stocked with medical supplies, and accepted the midwives' hanging of hammocks in these buildings next to the beds. And he created a communication and transport system that made ready hospital access a reality. When he revisited these centers from time to time, he saw that the medical supplies remained unopened, but the records the midwives kept showed very good outcomes. He began to pay attention to the ways in which these rural women gave birth, and eventually placed hammocks and an upright birthing chair in his own hospital. His was a model that worked, but it was dismantled after his death by obstetricians who did not share his open-minded attitudes and humanistic approach. He remains an inspiration today, and in 1999, his name was attached to a government award—the Galba de Araújo Award for Humanized Care in Childbirth, with one such award for each of Brazil's five regions.

In 2001 the Ministry of Health started a process of offering health professionals the possibility of becoming updated in humanized childbirth at the Center of Humanized Therapeutic Practices, in Ceres, in the state of Goiás. This center was one of the pioneers in the movement for the humanization of childbirth—its leaders were Lívia Martins Carneiro and Esther de Albuquerque Vilela. Their center was the first to receive the Galba de Araújo award for the Central-West. Since then, the center has become a reference point for humanized childbirth care for the Ministry of Health. This center began to offer a course dealing with the need to develop relational capabilities that would favor the physiological evolution of childbirth, giving emphasis to the quality of the therapeutic relationship. In addition, it intended to stimulate the practices of normal childbirth and breastfeeding and the adoption of humanized and noninvasive practices, respecting women's autonomy. But given the size of the country, this initiative had little impact because each course admitted only twenty to thirty professionals. To have a real impact on the maternal and neonatal mortality rates, it became necessary to plan the needed change in broader terms.

In 2004 the coordinators of the Women's Health Technical Area of the Ministry of Health proposed to create the series of seminars on Humanized Obstetric and Neonatal Care Based on Scientific Evidence that this chapter describes. The Technical Area asked the Health Secretariats of the states to indicate a hospital in each state attending more than 1,000 deliveries per year, including high-risk births, that was interested in improving the quality of care, committed to make the needed changes, willing to support other maternity services, and willing to include academic activities; this hospital would become the central focus for its state. Adopting the premise that those in positions of authority should be the first to become sensitized to humanized care, we invited to the seminars the directors of the maternities, as well as the heads of the obstetric wards, the neonatal wards, and the obstetric nurses from each of these hospitals.

For the seminar project, we sought the partnership of CLAP (the Latin American Center of Perinatology) linked to PAHO/WHO (the Pan American Health Organization/World Health Organization), DFID (U.K. Department for International Development), Febrasgo (the Brazilian Federation of Societies of Gynecology and Obstetrics), SBP (the Brazilian Association of Pediatrics), and Abenfo (the Brazilian Association of Midwives and Obstetric Nurses). We also sought partnership with places in which humanized care was already offered, such as the Center for the Humanization of Therapeutic Practices of Ceres-Goiás, the Sofia Feldman Hospital in Belo Horizonte–Minas Gerais, the Maternity School of Vila Nova Cachoeirinha, and the Santa Marcelina Hospital of Itaim Paulista, both in São Paulo.

The first two seminars took place in October and November 2004, with half of the state teams in São Paulo and the other half in Belo Horizonte. These cities were chosen for their geographic convenience and availability of air flights, and because they had model childbirth care services that were already humanistic. The seminar curriculum included presentations followed by debates about Ministry of Health policies; ethical and philosophical foundations of care; obstetric and neonatal practices based on scientific evidence; critical appraisal of type of birth care (vaginal or cesarean section); childbirth care in the different stages; puerperal care; care for the three main causes of maternal mortality: eclampsia, hemorrhage, and infection; prevention of the vertical transmission of HIV, hepatitis, and syphilis; care for the normal and the high-risk newborn; humanized care for women in situations of abortion and post-abortion; maternal-fetal iso-immunization; and care for adolescent pregnancies (see the sample seminar program schedule in Appendix 14.1). In this comprehensive way, we sought to incorporate the value of humanistic practice as a seamless way to support the pact goals of lowering mortality and improving overall health, showing that these approaches are inseparable because humanistic care is basic to preventing complications and emergencies. During those forty hours (over five days) of the seminar, the teams visited a model hospital and had to write a report or proposal developing two main objectives: (1) how they would reproduce these newly learned practices in their hospitals, and (2) and how they would reproduce the seminar in their states.

We found it amazing to witness the transformation that occurred in those five days. During the first two days, participants' resistance to the contents was visible. Some would sit at the back of the room, trying not to listen to the presentations. Credit must be given to the way Veronica Batista Gonçalves Reis, coordinator of this project at that time, handled the coordination of the whole process. Slowly, their resistance melted and turned into appreciation, and sometimes even enthusiastic adherence to the concepts being introduced. We were glad to receive a phone call, just one month after the first seminar, from Dr. Mário Gama Lima Júnior, director of the Maternity Carmela Dutra from Rio de Janeiro, reporting all the modifications they had already introduced in their hospital, such as all women having a chosen companion during labor and delivery, and changes to guarantee more privacy for women. He said that he knew more could be done in a longer time frame—this was only the beginning.

A few more months went by while we acquired the necessary funds to reproduce these seminars all over the country. A small amount was donated by DFID, but the majority of the resources came from the annual budget of the Ministry of Health. Also, it took a few months to organize the bureaucracy to administer such a portentous initiative: the goal was to involve at least 420 major maternity services and include every state in the country. The resources were transferred to the Institute Fernandes Figueira, a foundation of the National School of Public Health, in Rio de Janeiro, functionally linked to the Ministry of Health but autonomous. The Institute would offer courses all over the country and manage the administrative side of the seminars; the technical issues would be handled by the Ministry of Health's team.

Beginning in August 2005, twenty-eight more seminars took place, starting with Alagoas and the Federal District. During the state seminars, the Ministry of Health and state teams organized meetings with the state and capital Health Secretariats, the directors of the maternities whose teams were participating in the seminars, and local representatives of organizations such as Febrasgo, Abenfo, the feminist movement, ReHuNa, scientific associations, federal universities, and others, in order to establish how the advances in the shift of model of care would be monitored. At the end of each seminar, just as in the first two seminars, the maternity team would present its project publicly and receive some materials such as the book *A Guide to Effective Care in Pregnancy and Childbirth* by Enkin et al.; an institutional video on humanized care in the health care system beginning in the prenatal period, produced by the team of Ceres-GO and called *A Day of Life;* and copies of all the curricula and training materials from that seminar, so they could reproduce them in their regional seminars.

We hired some of the national pioneers in humanized childbirth care as Ministry of Health consultants in order to spread the concepts, the philosophy, and the practices of humanization: Anibal Faúndes, Edilsa Pinheiro Araújo, Esther Albuquerque Vilela, João Batista Marinho C. Lima, Lena Peres, Lívia Martins Carneiro, Marcos Augusto Bastos Dias, Marcos Leite dos Santos, Marcos Roberto Ymayo, Marilanda Lima, and Rivaldo Albuquerque Mendes. Each became responsible for the follow-up and support of the process in a few states. Their task was to become familiar with the state and the source-maternity teams and their projects, and to help them organize the seminars, implement new practices, overcome difficulties, and evaluate their processes. In addition, they served as instructors in nationwide seminars.

Bahia state had two seminars. Because its Health Secretariat was willing to speed up the process, they carried out the first one with their own funds in December 2005. The second one, one supported by federal funds, took place in July 2006 when the director of Itabuna hospital had the opportunity to present the results hospital staff had achieved in that short period.

In December 2005, during the Second International Conference on the Humanization of Childbirth in Rio de Janeiro, organized by ReHuNa, a meeting was held with all those involved in the first two seminars, where they presented some results of the first year. This meeting was also an opportunity for these medical professionals to participate in the larger conference and thus realize that there was much more involved in humanizing birth care than the evidence-based practices being fostered by the Ministry of Health: the humanization of birth is an international social movement with a strong foundation of caring individuals all over the world. Interestingly, instead of the traditional ceremonial table, the stage was arranged as a theatrical set: the organizers had brought furniture from their homes, and Bia Lessa, a well-known artist and sister of Heloísa Lessa, nurse-midwife and national coordinator of ReHuNa at that time, had displayed it in such a way that the stage looked like a cozy home, with a living room on the left side of the stage and a kitchen on the right. The purpose of this artistry was to express some of the core values behind the movement for the humanization of birth—family, friendly atmospheres, and relationship. The artists hoped that the conference participants would seek to incorporate these values into maternity care in their institutions.

This expressive decoration was continued at one of the first seminars of 2006 held in Natal—and what a surprise it was to participate in such a cozy environment! Although the seminar was held in the convention center of a hotel, the organizers had borrowed all they needed from the local furniture stores to match what they had witnessed as a new approach to seminars for humanized care. In the kitchen, located stage left, they had hung an image of the local patron saint with a ribbon tied around it the way people of the region do in their houses: this is their usual way to give thanks for a mercy received.

This project is considered a great success: by December 2006 this initiative had involved 457 maternities and 1,857 professionals in thirty national seminars, so we exceeded by almost 10% the 420 maternity hospitals that had been our original goal. Additional regional or municipal seminars were held in six states, involving around 100 or more institutions and around 800 professionals. Of course, we are aware that not all services are equally receptive, and that each state, or each service, will have its own process of change, at its own speed. However, the process is on the move, involving people all over the country.

Further developments include the necessary reforms the maternities will have to undergo in order to organize their infrastructure to offer humanized and evidence-based care. For instance, during the seminars, the teams from each hospital wrote descriptions of the changes they planned to implement. After their return, they had to adapt these proposals to the format required by the Ministry of Health in order to apply for funding. In other words, they could not "drop the ball"—they had to continue to work with what they had learned. The Ministry of Health reserved some funds for these reform projects and, at year's end 2006, twenty-seven maternity hospitals from seven states had applied: Amazonas (1 hospital), Ceará (1), Mato Grosso (1), Minas Gerais (2), Piauí (11), Rio de Janeiro (9), and Roraima (2). In the evaluation meeting held in December 2006, one of the proposals for future developments was to create a reference center on humanized care in each state that would offer ongoing practical training to professionals. By June 2007, an evaluation form had been developed and sent to all hospitals involved in the seminars in order to monitor the changes; we are presently receiving the last completed forms. Also, we are discussing the continuity of the process: not only how to continue with regional seminars until all the 4,055 hospitals are covered (or at least all the 590 major ones that attend more than 1,000 deliveries a year), but also how to continue updating professionals on humanized care. Because evidence-based practices have already been presented, we are planning some workshops on interpersonal relationships for 2009. This focus is much needed because laboring women are often disrespected. In addition, we plan a meeting with the Ministry of Education in order to discuss the contents of the obstetrics curricula in the medical and nursing undergraduate courses. Practices taught in these courses should be evidence-based.

WORKING WITH TRADITIONAL MIDWIVES

SCENARIO 2: BREVES

On a late afternoon in July 2006, a group of traditional midwives and their instructors (from the Health Ministry and the NGO Grupo Curumim, and a visiting Canadian midwife) traveled by two boats from the town of Breves to the town of Bagre, both located in the island of Marajó in the state of Pará, Amazon region, to participate in a four-day training for traditional midwives. The course was jointly organized by the Ministry of Health, the Health Secretariat of the state of Pará, several regional health municipalities, and the NGO Curumim Pregnancy and Childbirth, which has a great deal of experience in training traditional midwives. At a certain moment of this trip on this torrential and majestic Parauahu River, a tributary of the Amazon River, one of the boats failed and all its travelers were transferred to the other. So there they were: overcrowded, not enough lifesavers, during twilight, and without floodlights to show and lead their way; they could count only on the intense luminosity of the full moon. However difficult the conditions, they arrived at their destination. This scenario of insecurity and lack of infrastructure is part of daily life for the inhabitants of the Northern region.

The Amazon region has the greatest hydrographic basin of the planet and is the major Brazilian region in extension (5,217,423 square kilometers). Given its low population (21 million), it displays the lowest demographic density of the country: 4 inhabitants per square kilometer. Its large distances, its pattern of irregular population concentration, and the scarcity of means of travel and communication result in difficult access to goods and public services. Data on the indigenous people available from the National Foundation for the Indians (Funai) refer to a population of about 411,000 people, some living in reservations and others on the periphery of towns. They belong to about 220 ethnic groups and speak 180 languages. They have a precarious livelihood and little access to health services. These indigenous peoples are often exploited, considered subcitizens, pillaged, and not allowed to live according to their beliefs and traditions. Currently, they claim their right to self-determination and to live in their ancestral lands. In most of these communities, the midwife plays an important role. For population survival and preservation, it is fundamental to maintain and value midwifery traditions.

Among the Kalunga, one of the 2,000 Quilombola communities spread throughout Brazil, about 50% of all births are attended by traditional midwives. The Kalunga people live in an area of 230,000 hectares,[5] 330 kilometers[6] away from Brasilia, the capital of Brazil. Their community is distant and difficult to reach: one will not get to some villages by car—the alternatives are walking, going by boat, or riding a horse or a donkey. In these communities, the traditional midwives have a valued presence. The Quilombolas belong to a population segment of greatest social vulnerability and high degree of exclusion from goods and services. Traditional midwives are also important caregivers in the Northeast, mostly in the small villages, and also in the semidesert areas.

The program Working with Traditional Midwives was developed by taking into account the socioeconomic, cultural, and geographic diversity of the country, as well as the need to develop public policies that would correspond to the specificities of the rural, riverside, forest, desert, and other difficult-to-reach regions, in addition to the characteristics of the Indian and Quilombola population. It was launched in the year 2000 and has counted since then on the expertise of Grupo Curumim, an NGO that has created many teaching materials and a special didactic and experiential methodology for teaching traditional midwives. Other partners are the Institute for Sustainable Development Mamirauá/the state of Amazonas; the Center for the Humanization of Therapeutic Practices of the Hospital São Pio X; Ceres, Goiás; and others, as well as some state and municipal health secretariats.

By December 2006, 1,396 traditional midwives and 852 health professionals had been trained. The methodology adopted is participative, derived from Paulo Freire's[7] "pedagogy of problematization," (1996) in which the knowledge and experience of the participants is valued. The attitude of the instructors is important. They must take into account the traditional midwives' own knowledge and experience, and generate interaction between the empirical and intuitive wisdom the midwives' bring with the technical and scientific knowledge offered in the course. During the course, both participants and instructors also increase their understanding of themselves as individuals and as a group, of reality, and of their potential in a co-constructive process. This participative methodology makes use of different materials: the traditional midwives are encouraged to draw maps of their communities showing ways to get around, to use clay to model the female reproductive system, and to use the *Book of the Midwife* (*Livro da Parteira*, Grupo Curumim 2006), which contains pictures and drawings helpful to those with limited or no literacy. The topics addressed in this book include the female body; prenatal care; the exams that the midwife can and should perform; labor and positions for delivery; care for the newborn; materials and procedures for a clean childbirth; problems during pregnancy, childbirth, postpartum, and with the baby; what to do and how to refer women in case of problems; breastfeeding; and information on the use of medicinal herbs.

In the meetings, these traditional midwives tell their life stories and their experiences, and describe the hardships of working as a midwife outside the formal health care system—and they talk proudly of their trade. They speak of the nights without sleep, of their fright when a friend comes from far away to fetch them so they can help a woman in childbirth in a distant dwelling. They talk about the immense joy when all comes out well and the crises are over, and mothers and babies emerge healthy and full of strength. In spite of their devaluation by health care professionals and others, these traditional midwives are acknowledged and respected in the communities where they live and work, and they are often identified as leaders. As such, they become focal points for women's and children's health issues. In most settings, their work is not articulated with the formal health care system, and they have to work in isolation among precarious conditions. Their therapeutic resources include prayers and use of medicinal plants, massages, rituals, and magic spells. Most of their birth practices are noninvasive and educational, marked by emotional support and encouragement for the woman (and for her family members), and are culturally appropriate—in accordance with the beliefs, customs, and values of the woman receiving care. These midwives envelop the childbearing woman in a circle of support and transmit to her strength and security. Hegemonic views of such midwives delegitimate their traditional knowledge and associate them with ignorance, backwardness, and lack of hygiene. Thus, we find it both ironic and encouraging that, in fact, many of their practices encompass what scientific evidence now shows to be essential aspects of care: emotional support and respect for the woman, facilitating the physiology of the birth process through the use of upright positions, and encouraging bonding and breastfeeding. The purpose of "training" them includes bringing them up to date with evidence-based practice and reinforcing those customary practices that are already evidence-based.

The program Working with Traditional Midwives of the Brazilian Ministry of Health does not assume that the work of the traditional midwives is "alternative care for poor people." On the contrary, the developers of this program understand that home births attended by traditional midwives are safe and humanized options for care and need not to be eliminated but rather supported through channels of referral, transport, and ongoing education. Thus, part of our effort is to encourage the State and the medical profession to provide the necessary support by acknowledging and valuing the traditional midwives' work, improving their material and logistical conditions, and offering continuous education involving an exchange of knowledge between them and health care professionals.

It is fundamental that the work of traditional midwives be linked to the formal health care system. What happens when there is such integration is very interesting. For instance, just before the beginning of this project, Maués, a town in the state of Amazonas, had one of the highest neonatal mortality rates of the country. Change started immediately after the seminar conducted in the state. One of the consultants from the Ministry of Health, Marcos Leite dos Santos, had been advising the Health Secretariat of the municipality of Maués on the organization of a local maternity care system. This process had integrated urban traditional midwives into the system, and the local community health care agents had already identified almost sixty-five rural traditional midwives, defining clear references for risky cases. The results were outstanding: less than a year later, Maués displayed the very low neonatal mortality rate of 1.4/1,000. Next will come the Curumim training of these rural midwives and their own integration into the healthcare system, which is expected to produce further reductions, especially in maternal mortality. Recovery and preservation of traditional midwifery knowledge in interaction with technical-scientific knowledge is essential: this process contributes to the production of new knowledge and technology and greatly improved outcomes.

FINAL COMMENTS

For the proponents of the initiatives we have described in this chapter, it is evident that the determinants of avoidable maternal and neonatal mortality are complex and, as such, need complex interventions in order to effectively alter the current status. The main problem is the hegemonic technocratic model of care, and it will take time to reorient the paradigm: the last school of professional, direct-entry midwifery in Brazil was closed in 1972, and it was only in 2004 that a new one was opened at the University of São Paulo in response to growing awareness of the importance of autonomous professional midwifery. Midwifery culture has to be reinforced. Meanwhile, the Ministry of Health has funded courses for nurses in obstetrics in all states in order to enhance the multiprofessional approach to childbirth care. We have also funded courses for training doulas, under the leadership of Sofia Feldman Hospital's team, and have supported the construction and equipment of a number of birth centers. Seven of them are showing that a truly humanistic model of care is possible, but some others have been medically co-opted—always a danger when the technocratic model prevails. One of them, the freestanding birth center linked to the Federal University of Juiz de Fora, suspended care for childbirth in August 2007 by a determination of the university dean, and now offers only prenatal care and reproductive planning counseling. The Brazilian movement for humanization of childbirth, as well as other supporters, is pressing the university and the federal government. However, the university is linked to the Ministry of Education, has autonomous standing, and has shown little sensitivity to public opinion. The Ministry of Health was invited to mediate this conflict, and the birth center was expected to resume its activities by May 2008. Yet it did not happen, and in spite of the Ministry of Health's frequent statements in favor of reopening, in August 2008 the dean determined the definitive closure of that birth center.

Public policies to change childbirth in Brazil have to consider two lines of action: the one that promotes healthy and humanized childbirth care and the other that actively discourages unnecessary interventions, such as cesarean sections. Even though the official move is toward humanization, the inertia in the current status quo is demonstrated by the ascending curve of cesarean sections shown in Figure 14.1. Previous efforts to change the trend have had little impact; it is too early to tell how much impact our ongoing programs will have.

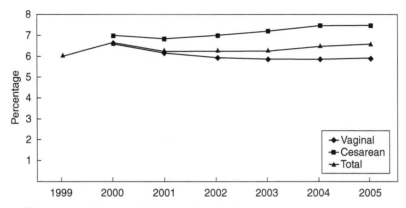

Figure 14.2. Preterm births associated with cesareans.

The WHO Latin America study by Villar et al. (2006) has shown how unnecessary cesareans affect maternal and perinatal mortality. WHO researchers studied 120 health institutions in eight Latin American countries, obtaining information on 97,095 deliveries out of 106,546 (91% coverage). They assessed maternal morbidity in relation to mostly severe conditions (blood transfusion and hysterectomy as severe hemorrhage, maternal admission to intensive care unit, maternal death, and maternal hospital stay for longer than seven days), constructing a summary "severe maternal morbidity and mortality index." For perinatal outcomes potentially affected by cesarean delivery, they investigated intrapartum fetal death, preterm delivery (up to thirty-seven weeks), admission to a neonatal intensive care unit for seven days or longer, and neonatal death before hospital discharge. Overall, the median cesarean rate was 33%; 49% were "elective" (planned in advance), 46% were intrapartum, and 5% were emergency without labor. *Both in the crude and in the adjusted analyses, an increase in the rate of cesarean delivery was associated with a significantly higher risk for severe maternal morbidity and mortality and postnatal treatment with antibiotics.* These findings also applied to perinatal outcomes: after adjustment for the case-mix of the populations served, the rate of cesarean delivery was positively associated with an increase in the rates of fetal death, number of infants admitted to the neonatal intensive care unit for seven days and more, and was borderline significant for neonatal death after adjusting for preterm delivery. Risk of preterm delivery and neonatal death rise when cesarean delivery rates rise outside the range of 10%–20% (in general, no hospital should have a rate higher than 15%, but in some regions with very high risk populations, slightly higher rates may be appropriate).

In Table 14.1, we see that those regions with higher cesarean rates also displayed higher proportions of low birth weight. In Figure 14.2 we see that the results of the study cited above are reflected in our own data: the ascending curve of preterm births in conjunction with cesareans gives reason for great concern. The Ministry of Health considers Brazil's high cesarean rates a serious public health problem, and on May 30, 2006, launched a campaign to reduce unnecessary cesareans; a new media campaign, in conjunction with the Supplementary Sector National Agency (which regulates HMOs), was launched in May 2008. Together with the seminars that promote healthy and humanized childbirth care, these campaigns may help sensitize public opinion in order to achieve the goal of changing childbirth.

Although many obstetricians initially resist this sort of change, there is a movement among them to become open to this new knowledge and what is being proposed. Some local sections of Febrasgo have organized meetings about humanized childbirth, inviting Ministry of Health consultants to speak to local obstetricians, who have listened with interest to this (for them) new approach. Such meetings have taken place so far in the states of Bahia, Rio Grande do Sul, and Santa Catarina—it is hoped these meetings will spread. Also, a series of large international conferences on the humanization of childbirth sponsored by ReHuNa, usually attended by more than 2,000 participants, and lectures around Brazil by international childbirth experts, including the lead editor of this volume, Robbie Davis-Floyd, that are well attended by obstetricians have helped redirect beliefs and attitudes. It is hoped this ongoing dissemination of knowledge will assist in altering obstetric practices.

This public sector movement also influences the private providers: in market economics, they have to compete by offering better services; as humanized care gains more space in the news, mother and baby magazines, and other media, private providers have to match that offering. Recently a few private hospitals of the interior of São Paulo introduced the use of tubs in labor. Also, some of the HMOs are beginning a campaign among their clients to influence their choices in the direction of normal birth. This interesting development is a result of many factors. First, the social movement for the humanization of birth has managed to get the media to pay attention to Brazil's shameful cesarean rates and non-humanistic childbirth care. Also, the supplementary sector, in which cesarean rates are about 80%, is coordinated by the Agencia Nacional de Saude Suplementar (ANS). The ANS is an agency of the Brazilian Ministry of Health, addressing public policy in the private sector and handling public health concerns; it has chosen the reduction of unnecessary cesareans as one of its priorities and is working with us to developing its strategy. In 2006 an NGO made up of health care consumers called Parto do Principio (a pun: *parto* means both "birth" and "I'm beginning from," and *principio* means both "beginning" and "principle") began working through the Public

Ministry—an agency of the judiciary that defends the rights of citizens—to challenge both the public and supplementary sectors to reduce unnecessary cesareans.

One of the results is that in May 2008, the ANS and the Department of Programmatic and Strategic Actions of the Ministry of Health launched a new campaign for normal birth, where a well-known model who gave birth vaginally to twins explains what it represented to her; besides, ANS has committed publicly to the reduction of its cesarean section rate from the current 80% to at most 60% by 2011—the Ministry of Health has defined that in the public sector, the current 30% rate will have to be reduced to 25% in the same period. And the international movement for the humanization of birth is a good partner—for example, one of its leaders, Michel Odent, gave a very convincing talk to the ANS on October 10, 2006, and the comments among the "cesareanist" physicians who attended indicated strong signs of change in their mentality. Also, the Ministry of Health negotiated an invitation for Odent to the Brazilian Congress of Gynecology and Obstetrics, held in Fortaleza in November 2007—a feat accomplished by the current Women's Health coordinator (until that point, the humanization of childbirth had not been a welcome subject in such meetings). Public awareness of the damage done by unnecessary intervention in birth in Brazil is definitely on the rise.

Maternal and neonatal mortality are problems that pertain to the whole society and so demand collective answers. The Pact for the Reduction of Maternal and Neonatal Mortality involves all levels of the government, as well as different organizations of civil society (see Appendices 14.2 and 14.3 for current lists of the professionals involved in the seminars and the main organizations committed to these goals). This movement to improve quality of care has "infiltrated" the whole healthcare system and has entered official government agendas: nowadays, all municipalities have to include in their annual plans what actions they will adopt to reduce the number of maternal and neonatal deaths.

The World Health Organization considers the Brazilian Pact for the Reduction of Maternal and Neonatal Mortality a model of social mobilization and articulation of government and civil society for the promotion of the Millennium Development Goals, as stated at the first UN conference on the subject (December 2004) and the third international roundtable promoted by the UN to discuss these goals. In addition, on December 11, 2006, the United Nations awarded the Pact for the Reduction of Maternal and Neonatal Mortality the prize for International Highlight in Social Mobilization and Dialogue to Promote the Millennium Development Goals. We may say it is a good start.

APPENDIX 14.1. PROGRAM OF THE SEMINARS: OUTLINE

Schedule		*Title of the Talk*	*Responsibility*
Day 1	Morning	1. Ministry of Health Guidelines for Obstetric and Neonatal Care	Ministry of Health Team
		2. Diagnostics of maternal health in the country and the Pact for the Reduction of Maternal and Neonatal Deaths[a]	
		3. Investigation of maternal and neonatal deaths	
	Afternoon	1. Ethical and philosophical foundations for the humanization of childbirth care	National Instructors
		2. Good practices: basis for scientifically based obstetric care	
Day 2	Morning	1. Critical appraisal of type of birth: vaginal or cesarean	National Instructors
		2. Care during labor (multiprofessional team, care by doctor and nurse, dealing with pain)	
	Afternoon	1. Care during the second stage	National Instructors
		2. Care during the third and fourth stages and the immediate puerperal period	
		3. Psychosocial support to women in the puerperal period	

[a]Occasionally, when a state has an organized follow-up of maternal and infant/perinatal deaths, it is presented by a Local Instructor.

APPENDIX 14.1 *(continued)*

Schedule		Title of the Talk	Responsibility
Day 3	Morning	1. Care for the normal newborn 2. Care for pathologies of the newborn	Local Instructors
	Afternoon	Visit to a maternity service	
Day 4	Morning	1. Hypertension in pregnancy and eclampsia 2. Hemorrhage in pregnancy and labor 3. Infections in gestation, in labor, and in the puerperal period 4. Discussion of clinical cases	1, 2, 3. Local Instructors 4. National Instructors
	Afternoon	1. Sickle cell anemia in gestation 2. Control of vertical transmission (HIV, hepatitis B, syphilis) and care to carriers during gestation 3. Strategies to humanize and improve the quality of care; preparation of the project	1. Ministry of Health Team or Local Istructors 2. Local Instructor 3. Ministry of Health and Health Secretariat of the State
Day 5	Morning	1. Maternal-fetal iso-immunization 2. Pregnancy in adolescents 3. Humanized care to unsafe abortion 4. Preparation of the project Instructors	1. Local Instructors 2. National or Local Instructors 3. Ministry of Health Team or National
	Afternoon	1. Presentation of the projects 2. Evaluation	Participants

APPENDIX 14.2. OFFICIAL PARTICIPANTS IN THE EFFORTS TO
REDUCE MATERNAL AND NEONATAL MORTALITY

Minister of Health

Humberto Costa (2003–05)/José Saraiva Felipe (2005–06)/Agenor
Álvares (2006–07)/José Gomes Temporão (2007–)

Secretary of Health Care

Jorge Solla (2003–05)/José Gomes Temporão (2005–07)/José Carvalho
de Noronha (2007–)

Director of the Department of Programmatic and Strategic Actions

Tereza de Jesus Campos Neta (2003–05)/Cristina Boaretto and Katia
Ratto (2005–07)/Adson Roberto França Santos (2007–)

Coordinator of the Women's Health Program

Maria José de Oliveira Araújo (2003–2007)/Regina Coeli Viola (2007–)

Coordinator of the Children's Health Program

Aléxia Luciana Ferreira (2003–05)/Ana Cecília Lins Sucupira (2005–
07)/Elsa Regina Justo Giugliani (2007–)

Coordinator of the Health of Adolescents and Youth Program

Thereza De Lamare Franco Netto (2003–)

Ministry of Health Technical Team Working on the Seminars Project

Ana Margareth Gomes Leite/Daphne Rattner/Isa Paula Hamouche
Abreu/Márcia CavalcanteVinhas Lucas/Regina Coeli Viola/Rurany
Ester Silva/Verônica Batista Gonçalves Reis/Tereza Passarella

Instructors for the 2004 Seminars[a]

Adson França/Ana Lúcia Ferraz Almstaden/Anatália Lopes Basile/Aléxia
Ferreira/Carlos Eduardo Correa/Cristião Rosas/Daphne Rattner/

NOTE: The list will always be incomplete, since there are partners contributing
to this effort all over the country. So far, almost 300 events have been held since
the pact was launched March 8, 2004. Twenty-five out of twenty-six states and the
Federal district have adhered to the pact.

[a]After the two seminars in 2004, twenty-eight other national seminars were held,
with both national and local instructors. For the sake of economy, we acknowledge
only the participants in the initial effort.

Eduardo Baiochi/Eduardo Campos/Ester Albuquerque Vilela/
Fernando Althabe (CLAP-PAHO-WHO)/Fernando Barros
(CLAP-PAHO-WHO)/Isa Paula Hamouche Abreu/ Ivo Lopes/Julio
Javier Spindola (PAHO)/João Alécio Juliano Perfeito/João Batista
Marinho Lima/José Carlos Reichelman/José Orleans/ Marcos Leite
dos Santos/Marcos Roberto Ymayo/Maria José de Oliveira Araújo/
Mirian Rego Leão/Nadia Zanon/ Osmar Ribeiro Colas/Regina
Coeli Viola/Tereza Campos Neta/Tereza Passarella/Verônica Batista
Gonçalves Reis/Vilma Nishi

External Counselors for the Seminars Project

Anibal Faúndes/Edilsa Pinheiro Araújo/Esther Albuquerque Vilela/João
Batista Marinho C. Lima/Lena Peres/Lívia Martins Carneiro/
Marcos Augusto Bastos Dias/Marcos Leite dos Santos/ Marcos
Roberto Ymayo/Marilanda Lima/Rivaldo Albuquerque Mendes

Partners in the Organization of the 2004 Seminars

CLAP (Latin American Center of Perinatology linked to PAHO/WHO)
DFID (U.K. Department for International Development)
Febrasgo (Brazilian Federation of Societies of Gynecology and Obstetrics)
SBP (Brazilian Association of Pediatrics)
Abenfo (Brazilian Association of Midwives and Obstetric Nurses)
Center for the Humanization of Therapeutic Practices of Ceres-Goiás
Sofia Feldman Hospital
Maternity School of Vila Nova Cachoeirinha
Santa Marcelina Hospital of Itaim Paulista

NGO Partner Working with Traditional Midwives

Curumim Gestação e Parto

APPENDIX 14.3. PARTNERS IN THE PACT FOR THE REDUCTION
OF MATERNAL AND NEONATAL MORTALITY

National Coordinator

Adson Roberto França Santos

Inside the Ministry of Health

Secretariat of Health Care (SAS): Children's Health Technical Area, Women's
Health Technical Area and Adolescent and Youth Health Technical Area
Secretariat of Health Surveillance (SVS)
Secretariat of Strategic and Participant Management (SEGEP)

Secretariat of Management of Work and Health Education (SGTES)
Department of Indigenous Health of the Foundation of Indigenous
    Health (FUNASA)
National Agency for the Supplementary Health Sector (ANS)
National Policy for the Humanization of Health Services (PNH)

Other Ministries

Special Secretariat of Policies for Women (SEPM)
Special Secretariat of Policies for the Promotion of Race Equality
    (SEPPIR)
Special Secretariat of Human Rights (SEDH)
Councils

National Council of State Health Secretaries (CONASS)

National Council of Municipal Health Secretaries (CONASEMS)
National Council of the Rights of Adolescents and Youth (CONANDA)
Federal Council of Medicine (CFM)

Professional Associations

Brazilian Medical Association (AMB)
Brazilian Federation of the Associations of Gynecology and Obstetrics
    (Febrasgo)
Brazilian Society of Pediatrics (SBP)
Brazilian Association of Nursing (ABEN)
Brazilian Association of Obstetric Nurses (Abenfo)
National Federation of Physicians (FENAM)

Representatives of Social Organizations

Brazilian Feminist Network of Health, and Sexual and Reproductive
    Rights (RedeSaude)
Brazilian Articulation of Women (AMB)
Confederation of Women of Brazil
Articulation of the Organizations of Brazilian Black Women
Brazilian Network for the Humanization of Childbirth
    (ReHuNa)
National Network of Traditional Midwives (RNPT)
National Network of Human Milk Banks
Children's Pastoral (linked to the Catholic Church)
Brazilian Association of Graduate Studies in Collective Health
    (ABRASCO)

Invited Members

United Nations Population Fund (UNFPA)
Pan American Health Organization (PAHO)
United Nations Children's Fund (UNICEF)
Cochrane Center of Brazil/ Federal University of São Paulo
    (Cochrane-UNIFESP)
International Baby Food Action Network (IBFAN Brasil)
World Alliance for Breastfeeding Action (WABA Brasil)

ACKNOWLEDGMENTS

The authors wish to thank Monika Von Koss, Heinrich Rattner, Paula Viana, Marcos Leite dos Santos, and volume editors Robbie Davis-Floyd and Betty-Anne Daviss for their careful reading and thoughtful suggestions.

NOTES

1. The use of a partogram is recommended by WHO and the United Nations Population Fund (UNFPA) as part of basic, safe obstetric/midwifery practice in all labors, especially in settings with high maternal mortality. (See *Integrated Management of Pregnancy and Childbirth: Pregnancy, Childbirth, Postpartum and Newborn Care: A Guide for Essential Practice 2006.*) There are two kinds of partograms. The one used primarily in Europe tracks maternal heart rate; blood pressure; length, frequency, and strength of contractions; rupture of membranes; cervical dilation; drugs administered; and the baby's heart rate. The Latin American partogram developed by CLAP also takes into consideration maternal parity and position during labor and thus is more tailored to the individual woman. PAHO/CLAP and the International MotherBaby Childbirth Initiative recommend use of the latter. See http://www. cedip.cl/Guias/Guia2003/capitulo08.swf; R. Schwarcz, A. G. Diaz, and F. Nieto, "Partograma con curvas de alerta: guía para la vigilancia del parto," Salud Perinatal, *Boletín del CLAP-OPS/OMS* 2.8:93–96, 1987; CLAP-OPS-OMS, *Perinatales Techniques,* 1990 [Scientific publication CLAP, Number 1202], Montevideo, Uruguay; Evaluación del trabajo de parto con Curva de alerta. (This endnote is excerpted from the International MotherBaby Childbirth Initiative (www.imbci.org)).

2. Between latitudes 5°11'2" and −33°44'32" and between longitudes −34°47'30" and −73°58'32".

3. There are, though, a few initiatives of reforestation.

4. For 2004, the country's maternal mortality was estimated to be 74.5/100,000 live births and the neonatal mortality was 18.3/1,000 live births. In developed countries the maternal mortality is expected to be fewer than 20/100,000 live births and the total infant mortality rate is under 10/1,000 live births. These indices mean approximately 2,000 maternal deaths and 38,000 infant deaths each year in Brazil. The neonatal period extends from birth to twenty-eight days of life, and maternal mortality includes deaths from pregnancy up to forty-two days after childbirth or abortion.

5. Hectare: in the metric system, a unit of surface, or land, measure equal to 100 ares, or 10,000 square meters; equivalent to 2.471 acres.

6. Or 206 miles.

7. Paulo Freire (1921–97) was an internationally renowned Brazilian pedagogue who proposed that learning is also a political practice: it depends on how knowledge is transmitted—or constructed jointly by teacher and students, the teacher being the facilitator of the process. His most famous books are *Educação como prática de liberdade* [Education as Practice of Freedom], *Pedagogia do Oprimido* [Pedagogy of the Oppressed], *Pedagogia da Esperança* [Pedagogy of Hope], *A importância do ato de ler* [The Importance of Reading], and *Pedagogia da Autonomia* [Pedagogy of Autonomy].

REFERENCES

Araújo, Maria José Oliveira, and Verônica Batista Gonçalves dos Reis (org.) 2005. Anais dos Seminários Nacionais sobre Assistência Obstétrica e Neonatal Humanizada baseada em Evidências Científicas. Brasília: Ministério da Saúde.

Barbosa, Gisele Peixoto, Karen Giffin, Antonia Angulo-Tuesta, Andrea de Souza Gama, Dóra Chor, Eleonora D'Orsi, and Ana Cristina Gonçalves Vaz dos Reis. 2003. "Parto cesárea: quem o deseja? Em quais circunstâncias? [Cesarean Sections: Who Wants Them and under What Circumstances?]" *Cadernos de Saúde Pública* 19:1611–20.

Behague, Dominique P., Cesar G. Victora, and Fernando C. Barros. 2002. "Consumer Demand for Caesarean Sections in Brazil: Informed Decision Making, Patient Choice, or Social Inequality? A Population Based Birth Cohort Study Linking Ethnographic and Epidemiological Methods." *British Medical Journal* 324:942–47.

Dalsgaard, Anne Line. 2000. "Matters of Life and Longing—Female Sterilization in Northern Brazil." Ph.D. dissertation, University of Copenhagen.

Davis-Floyd, Robbie, 2004 (orig. pub. 1992). Birth as an American Rite of Passage, 2nd edition. Berkeley and London: University of California Press.

Faundes, Anibal E., and José Guilherme Cecatti. 1991. "Operação Cesária no Brasil: Incidência, Tendência, Causas, Consequência e Propostas da Ação." *Cadernos de Saúde Pública* 7.2: 150–73.

Freire, Paulo. 1996. *Pedagogia da autonomia: saberes necessários à prática educativa*. São Paulo: Paz e Terra (Coleção Leitura).

Hospital Manoel Novaes. 2006. "Projeto Implantação do conceito de Atenção Obstétrica Humanizada." PowerPoint presentation.

Hotimsky, Sonia N., Daphne Rattner, Sonia Isoyama Venancio, Cláudia Maria Bógus, and Marinês Martins de Miranda. 2002. "O parto como eu vejo . . . ou como o desejo? Expectativas de gestantes, usuárias do SUS, acerca do parto e da assistência obstétrica" [Childbirth As I See It . . . Or As I Wish It Was? Expectations of Pregnant Women Towards Childbirth and Obstetric Care in Public Health Care System]. *Cadernos de Saúde Pública* 18:1303–11.

Ministério da Saúde. 2000. Grupo Curumim, Gestação e Parto (ONG). *Trabalhando com Parteiras Tradicionais*. 2 ed. Atual. E. revisada. Brasília: Editora do Ministério da Saúde.

————. 2004a. *Projeto de capacitação em atenção humanizada—2004. Documento de trabalho.* Brasília: Ministério da Saúde (mimeo).

————. 2004b. *Seminários Nacionais sobre atenção obstétrica e neonatal humanizada baseada em evidências científicas. Documento de trabalho.* Brasília: Ministério da Saúde (mimeo).

————. 2005. *Proposta Preliminar para a concretização do Trabalho do Grupo de Consultores (as). Documento de trabalho.* Brasília: Ministério da Saúde (mimeo).

————. 2006a. *Atenção à Saúde da Mulher. Gestão orçamentária e evolução dos principais gastos no período 2003 a 2006.* SUS—BRASIL. Brasília: Ministério da Saúde (mimeo).

————. 2006b. *Estudo da mortalidade de mulheres de 10 a 49 anos, com ênfase na mortalidade materna: relatório final.* Brasília: Editora do Ministério da Saúde.

————. 2006c. Grupo Curumim, Gestação e Parto (ONG). *Livro da Parteira.* Brasília: Ministério da Saúde.

————. 2006d. *Estudo da mortalidade de mulheres de 10 a 49 anos, com ênfase na mortalidade materna: relatório final.* Brasília: Ministério da Saúde.

————. 2007. *Área Técnica de Saúde da Mulher—Relatório de gestão 2003–2006: Política Nacional de Atenção Integral à Saúde da Mulher.* Brasília: Ministério da Saúde.

————. In press. Trabalhando com parteiras tradicionais/Desenvolvimento de tecnologias para assistência ao parto e nascimento domiciliar: A experiência do Ministério da Saúde de 2000–2005. Brasília: Ministério da Saúde.

Peres, Lena. 2006. "Relatório Final dos Seminários de Atenção Obstétrica e Neonatal Baseada em Evidências Científicas—Sem AON." PowerPoint presentation.

Potter, Joseph E., Elza Berquó, Ignez H. O. Perpétuo, Ondina Fachel Leal, Kristine Hopkins, Marta Rovery Souza, and Maria Célia de Carvalho Formiga. 2001. "Unwanted Caesarean Sections among Public and Private Patients in Brazil: Prospective Study." *British Medical Journal* 323:1155–58.

Rattner, Daphne. 2001. "Quality of Care in Childbirth: Seeking a Comprehensive Approach." Doctoral dissertation, University of North Carolina, Chapel Hill.

Villar, José, Eliette Valladares, Daniel Wojdyla, Nelly Zavaleta, Guillermo Carroli, Alejandro Velazco, Archana Shah, Liana Campodónico, Vicente Bataglia, Anibal Faundes, Ana Langer, Alberto Narváez, Allan Donner, Mariana Romero, Sofia Reynoso, Karla Simônia de Pádua, Daniel Giordan, Marius Kublickas, Arnaldo Acosta. 2006. "Caesarean Delivery Rates and Pregnancy Outcomes: The 2005 WHO Global Survey on Maternal and Perinatal Health in Latin America." *Lancet* 367:1819–29.

WHO. 2003. *Integrated Management of Pregnancy and Childbirth. Pregnancy, Childbirth, Postpartum and Newborn Care: A guide for Essential Practice.* Geneva: World Health Organization.

Chapter 15

"Orchestrating Normal"
The Conduct of Midwifery in the United States

Holly Powell Kennedy

Everybody whose life you touch, you have an opportunity to leave something positive or leave something negative... that's why you just have to give, give her something. You know, a "take home"... her parting gift should be more than well, I had good care and... a good baby. You know—something for her head, something for her heart, something for her soul.
Nurse-midwife (Kennedy, Davis, and Erickson-Owens 2006: 89)

INTRODUCTION

The focus of this book is to present what is working well for birth around the world, rather than what is not. The purpose of this chapter is to provide a lens with which to examine the midwifery model of care in the United States through a synthesis of my research program about the work of midwives and studies done by other U.S. colleagues. The model I describe is meant to stimulate reflection, research, and policy changes on the most effective and satisfying ways we can work "with women" during childbirth.

It is essential for the reader of this chapter to understand my background and perspective, because it shapes and colors my research. I am a certified nurse-midwife/researcher who teaches midwives, advanced practice nurses, and doctoral students. In 1978, as a family nurse practitioner intern at the Frontier Nursing Service in the mountains of Kentucky, I stumbled onto the midwifery model of care. I was stunned—it was different from than anything I had seen before in nursing. Because of that pivotal experience, I became a midwife, and just celebrated my twenty-fourth anniversary of working with women and their families. Understanding my history is important because I came to childbirth afraid of it—until I went to midwifery school, I had never seen a birth without bright lights or technology. The environments in which I had observed birth all had the aura of "critical" care. It took years to dispel those fears, and even today, vestigial memories can creep in when I am tired.

Throughout my years of practice, I have worked on local and national levels to support midwifery as a model that should be the standard of care for all women in the United States. During those years, some intensely political, I became increasingly aware that there were profound misconceptions and knowledge gaps among those I was trying to convince. The first was the lack of studies to link the actual work (or processes of care) of midwives with perinatal and women's health outcomes. We knew that midwifery outcomes were excellent compared with medicine (Harvey et al. 1996; MacDorman and Singh, 1998; Oakley et al. 1995), but we had not identified or described the reasons for this very well. The second gap was why midwives were not particularly esteemed or sought after in many communities. To this day I receive comments from people who, upon learning my occupation, say "I didn't think that was legal." These two issues fueled my passion to create a research program dedicated to describing the work of midwives and linking it to outcomes. I think back to my early introduction to midwifery and realize that I did not understand fully what I saw—I just knew there was something special about the interaction between the midwife and each woman. But it was difficult to describe; it seemed almost invisible. That is what this chapter is about—describing the often invisible (and sometimes disparaged) work of midwives as a model of care that represents what all women deserve during the powerful and life-altering time in their lives that is pregnancy and birth.

MIDWIFERY IN THE UNITED STATES

The history of midwifery in the United States is rich, unique, and far too complex to fully describe in this chapter. However, a brief overview of midwifery's past is essential to describe midwives' current work within the culture of birth in the United States. We reflect those roots in our actions, our writings, and our day-to-day work with women giving birth and across their lifespan.

Little is known about the work of indigenous midwives prior to the colonization of North America (Bushnell 1981). Early midwives came to the United States as immigrants or slaves and cared for women from their own communities during the first 250 years of settlement (Rooks 1997). Each future midwife was usually an informal apprentice to a community midwife. The diary of Martha Ballard, a colonial midwife in rural Maine, portrays birth and midwifery as part of everyday life (Ulrich 1990). Her description of her work as a midwife is one of support for the woman and, generally, noninterference in the birth process. Midwifery then, as it is today, was set against the social backdrop of current medical thought, religion, and politics. Gradually, traditional midwifery was almost eliminated because of decreased immigration, acculturation, and medical oppression (Dawley 2003). African American traditional midwives in the South, also called granny midwives, were unregulated until the mid-20th century and were also eventually eliminated (Dougherty 1978; Logan 1989).

Nursing was combined with midwifery early in the 20th century by health care reformers concerned about high infant mortality rates among the poor. This model proved to be highly successful in demonstration projects such as the Frontier Nursing Service (Kentucky) and the Maternity Center Association (New York City). That combination continues today as the most common route to midwifery in the United States (Dawley 2003). The American College of Nurse-Midwives (ACNM) was incorporated in 1955. Currently, over 11,000 midwives have been certified through the American Midwifery Certification Board (AMCB, formerly the ACNM Certification Council)–a number that has doubled in the past ten to twelve years. (ACNM 2006b). Approximately 7.4% of all 2005 births (11.2.% of spontaneous vaginal births) in the United States were attended by certified nurse-midwives (CNMs) or certified midwives (CMs) (Martin et al. 2007). The majority attend births in hospitals (Schuiling, Sipe, and Fullerton 2005). Nurse-midwifery is legal and regulated in all fifty states and Puerto Rico. CNMs and CMs continue to care for vulnerable women in many regions of the country.

Although midwifery experienced a rebirth by joining forces with nursing during the 20th century, that fusion does not represent a complete picture of the profession in the United States. Direct-entry midwives (DEMs), often called lay midwives in the past, do not come into the profession through nursing. In 1982 DEMs combined with some CNMs to establish the Midwives Alliance of North America (MANA), an organization with a goal to represent all midwives, not just those who were nurse-midwives. There are approximately 1,300–2,300 practicing DEMS according to MANA (2005a). DEMs who seek certification do so through the North American Registry of Midwives (NARM). This organization certifies applicants as certified professional midwives (CPMs). Direct-entry midwives are recognized by laws and regulatory statutes in twenty-four states (MANA 2005b). The vast majority of DEMs attend births at homes.

Both the ACNM and MANA are committed to the health and well-being of mothers and their babies. Both believe that midwifery is one way to achieve that goal. Both believe that birth is a normal event that rarely needs medical intervention. A fundamental difference between the two organizations is the route to credentialing as a midwife. MANA and NARM recognize multiple paths to midwifery knowledge, including self-study, apprenticeship, formal schooling, and primary experience in out-of-hospital birth settings (NARM 2004). The AMCB requires candidates for the certification exam to demonstrate satisfactory completion of a program in nurse-midwifery (or in a master's program, satisfactory completion of all basic theoretical and clinical requirements of the nurse-midwifery component) accredited by or with pre-accreditation status from the ACNM Division of Accreditation (ACNM DOA) (AMCB 2005). The ACNM DOA requires graduates to hold at least a baccalaureate degree. Of those midwives certified by the AMCB between 2003 and 2005, 77% held a master's degree (B. Graves, AMCB, July 16, 2006, personal communication), and 4.5% of ACNM members have earned a doctorate (Schuiling, Sipe, and Fullerton 2005). The relationship between ACNM and MANA is reflected in the existence of the "Bridge Club," formed "out of a need for mutual understanding, respect and unity among all midwives . . . whose philosophies vary, but who embrace the concept of building bridges, midwife-to-midwife" (MANA 2005c).

Why is this background important to this chapter? Midwifery practice in the United States is multifaceted, but midwifery services and birth settings are not accessible to all women, because of various barriers, including insurance, financial considerations, legal restrictions, and social constraints (Miller 1997). Midwifery could be seen to reflect the experience of oppressed groups because of the gender of the majority of its members as well as of the women it serves.

ACNM and MANA are working hard to create positive change for midwifery within the existing dominant health care arena—at home, in birth centers, and in the hospital. That being said, the tensions between the midwife groups represent one small part of the challenges of being a midwife in the United States, regardless of type. American midwives practice in a country in which the dominant worldview of birth (held by both medical practitioners and women) is as an event with high potential for pathology; it is deemed "normal" only in retrospect. Davis-Floyd (2004a) refers to this worldview as the "technocratic model of birth." Against this backdrop, midwives must balance their alternative "midwifery model of care," which stems from a very different and minority worldview of birth in the United States. Their challenge is to provide the best clinical care supported by a midwifery philosophy; to do so, they must intricately position themselves within health care settings as respected providers. Both goals shape and influence their daily conduct of the practice of midwifery. This chapter includes data derived from all kinds of midwives in all kinds of birth settings in the United States. Therefore, instead of differentiating between types of midwives, I will use only "midwife." The birth model I present, based on research, is a reflection of what I believe the majority of midwives in the United States strive for within the challenges of their specific practice settings and communities.

A MODEL OF MIDWIFERY CARE:
THE VOICES OF WOMEN AND MIDWIVES

Part of the work I present in this chapter represents research studies, primarily qualitative in design, in which my colleagues and I examined the work of midwives through various lenses, including phenomenology, Delphi, narrative analysis, survey, metasynthesis, and concept analysis. We conducted most of the studies directly with women and midwives, both to explore midwifery practice and to understand what it is like to be a recipient of that care. Again, the samples represent all kinds of midwives and all kinds of birth settings. A number of studies focused on describing exemplary practice (Kennedy 1995; 1999; 2000; Kennedy and MacDonald 2002; Kennedy et al. 2004; Kennedy and Shannon 2004). A qualitative analysis of textual data from a large survey of ACNM midwives about managed care provided a description of real world difficulties in practice today (McCloskey et al. 2002). Finally, two projects synthesized existing qualitative studies to establish the current state of knowledge about the work of midwives in the United States (Kennedy, Rousseau, and Kane Low 2003; Kennedy, Levi, and Kane Low, 2005).

"ORCHESTRATING NORMAL":
CONDUCTING THE WORK OF MIDWIFERY

So what have we learned through all this research? The practice of U.S. midwifery is deeply rooted in a belief in the *normalcy* of pregnancy and birth as a physiologic event that is more likely to be healthy than pathologic. It is this belief in normal that most likely separates the midwife who practices midwifery from the midwife or physician who practices obstetrics. In other words, this is a model of practice philosophically oriented in a belief system rather than in a specific professional discipline. This belief in normal lays the foundation for the work of the midwife within the culture of Western medicine. A presiding focus of midwifery care is the support of normalcy during pregnancy, labor, and birth.

The majority of qualitative studies used interview and/or narrative data in which midwives and women talked about their practice and experiences. The participants often invoked metaphors to describe an environment of caring, and those metaphors had a great deal to do with *place*, with both physical and psychological meanings. Theoretically, these metaphors are closely tied to the medical geography literature. Theorists from this discipline suggest that by understanding, working with, and shaping the environment, a person can be (stay) healthy or heal when needed (Gesler and Kearns 2002). Therefore, the model of birth care presented in this chapter is visualized as a geographical terrain to be navigated (Kennedy et al. 2004). The model involves two major processes of care. The first process of care is developing a relationship between the midwife and the woman—it is foundational and mutual. The second process of care is "orchestration"—the conduct of the midwife's work with the woman to meet her needs within the existing health care system. Outcomes of Western perinatal medicine are often narrowly conceptualized to include only those that can be physically measured. But we describe the overarching outcomes of care more broadly as "life journeys" because the participants stressed achievements that went far beyond usual perinatal measures. Optimal health of the woman and infant is clearly the summit for both obstetrical and midwifery models, but during the journey other outcomes are achieved by the woman, including trust, power, satisfaction, as well as growth and pride for the midwife.

The Relationship between the Midwife and the Woman as Bedrock and Foundation

The first process is rooted in the power of relationship. Women continually described how the midwife listened to them. They felt respected and valued, and developed a trust and alliance with the midwife. A dominant theme was of a partnership based on mutuality and honesty. Mutuality meant that both the midwife and woman held information valuable to the partnership. It is through this relationship that the midwife worked to create an environment conducive to meeting the needs of the woman and her family. Relationship building usually required time, caring, communication skills, intimacy, and at times disclosure. It was supported by a nonjudgmental attitude, compassion, and integrity, among other qualities. One woman commented, "They took the time to know where I was, what I was doing, what my schedule needed to be and what they needed to accommodate me, instead of me accommodating them" (Kennedy 1995: 415).

Continued exploration revealed that this relationship is foundational to truly understanding the woman in the context of her life, which informs the midwife, who can then provide more effective care. It means listening with all of the senses, intuiting what is behind what the woman says (or not) and following up on that—difficult to do if there is not an established relationship.

Story after story from midwives and mothers demonstrated the nature of these relationships. Many of them indicated continuity of care with women, but not always. Not all of the women said they were perfect relationships, and at times a participant said that she would have liked some things about the midwife to be different. However, in general, most of the women valued the relationship and felt a loss when the pregnancy and birth were completed: "I tell you, I wasn't ready to do that . . . she knew me, she knew my family . . . her excitement was like it was her first delivery too" (Kennedy et al. 2004: 18). One woman sent a letter to her midwife four years after her birth commenting on how it felt to her: "I was just 19 when I had [my daughter], but you treated me with respect and kindness. I want you to know how much that meant to me, and still means to me today." These findings are similar to those recounted by Johnson and Davis-Floyd (2006), in which context and the women's desires and definition of the situation are honored, and relationships are foundational to knowledge of the woman.

Developing the relationship was not without conflict for the midwife. Midwives commented about their frustration with the current health care system that does not see the value in the *time* it takes to practice midwifery effectively and to develop that relationship. One midwife said, "It puts more pressure on providers to work faster, and [there is] greater antagonism among providers who are judged on speed" (McCloskey et al. 2002: 131). The difficulties grew when midwives were called to care for women who did not seek the service because of a similar philosophy about birth, but were simply assigned to their clinic, and midwives voiced internal struggles about how women made their choices. Some midwives said they could not care for women who wanted certain birth options, such as medicated births or epidurals, and referred them to other providers (Annandale 1987). Others continued to work with women, even when their values were conflicting. "I had a hard time letting go of the fact that people don't necessarily feel like giving birth as something that should be a challenge. They say, 'I want an epidural, why would anyone want to go through that pain?' . . . So, I've had to give up some of that thinking—you know, [that] this is the *right* way—you should want to feel that pain and feel proud of yourself after you give birth . . . being able to support people in their choices, though they might not have been my choices" (Kennedy at al. 2004: 17).

Building the relationship is an intricate process; it means connecting with everyone in the room. Our assessment strategies revealed some of the "invisible" nature of the midwife's work. One midwife who attends birth in the woman's home noted that her work did not look like "doing," and described it as the "critical art of doing *nothing* well," a specific skill that must be developed. She said, "As a community midwife, I sit for many long hours doing this 'nothing,' silently observing while listening to the parents talk about their hopes and dreams, fears and frustrations" (Kennedy 2000: 12). Davis-Floyd and Davis described it as more than a connection among the mother and family and midwives—as a web "connecting each individual to the deepest essence of herself" (1996: 246).

Although it is possible for a midwife to establish a relationship with a woman in labor when meeting her for the first time, prior knowledge of her through a longer-term, trusting relationship is an asset during the labor and birth. The importance of this relationship became even more apparent as midwives described their prior knowledge of the woman to influence "how" they provided care and navigated the health care system as her advocate during labor and birth.

Orchestration as a Means of Navigating the Terrain and Culture of Western Medicine

Many midwives talked about the "art" of their care. The definition of "art" is multifaceted; it includes (1) scholarship, learning, and science; (2) skill in applying the principles of a special science; (3) human skill as an agent; and (4) skill in doing anything as the result of knowledge and practice (*Oxford English Dictionary* s.v. "art"). Each of these can be seen in the second process, which reflects how midwives "orchestrate" their care. We chose the word "orchestrate," defined as "to combine harmoniously (as in instruments) to produce a desired effect" (*Oxford English Dictionary* s.v. "orchestrate") because it reflected the art and action relayed in the stories. The midwives described a strong and well-developed knowledge base combined with a skill set that enabled them to provide excellent clinical care, as well as the capacity to maneuver within the health care system as an advocate and conduit. Orchestration contained several elements, including navigating normalcy, understanding the woman's environment, and use of self as instrument.

Navigating Normalcy

Midwives described their goal to create an environment in which normalcy was preserved, the woman's desires were met, and the woman was kept safe along the way. Navigation implies a careful assessment of the best route through the environment, harking back to the geographic roots of the model. They often used the symbolic language of art as they described the "dance" of labor and "juggling" the health care team. "I read the tempo, the dance of the labor, and who's in sync and who's out of step. [Then] just very subtly and in a low key way redirect it, or repace it, and hopefully bring it to a place where the mom is getting what she needs" (Kennedy et al. 2004: 19).

The first challenge is the preservation of normalcy within a circle of safety. The struggle often lies in the fact that defining "normalcy" and "safety" can mean vastly different things depending on the worldview of the beholder—the woman, her family, nurses, physicians, or midwives themselves. The work is to manage all of that, as one midwife describes:

> I've always felt that my client or patient is the mother, father and the baby. They *all* are, kind of as a unit. But over the years I think I've learned that it's anybody who happens to be there, including the nurses, including my

consultant . . . truth be told when I can keep the nurses and consultants thinking as positively as I am—not creating a doubt, not letting in doubts when there aren't any there. So I'll do people stuff, managing the social environment, I'm really aware of things that I can look at in the environment and know that they need to be changed.

Influencing the worldview of health care providers to visualize birth as normal is not easy. As in my own experiences before becoming a midwife, many providers have never seen a birth fully powered by the woman, and have never seen or believed in the strength of women. One of the midwives described her work with nurses who had never heard birth cries because their patients were all "epiduralized." The midwife had to help the nurses learn to let go of their reliance on the electronic fetal monitor and to trust birth and to trust her:

> When there was a nurse who was assigned to a patient that I had, who was very uncomfortable with the patient off the monitor, my initial reaction was to provide education to the family that the nurse could [*over*] *hear*. . . . It was usually *through the patient* so that it wasn't a trigger for the nurse who was already anxious about the lack of technology . . . *and* I didn't leave [the room]. . . . That probably took a year or so for most of them to observe. All the midwives modeled that in a way that was very consistent, philosophically the same, and became inclusive of bringing [the nurses] into the model. (Kennedy and Shannon 2004: 556)

The process of keeping birth normal required a continual and vigilant stance by the midwife, day in and day out. It meant constantly working with the setting to hold technology and interventions at bay and to reassure all that what they were seeing was normal. "So, what I have found I need to continue to do is articulate how well the mom is doing . . . if I slip and stay silent—things get done [that shouldn't]. . . because I want everyone in that room to continuously hear that this is normal . . . the silence—that road gives the residents, interns, nurses the aptitude to fill it with their anxiety" (Kennedy 2002: 1760).

The midwives found they had to constantly relay the message that birth is normal to anyone who would listen to them. Midwives conveyed that message to women, starting early on in describing the growth of the baby, the mother's pelvis, and how well nature had designed her body to do the work of birth: "talking about normalcy—what our bodies are meant to do and can't do. . . . Just like reaffirming that what they're doing [are] all the right things, in the right passage—sometimes there is a slowdown here, this is normal and talking about normalcy as opposed to thing that are abnormal" (Kennedy and Shannon 2004: 556).

Helping women trust and believe in the power of their bodies ultimately becomes a journey to an end, as well as to a beginning life as a mother.

One woman who had birthed three times in the hospital asked the midwife at her subsequent home birth to tell her when to push. The midwife said to her, "No, your body will tell (Kennedy and Shannon 2004: 557).The woman was stunned when she felt the power of her body commenting to the midwife that she could not believe, after having three babies, that she never knew how this worked and how it felt. The midwife chose this story to tell because it demonstrated to her how important it is for women to discover what their bodies can do. (Johnson and Davis-Floyd (2006) describe this process as keeping the woman as the central actor—when she remains central and not peripheral in the birth, the experience can become transformational in her life.

Understanding the Woman's Environment: Working with It and with Her

Most midwives talked about the context of the woman's life and its influence on labor and birth. Multiple stories described long or unusual labors that took skill and sometimes intuition to figure out what was really happening. One midwife said she thought that often when labor stalled that, "it is not dystocia of the part; it is a dystocia of life" (Kennedy and Shannon 2004: 557). Midwives likened this process of discovery to "teasing membranes" in third stage—"you have to be careful or [the sac] will break." One midwife provided insight into the skill it takes to validate women's needs to express their fears and concerns when she described how a first-time mom with a fair amount of the baby's head showing in second stage said, "I can't do it!" The midwife said that as long as the baby is fine, she encourages women to take a break when this kind of doubt arises. Her experience is that they stop and regroup, and a couple of contractions later, they muster up the strength and push their baby out.

> But this woman really surprised me and she said, "I'm scared." I said, "What are you scared of?" She said, "Well, I'm afraid it's really going to hurt when I push the baby out and I think maybe I should have some medication." I said, "Well, you know it's an option . . . Then she said, "Well, I'm afraid I'm not going to be a good mother." I started to think, "Oh boy, there's going to be a long list here." I said, "What else are you afraid of?" She said, "I'm really afraid we're not going to manage financially when this baby's born, and I'm afraid that motherhood is going to just turn my life upside down and I'm not going to have any control over things anymore, and I won't be good at it. . . ." Well this went on for 45 minutes. I was flabbergasted and every contraction she just blew through it—didn't push, and the baby didn't come out.

The woman decided to have a small amount of medication and then proceeded to give birth to the baby before it was administered. Reflecting on the story, the midwife felt the woman just needed to talk out her fears and options, be heard, and make choices. She said the woman went on to be delighted in her motherhood and that the nurses at her hospital still talk about this birth.

This example illustrates the power of encouraging women to express their fears, of *listening to women,* and shows how midwives can create a nurturing environment in which women feel free to speak and to deal with labor as they need to. Sometimes this means simply being present and listening. Other times it means changing the physical and/or emotional space in the room.

> So when I go into a room, I look at where people are, I look at who's physically standing near the mom, I look at who's touching her, who's establishing eye contact with her, the tone of voice people are using with her. If they are tuned in and their voice is pitched and their words are chosen in a way that shows an awareness of the work she's doing and an awareness of who she is and what her strengths and weaknesses are, I try to use that. I try to use that to my best advantage in helping her. If I've got that black hole of fear in the room, that's probably the person I'm going to go over to and sit next to and maybe touch their hand or put my arm around their shoulder and say, "Are you OK? You know things are really going well here but you look really worried." Sometimes just by my doing that you can just feel "Oh, OK. Somebody says it's OK. Somebody says this is all right, that this is good."

The power of understanding the context of the woman's life cannot be underestimated. Using this power did not mean that midwives viewed themselves as psychologists or therapists. However, consistently in my studies and in those analyzed in the metasynthesis, midwives reported how valuable it was to know what was important to women in their lives—their fears, their strengths, and their past. This knowledge enabled them to provide a fully holistic approach to their care of women and their families.

The Midwife as an Instrument of Care: Presence and Advocacy

During my analysis of the stories and data, it became clear that in the midwifery model, the midwife is an "instrument" of care. In other words, as midwives navigated the terrain of normal birth supporting the women's power, they themselves constituted the primary medium of care. In navigation, as in many instruments used in health care, it is vital to assess validity and reliability. In my studies, the validity of the "midwife as instrument" was demonstrated in midwives' attention to detail and vigilance in their care. Midwives observed, measured, assessed, consulted, and did all they could to ensure that the pregnancy and birth were normal. Even though their model of care focuses on normalcy, they did not just assume that things would be normal. One midwife said, "Certainly assessment is important in the entire process of what I do. I'm always assessing what the woman is saying, watching non-verbal language, listening acutely to what she isn't saying." Women also noted the thoroughness of this assessment: "One thing that stood out was the excellence of the medical care, from purely a medical standpoint—I don't think I've ever had anyone check my thyroid before" (Kennedy 2000: 9).

One definition of "instrument" in the *Oxford English Dictionary* (s.v. "instrument") is "anything that serves or contributes to the accomplishment of a purpose or end." Whether it is at the bedside through the therapeutic use of presence, or battling behind the closed doors of the obstetrical chief's office, the midwife negotiates to achieve the best outcome possible. Several stories illustrated how midwives used their "presence" to "orchestrate" various scenarios to such ends.

Presence as a midwife is a purposeful action. One woman told me, "She was right there and it was as if she was going to have this child right along with me and I found a lot of comfort—physically and mentally—in that" (Kennedy 1995: 415). One midwife told a story of a young adolescent's reaction to the birth midwife knitting during her labor. During postpartum care, a midwife asked the young woman how her labor had been. She said, "Well, I thought I was going to die because of the pain. But every time I looked up [the midwife] was knitting. And I figured I couldn't be going to die if she was knitting. Because if was going to die she'd be doing something!" I interviewed the birth midwife later about this story, and she said this young woman worked beautifully with her labor and did not need anything but her presence. She said she specifically uses knitting as part of her presence in the room to reassure all who are there. "I knit with women in labor. It's my way . . . of telling everyone who is willing to pay attention, that labor is normal" (Kennedy and Shannon 2004: 557).

Advocacy for women and normal birth is another way that midwives use themselves as instruments to achieve their goals. Advocacy entails a wide range of actions. Sometimes it means working to get a birth tub into a labor room, other times to promote a care plan that seems outside the realm of "normal" obstetrics as usually practiced in the United States. Midwives often become advocates in challenging clinical cases when a woman is asking for something "different." Some midwives described advocacy in terms of serving as a conduit, like a channel to conduct water. You visualize the conduction, such as water over a dam, but you do not see the channel itself. From such perspectives, midwives work to navigate the health care system in the interest of the woman in ways that support the woman's power and achievements, while the midwife remains a background presence during the labor and birth. One midwife said, "I see myself as a guide on a canoe trip, ready to grab a paddle if we hit a snag, but otherwise watching the water and the paddler's ability to navigate, giving encouragement and suggestions as needed." A midwifery client echoed this metaphor when describing her birth: "It was a searing, forever-to-be-etched experience, and my midwife stood out as someone who rode the river with me" (Kennedy 2000: 10).

Midwives' advocacy for women is often invisible to many, as it is usually carried out behind closed doors in order to change systems, opinions, and rules. This intricate and often political process requires personal account-ability, tenacity, and courage. Sometimes it means using evidence to sup-port decreasing the use of technology, such as intermittent auscultation of the fetal heart tones during labor instead of continuous electronic moni-toring. Other times it means helping one individual achieve a special birth by bending hospital rules. It always means balancing the worldviews of the midwife and the Western medical practitioner to find the best way to meet each woman's individual needs.

Life Journeys: The Summit Is in the Journey

The obstetrical world most often measures perinatal success by practice statistics such as morbidity and mortality rates for mothers and infants. Such purely numerical measurements indicate the value of midwifery care, as a number of epidemiological studies show (Harvey et al. 1996; MacDorman and Singh 1998; Oakley et al. 1995; Johnson and Daviss 2005). These studies reveal that U. S. midwives practicing both inside and outside the hospital use fewer drugs and other interventions than do obste-tricians and that they achieve rates of perinatal mortality equal to those achieved by obstetricians attending low-risk births, lower rates of maternal and infant morbidity, higher rates of maternal satisfaction, and higher rates of breastfeeding. Yet midwives are very aware that such measurements are an incomplete reflection of the full range of outcomes of pregnancy and birth, insisting that outcomes of care go well beyond the physical birth. Women told stories of growth and healing. Midwives told similar stories of watching the women they cared for achieving a powerful voice, a sense of victory, and wonderful memories for a lifetime, speaking of the importance of "optimal care."

The following narrative provides a poignant example of the long-last-ing power and memories that can be created during a woman's birth. Sixteen years after this midwife attended the birth of an adolescent woman, a young man walked into a clinic with his aunt and requested to see her. The midwife recalled, "After so many years I had forgotten this lady. [She—the young man's mother—] had developed breast cancer and she had died. One of the things she had asked [her son] was to come find me and go over the story about how he was born. The sister . . . brought him to me so we could grieve together. So we sat in my office and cried, and told him the story of how he was born. It's amazing to me that someone should remem-ber you so many years later" (Kennedy et al. 2004: 20).

The midwife said she remembered little about this young woman except that she had wanted her birth to be natural and for her family to be there. She had advocated for a family birth during an era when that was less common in the hospital. That woman must have experienced an important connection during her transition to motherhood and family birth experience with that midwife. It was so powerful that she wanted her adolescent son to have that same kind of help and support in his transition to life without his mother. The midwife was both amazed and touched by the impact of her actions for this family. Other midwives in my studies have also talked specifically of the importance of recognizing and achieving each woman's potential and power during her birth experience.

In one of my studies (Kennedy 2000), which sampled sixty-four midwives identified by midwifery leaders as exemplary and who reported a cesarean birth rate of 6% in their practices, the most important outcome identified by the midwife participants was "optimal health of the mother and/or infant in the given situation" (Kennedy 2000: 8). This statement indicates some flexibility in midwives' definition of optimal. For example, a woman who experiences an intrauterine fetal demise is in no less need of a caring birth that meets her own unique needs. One woman told a story of a difficult hospital birth in which she was not attended by a midwife. She credited the nurse with saving her from a cesarean delivery, but also recounted the intense pain of hearing her baby cry and cry and not being allowed to comfort him during multiple blood tests. She chose a midwife for her next birth at home. She said, "I also had a lot of doubt about myself and my capability of having a natural birth. . . . I felt like a failure after that first birth. . . . And I think [the midwife] sort of sensed that. . . . She said, 'I think you're holding back' . . . I told her I was afraid that I couldn't do it. . . . She reassured me that I could." This mother went on to have her second baby at home. After the birth she said, "That was a really healing thing for me because he was able to go right to my stomach . . . nurse immediately and he didn't cry" (Kennedy et al. 2004: 19). Another woman described the experience of giving birth unexpectedly to an infant with Down syndrome:

> As an experienced mom, I looked for a midwife who would not feel threatened that I wanted to be ultimately responsible for medical choices. I did not, however, anticipate how life enhancing her role would be postpartum. I have no regrets about my birth experience, and have fallen in love with my baby. . . . I often reflect with a deep sense of gratefulness for all the people involved in her birth . . . for the loving kindness and sensitivity to our pain. It helped me to marshal my maternal instincts when everything in me wanted to escape. A midwife's impact here . . . has lifelong repercussions. Unforgettable moments are created. (Kennedy 1999: 82)

This street goes both ways. Midwives' attendance at birth has a powerful impact not only on the women they serve, but also on the life journeys of the midwives themselves. On one hand, midwives described their growth and pride in their work, but they also described how the work took a toll as they tried to balance their personal and professional lives, and struggled with the stresses generated when the midwifery model of care collides with the majority worldview or technocratic model of birth.

NAVIGATION WHEN WORLDVIEWS COLLIDE

Earlier in this chapter, I stated that a belief in normal birth separates those who practice midwifery from those who practice obstetrics and lays the foundation for the work of midwives. The dominant culture of Western medicine in the United States is a rocky terrain for a midwife to negotiate, and is often a collision course between the two worldviews of birth. The midwives in these studies demonstrated a clear, feminist stance—they saw the woman "in charge"—it is her birth and the midwife is the "guest" in the setting. The core competencies for midwifery practice reflect this philosophy of partnering with women in health care (ACNM 2002) and recognize that the woman is a "direct care provider for herself and her unborn baby; thus the most important determinant of a healthy pregnancy is the mother herself" (MANA 1994). This philosophy diverges greatly from the patriarchal atmosphere prevalent in most United States birth settings.

In our recent metasynthesis of qualitative research about midwifery practice in the United States (Kennedy, Levi, and Kane Low 2005), the single most dominant theme that emerged was "practice conflict," which Annandale (1987) described as a social conflict that reveals the reality of navigating institutional conflict. She identified "management expediency" as that which allows midwives to operate in this context while recognizing that obstetrical ideology is omnipresent and highly influences their decision-making.

Scoggins (1995) found that nurse-midwives believed that nurses were often highly territorial and did not accept the midwives as professionals. Many midwives attributed this to nurses' lack of power, but also believed that nurses often did not understand the midwife's role or training, leading to resentment and at times, sabotage. "A bunch of very jaded high-tech nurses who were resistant . . . would go behind our back and say 'this looks like a late' or things like that and would bring things up to the docs without bringing it up to us first. They wanted to put your butt on the line just for the thrill of trying to figure out how they could sabotage you and make you look like a fool. You always had to watch your back" (quoted in Scoggins 1995: 78).

Nurse/midwife conflicts often result from disagreements about the management of labor and birth. For example, most midwives will try to avoid technological interference and will support the natural processes of birth. The nurse might see this approach as dangerous. This disagreement and collision of worldviews can result in hostile and confrontational behavior in front of laboring women. Cragin (1998) found that the practice of midwifery meant stretching the definitions of normal childbirth to the limits, which became the intersection where midwifery practice engages with biomedicine. Examples include stretching imposed time limits such as due dates, length of labor, and length of time allowed for membranes to remain ruptured before birth. Other times it means stretching and changing rules or policies, such as how women are monitored during labor. Many of these rules are built around tradition rather than evidence—"it's how it's always been done"—as the operational focus.

Navigating the dual terrains of the midwifery and medical worldviews means that midwives sometimes have to hide some of their alternative practices in order to fit into the dominant culture. Gorman (1999) noted that CNMs who used alternatives were sometimes seen as being on the fringes of their own profession. They occasionally concealed their actions in order to keep their jobs in hospitals and birth centers. Those midwives who appeared radical did not last long. Balancing a practice with physicians meant at times having to comply with the technocratic model. On occasion, midwives would have to mask their beliefs while they worked to protect their clients from medical interference. It is a high-wire act: "I have had to give up some of the things . . . you have to be careful to make them think you're not on the fringes" (Gorman 1999: 87).

Lentz described the hostility meted to midwives who attend home birth: "Once physicians know my women are going to have a home birth with a lay midwife, they don't want anything to do with her; he will even tell her not to call him if there are problems" (1996: 232). Home birth midwives also talked about efforts to discredit their practice, such as being reported to the health department when they did the right thing by transporting a laboring woman who needed medical care. Those midwives described the contempt they experienced from nurses and physicians, an attitude of "you don't know 'nothing'—you're stupid—you have no education" (233). Recounting stories of home-to-hospital transfer, Davis-Floyd (2004b) describes how this obstetrical disregard for midwives' knowledge and information can result in "fractured articulations" that too often lead to tragic outcomes.

Some of the midwives interviewed experienced the midwifery model and the medical/technocratic model as polar opposites. However, there were also examples of blending and merging the worldviews among and between groups of midwives. This blending was evident in the variation in midwifery practices, as well as in midwives' approaches to education. Their views on education depended upon their beliefs about what knowledge was necessary to attend births safely. Gorman (1999) found that DEMs did not believe that nursing was important to become a midwife and felt that nurse-midwifery was a dependent profession in the hospital hierarchy. One midwife talked about the change that happened after she obtained the requisite education to become state-licensed: "[It] has made me transport people that I wouldn't have, that I normally would have been more willing to just stay at home . . . [licensing] has made me be paranoid about certain areas—meconium staining, prolonged labor, and postpartum hemorrhage and using any kind of herb at all that I could have in the past" (Weitz and Sullivan 1985: 51).

This conflict and collision between worldviews takes a toll. For some midwives it even meant compromising on how they practice and make an economic living. "To cope with such a large practice, a midwife would have to limit the amount of time spent with each client and routinize care. The midwife with the largest volume of practice essentially has done so . . . although she takes pride in her successful business; the other midwives have stigmatized her for no longer providing family-centered holistic care, rather than emulating her financial success. The balance between commitment to family-centered holistic midwifery and profit for services rendered is not easily achieved" (Weitz and Sullivan 1985: 47).

McCloskey et al. received similar comments from midwives in busy practices. "We are seeing women with more complex medical/social problems. There is less time for teaching, personalized care, and a greater number of clients both at the office and in labor and delivery" (2002: 131).

Only a few studies represented the voices of physicians, and those discussions were not about philosophy but more about their experiences of collaborating with midwives. Miller (1997) noted that collaborative practice with physicians does not take place in a vacuum—it is affected by legislative, institutional, economic, social, political, professional, historical, and institutional variables. She described both positive and negative experiences in those relationships. Physicians who felt "dumped on" were quite clear about the experience. One said, "How did they expect me to feel? The midwives in our practice talked about being so sensitive, so caring, yet they cut me off in front of patients, wouldn't even let me come into the room . . . I felt like I was always the bad guy—who wants to work in a situation like that?" (Miller 1997: 304). Yet those who described successful collaborative midwife/physician relationships saw each other as confident and expert practitioners: "When I started, Dr. X didn't really understand what a midwife could do. It took a lot of talking and a lot of nights working together for her to understand my abilities. I guess the highest compliment came when she chose me, the only midwife, out of all the docs in the practice to deliver her baby" (Miller 1997: 303).

Miller (1997) identified several elements essential for successful collaborative practice:

- Open communication and information on all levels
- Decision making by consensus
- Role clarity
- Agreements to work toward creating systems and pathways for collaboration
- Similar financial rewards and advantages
- Nonhierarchical structures and rotating leadership

She did not specifically outline the need for clarity on philosophy; rather, it was implied. One of her midwife interviewees said, "All this stuff has to be worked out and worked through. You need to lay down rules of human behavior, truthfully, between all people . . . we need folks who can fight it out, stand their ground—make their methods and rationales understood. Passive-aggressives need not apply to our practice" (Miller 1997: 304). This statement suggests the critical need for midwives to ground their practice using the best scientific evidence available, in addition to the woman's desires and their clinical judgment, to argue for their practice decisions.

Midwife Elizabeth Davis summed up the delicate articulation between woman and midwife well: "So you know, the choreography of the woman's expression of need . . . it's a fine line—permission to have your birth be whatever it is going to be, and the midwife's skill and also her need to have a safe outcome. I think really most of us struggle with that" (Davis-Floyd and Davis 1996: 265). In the end, it appears that U.S. midwives manage conflict through a skillful "dance" aimed at constructing a practice that articulates with the majority worldview of birth, while artfully preserving and protecting the philosophical worldview of midwifery.

THE FUTURE OF MIDWIFERY IN THE UNITED STATES: SWIMMING UPSTREAM OR CATCHING A WAVE?

This chapter has provided a description of the midwifery model in the United States drawn from multiple studies. The work of midwives is complex and very much an uphill battle. As noted by one of the midwives, the majority worldview of Western medicine about birth is also shared by many women. This adds to the struggle as midwives work to provide the best care and then find it not accepted by the very women they believe it would benefit. "The midwives feel that they must constantly struggle to force such clients to take back responsibility for their births . . . the lack of a shared set of values between client and midwife may increase the psychological distance between them" (Weitz and Sullivan 1985: 50).

Women are the ones who ultimately can demand a change in birth attendants. They can insist on midwifery as the primary model of care in the
United States. However, they have to believe it is best for them. And they
have to want it. That is not the current tide of belief in the United States. For
example, the chapter on labor and delivery in the bestseller *What to Expect
When You're Expecting* (Murkoff, Eisenberg, and Hathaway 2002) focuses on
concerns and provides an impression of birth as a risky event, with minimal
language about women's strength or competence to birth. "Your baby will
be squeezed, compressed, pushed, and molded . . . there is an element of
risk in this stressful journey" (347). Considerable attention (three and one-
half pages) is given to induction of labor, with a side bar box for emphasis
titled, "Giving Mother Nature a Boost" (342). This focus contrasts sharply
with the description of labor in a less widely circulated book by England and
Horowitz (1998). "There are three things that are givens about labor: It's
hard work, it hurts a lot, and you can do it. That's the bottom line. All the
rest you learn about is icing on the cake" (120). If you were pregnant for
the first time, how would you know which to believe or choose?

Where do we go from here? I believe there are several areas to explore and
understand before significant change can happen. One is research to answer
essential questions about supporting normal birth in the United States. How
do we measure the influence of the philosophy of midwifery practice on
perinatal and long-term health outcomes? How does fear about potential
pathology, common to the medical worldview of birth, creep into the decision-
making equation and the outcomes? Exciting and hopeful work is being produced by the Optimality Working Group in the United States (Judith Fullerton
April 27, 2008, personal communication). This group is making progress in
examining birth outcomes from an "optimality" stance rather than one that
is solely risk based. It demands an accounting of care processes in addition to
outcome, suggesting they are highly related. Optimality has been specifically
defined for perinatal health as "the maximal perinatal outcome with minimal
intervention placed against the dynamic context of the woman's social, medical, and obstetric history" (Kennedy 2004: 766). The concept and measurement of optimality suggests a route toward accounting for the midwife as an
"instrument" of care, and needs to be more fully studied.

Research on specific practices used by midwives will also make inroads in
our knowledge about normal birth. We know that the presence of midwives
in hospitals has challenged and changed practices. For example, twenty years
ago, it was common for the baby to be whisked off for assessment in a separate corner of the room or the nursery without being given to the mother.
In my early days as a midwife attending birth in the hospital, few of my physician colleagues delivered a baby without an episiotomy. I can vividly recall
the obstetrician standing behind me, picking up the scissors and saying, "If
you don't cut, I will!" Now, in that same hospital, residents are taught by

midwives how to protect the perineum and avoid episiotomy. Research such as that of Albers et al. (2005) on promoting perineal integrity is important in documenting the safety and efficacy of these and other practices.

Research on how midwives stretch the "boundaries of normal"—on how they "normalize uniqueness" (Davis-Floyd and Davis 1996)—is essential. The first step is working with midwives to define what they do that is different from mainstream obstetrics. Some of these elements of difference have already been well documented, such as presence. But what other boundaries do we stretch? An example of how effective research can help clinicians begin to question "traditional" practice is Judith Mercer's work on delayed cord clamping (Mercer et al. 2006). She described a birth of an infant she attended at home many years ago with a very tight double nuchal cord that she did not cut and clamp (Mercer and Skovgaard 2004). The infant was pale and without tone, reflexes, or respiratory effort, but had a heart rate over 100. With stimulation at the mother's perineum, the infant pinked up, developed normal tone, and began to breathe gently. The cord was not cut and clamped during the resuscitation. Mercer believed that the infant's resuscitation was enhanced because of its ability to re-perfuse through an intact cord, even though in almost all hospitals, the infant would have been severed immediately from the placenta and taken to another place for evaluation. That experience was an inductive scientific moment for Mercer, and she has devoted her research to this topic. Working with a cohort of very-low-birth-weight infants, she demonstrated through randomized controlled trials that delayed cord clamping is protective (Mercer et al. 2006). The fact that she was able to accomplish this kind of study in a tertiary teaching institution places her as a midwifery pioneer in research on the support of normal birth. Work in other areas like this must continue and receive creative press coverage that helps the public question the care they are receiving.

Another path is likely to be as important: how do we convince women that they, and not practitioners, own birth? They are the ones who must make the decisions that will support their bodies' abilities to bear children under their own power. We must work to help women question the growing overuse of technology in childbirth. We must find creative ways to disseminate the message that their bodies are to be trusted—that birth is a healthy and achievable event within their personal power. It is essential to help them to question the growing trend toward routine elective cesarean delivery (ACNM 2006a). They must also know that memories of birth experiences last a lifetime and can enhance their lives or become a lifelong source of trauma (Beck 2004). Midwives have a role in creating and disseminating that message. And we have a responsibility to challenge the dominant worldview whenever we encounter it, in whatever way we can. That challenge must be one that understands, gently exposes, and teaches women, physicians, nurses, midwives, and all who participate in birth that birth is a powerful event that should be attended with respect and knowledge, and in partnership with the woman.

Finally, we must examine how we are teaching midwifery students. Lange and Kennedy (2006) recently published a study that exposes the dissonance students feel between what they are taught in school about midwifery philosophy and practice and their perceptions of what they see in their student clinical experiences. Half of the students perceived a lack of congruence between "ideal" and actual" practice in the support of normal birth. Placing nurse-midwifery students in home birth settings is exceptionally difficult because of malpractice constraints, and it is increasingly difficult for students to observe a completely noninterventive birth in the hospital setting. But experiences with birth in home and birth center settings, as well as exposure to hospital settings that support normalcy and women's power, are essential in helping students learn what midwifery and birth are really about. Midwives and physicians who have observed out-of-hospital births find the experience profoundly different from attending in-hospital births and highly instructive in their efforts to learn about normal birth, because of the lack of intervention and the freedom of the mother to move and find her own positions of comfort. This approach contrasts markedly with most in-hospital environments, where 80% of women experience continuous fetal monitoring (Parer 2003).

Despite the conflicts reflecting the how midwives navigate the challenging terrain of caring for women within the dominant Western medical culture, their model is effective. Midwives orchestrate care through relationships with women and through navigating the environment to support normal birth. They work with women within the context of their lives. Midwives use themselves as instruments of care through presence and advocacy. The outcomes of the midwifery model include those valued by the dominant worldview of Western medicine, but they expand beyond those statistical measures toward life journeys for both the mother and the midwife. This book is one way to begin—a gathering of information about models that work. With this information, all of those who are invested in the culture and worldview of the midwifery model can begin to fracture the dominant ethos and celebrate women and birth.

ACKNOWLEDGMENTS

Many, many thanks to those who have assisted me in this journey:

Research Participants: The midwives and recipients of midwifery care who freely shared their time and thoughts.
Data collectors and analysts: Deb Erickson-Owens, Jo Anne P. Davis, Emily MacDonald, Maureen Shannon, Usa Chuahorm, Kathryn Kravetz, Lisa Kane Low, and Amy Levi.
Consultants: The Optimality-Index Working Group, Judith Fullerton, and Patricia Aikins Murphy.

Funders: University of Rhode Island Foundation; ACNM/Ortho-McNeil Graduate Fellowship; Rhode Island Chapter of the ACNM; Sigma Theta Tau—Alpha Eta Chapter; University of California–San Francisco School of Nursing; and University of California–San Francisco Academic Senate.

And last, but not least: Jeanne DeJoseph, CNM, PhD, for her wise counsel, empathic heart and ear, and superb editorial skills—she is the Goddess on my shoulder!

REFERENCES

ACNM. 1999. *ACNM Membership Survey.* www.acnm.org. Accessed June 24, 2005.

———. 2002. *ACNM Core Competencies for Basic Midwifery Practice.* Silver Spring, MD: American College of Nurse-Midwives. http://www.acnm.org/display.cfm?id=484. Accessed April 15, 2006.

———. 2006a. *American College of Nurse-Midwives Calls for Accurate Reporting on New NIH Findings about Cesarean Delivery. Recent NIH Conference Is Not a License for Doctors to Offer C-Section on Demand.* Press release. Silver Spring, MD: American College of Nurse-Midwives. http://www.midwife.org/news.cfm?id=916. Accessed April 16, 2006.

———. 2006b. *American College of Nurse-Midwives Essential Facts about Midwives – Updated 2008.* Silver Spring, MD: American College of Nurse-Midwives. http://www. acnm.org/siteFiles/news/news/Essential_Facts_about_Midwives.pdf. Accessed November, 22, 2008.

AMCB. 2005. *American Midwifery Certification Board: Candidate Booklet.* http://www. amcbmidwife.org/c/94/candidate-booklet.

Albers, L. L, K. D. Sedler, E. J. Bedrick, D. Teaf, and P. Peralta. 2005. "Midwifery Care Measures in the Second Stage of Labor and Reduction of Genital Tract Trauma at Birth: A Randomized Trial." *Journal of Midwifery and Women's Health* 50.5:365–72.

Annandale, E. C. 1987. "Restructuring Maternity Care: Practice Behavior in a Midwife-Run Birth Center." Ph.D. thesis, Brown University, Providence, RI.

Beck, C. T. 2004. "Post-Traumatic Stress Disorder due to Childbirth: The Aftermath." *Nursing Research* 53.4:216–24.

Bushnell, J. M. 1981. "Northwest Coast American Indian's Beliefs about Childbirth." *Issues in Health Care of Women* 4.4:249–61.

Cragin, L. 1998. "Midwifery Practice at the Edges of Normal Birth: 'I Might Be Able to Be a Little More Out There Because They Trust Me.'" Pilot study, University of California–San Francisco.

Davis-Floyd, R. 2004a. *Birth as an American Rite of Passage,* 2nd ed. Berkeley, CA: University of California Press.

———. 2004b. "Home Birth Emergencies in the United States: The Trouble with Transport." In *Unhealthy Health Policy: A Critical Anthropological Examination,* edited by A. Castro and M. Singer, 329–350. Walnut Creek, CA: AltaMira Press.

Davis-Floyd, R., and E. Davis. 1996. "Intuition as Authoritative Knowledge in Midwifery and Home Birth." *Medical Anthropology Quarterly* 10.2:237–69.

Dawley, K. 2003. "Origins of Nurse-Midwifery in the United States and Its Expansion in the 1940s." *Journal of Midwifery and Women's Health* 48.2:86–95.

Dougherty, M.C. 1978. "Southern Lay Midwives as Ritual Specialists. In *Women in Ritual and Symbolic Roles*, edited by J. Hoch-Smith and A. Spring. New York: Plenum Press.

England, P., and R. Horowitz. 1998. *Birthing from Within: An Extra-Ordinary Guide to Childbirth Preparation*. Albuquerque, NM: Partera Press.

Fullerton, J. 2005. *The Optimality Working Group*. Silver Spring, MD: American College of Nurse-Midwives Division of Research. http://www.acnm.org/about. cfm?id=255. Accessed April 15, 2006.

Gesler, W.M., and R.A. Kearns. 2002. *Culture/Place/Health*. New York: Routledge.

Gorman, M.M. 1999. "A Description of the Beliefs, Practices and Pathways to Birth of Certified Nurse-Midwives and Direct Entry Midwives." Ph.D. thesis, Wayne State University, Detroit, MI.

Harvey, S., J. Jarrell, R. Brant, C. Stainton, and D. Rach. 1996. "A Randomized Controlled Trial of Midwifery Care. *Birth* 23.3:128–35.

Johnson, C.B., and R. Davis-Floyd. 2006. "Why Midwives Matter: Overcoming Barriers to Caretake the Power of Birth." In *Mainstreaming Midwives: The Politics of Change*, edited by R. Davis-Floyd and C. B. Johnson, 507–40. New York: Routledge.

Johnson, K.C., and B.-A. Daviss. 2005. "Outcomes of Planned Home Births with Certified Professional Midwives: A Large Prospective Study in North America." *British Medical Journal* 330.7505:1416. www.bmj.com.

Kennedy, H.P. 1995. "The Essence of Midwifery Care: The Woman's Story." *Journal of Nurse-Midwifery* 40.5:410–17.

———. 1999. "Linking Midwifery Practice to Outcomes: A Delphi Study." Ph.D. thesis, University of Rhode Island, Kingston.

———. 2000. "A Model of Exemplary Midwifery Practice: Results of a Delphi Study. *Journal of Midwifery and Women's Health* 45.1:4–19.

———. 2002. "The Midwife as an 'Instrument' of Care. *American Journal of Public Health* 92.11:1759–60.

———. 2004. "A Concept Analysis of 'Optimality' in Perinatal Health. *Proceedings of the American Academy of Nursing State of the Science Congress*, Washington, DC, October.

Kennedy, H.P., J.A.P. Davis, and D. Erickson-Owens. 2006. "Voices of Diversity in Midwifery: A Qualitative Study. *Journal of Midwifery and Women's Health* 51: 85–90.

Kennedy, H.P., A.L. Levi, and L. Kane Low. 2005. "A Metasynthesis of Midwifery Knowledge in the United States." *Proceedings of the Triennial Congress of the International Confederation of Midwives*, Brisbane, AU, July 24–28.

Kennedy, H.P., and E. MacDonald. 2002. "Altered Consciousness in Childbirth: Potential Clues to PTSD?" *Journal of Midwifery and Women's Health* 4:380–83.

Kennedy, H.P., A.L. Rousseau (Levi), and L. Kane Low. 2003. "An Exploratory Metasynthesis of Midwifery Practice in the U.S." *Midwifery* 19:205–14.

Kennedy, H.P., and M.T. Shannon. 2004. "Keeping Birth Normal: Research Findings on Midwifery Care during Childbirth." *Journal of Obstetric, Gynecologic, and Neonatal Nursing* 33:554–60.

Kennedy, H.P., M.T. Shannon, U. Chuahorm, and M.K. Kravetz. 2004. "The Landscape of Midwifery Care: A Narrative Study." *Journal of Midwifery and Women's Health* 49.1:14–23.

Lange, G., and Kennedy, H.P. 2006. "Student Perceptions of Ideal and Actual Midwifery Practice." *Journal of Midwifery and Women's Health* 51.2:71–77.

Lentz, J.R. 1996. "Times Past—Times Present: The Midwife." Ph.D. thesis, Rice University, Houston, TX.

Logan, O.L. 1989. *Motherwit: An Alabama Midwife's Story.* New York: Penguin Books.

MacDorman, M.F., and G.K. Singh. 1998. "Midwifery Care, Social and Medical Risk Factors, and Birth Outcomes in the USA." *Journal of Epidemiology and Community Health* 52.5:310–17.

MANA. 1994. *Core Competencies for Basic Midwifery Practice.* Midwives Alliance of North America. http://www.mana.org/manacore.html. Accessed April 15, 2006.

———. 2005a. *Numbers of Midwives.* Midwives Alliance of North America. http://www.mana.org/press.html. Accessed November, 22, 2008.

———. 2005b. *Direct-Entry Midwifery State-by-State Legal Status* (Updated 4-25-2007). Midwives Alliance of North America. http://mana.org/statechart.html. Accessed November 22, 2008.

———. 2005c. MANA-ACNM Bridge Club. Midwives Alliance of North America. http://mana.org/bridgeclub.html. Accessed November 22, 2008.

Martin, J.A., B.E. Hamilton, P.D. Sutton, S.J. Ventura, F. Menacker, S. Kirmeyer, and M.L. Munson. 2007. "Births: Final Data for 2005." *National Vital Statistics Reports* 56.6.

McCloskey, L., H.P. Kennedy, E.R. Declercq, and D.R. Williams. 2002. "Nurse-Midwives and the Maternal and Child Health Safety Net in the Era of Managed Care: Reports from the Field. *Maternal and Child Health Journal* 6:127–36.

Mercer, J., and R. Skovgaard. 2004. "Fetal to Neonatal Transition: First Do No Harm." In *Normal Childbirth: Evidence and Debate,* edited by S. Downe, pp. 141–160. New York: Churchill Livingstone.

Mercer, J.S., B.R. Vohr, M.M. Mcgrath, J.F. Padbury, M. Wallach, and W. Oh. 2006. "Delayed Cord Clamping in Very Preterm Infants Reduces the Incidence of Intraventricular Hemorrhage and Late-Onset Sepsis: A Randomized Controlled Trial. *Pediatrics* 117.4:1235–42.

Miller, S. 1997. "Midwives' and Physicians' Experiences in Collaborative Practice: A Qualitative Study." *Women's Health Issues* 7.5:301–8.

Murkoff, H., A. Eisenberg, and S. Hathaway. 2002. *What to Expect When You're Expecting,* 3rd ed. New York: Workman.

NARM. 2004. *How to Become a CPM.* North American Registry of Midwives. http://www.narm.org/htb.htm#mission. Accessed May 28, 2005.

Oakley, D., M.E. Murray, T. Murtland, R. Hayashi, F. Anderson, F. Mayes, and J. Rooks. 1995. "Comparisons of Outcomes of Maternity Care by Obstetricians and Certified Nurse-Midwives." *Obstetrics and Gynecology* 88.5:823–29.

Parer, J.T. 2003. "Electronic Fetal Heart Rate Monitoring: A Story of Survival." *Obstetrical and Gynecology Survey* 58.9:561–3.

Rooks, J.P. 1997. *Midwifery and Childbirth in America.* Philadelphia: Temple University Press.

Schuiling, K.D., T.A. Sipe, and J. Fullerton. 2005. "Findings from the Analysis of the American College of Nurse-Midwives Membership Surveys: 2000–2003." *Journal of Midwifery and Women's Health* 50.1:8–15.

Scoggins, J.P. 1995. "The Occupational Identity of Nurse-Midwives in Relation to Nursing, Medicine, and Midwifery." Ph.D. thesis, University of Arizona, Tempe.

Ulrich, L.T. 1990. *A Midwife's Tale: The Life of Martha Ballard based on her Diary, 1785–1812.* New York: Knopf/Random House.

Weitz, R., and S. Sullivan. 1985. "Licensed Lay Midwifery and the Medical Model of Childbirth. *Sociology of Health and Illness* 7.1:36–54.

Conclusion

Robbie Davis-Floyd, Lesley Barclay, Betty-Anne Daviss, and Jan Tritten

In developed countries it has been demonstrated that the development of a nation-wide system of integrated midwives is the single most important factor in reducing maternal mortality.

> JERKER LILJESTRAND, Co-chair, Safe Motherhood Program, FIGO (Presentation at the Meetings of the International Federation of Latin American and Caribbean Obstetricians and Gynecologists, May 2005)

The "medical model" shows us pregnancy and birth through the perspective of technological society, and from men's eyes. Birthing women are thus objects upon whom certain procedures must be done. The alternative model . . . which I will call "the midwifery model" . . . is a woman's perspective on birth, in which women are the subjects, the doers, the givers of birth.

> BARBARA KATZ ROTHMAN, *In Labor: Women and Power in the Birthplace* (1982: 34)

THE IMPORTANCE OF IDEOLOGY: WHAT'S IN A NAME?

In 2002 Ellen Hodnett carried out a systematic review of 137 reports on factors influencing women's evaluations of their childbirth experiences. Her objective was to summarize what was known about satisfaction with childbirth, with particular attention to the roles of pain and pain relief. The reports included in Hodnett's review included descriptive studies, randomized controlled trials, and reviews of intrapartum interventions. The results were as follows: "Four factors—personal expectations, the amount of support from caregivers, the quality of the caregiver-patient relationship, and involvement in decision making—appear to be so important that they override the influences of age, socioeconomic status, ethnicity, childbirth preparation, the physical birth environment, pain, immobility, medical interventions, and continuity of care, when women evaluate their childbirth experiences." The review's conclusion is that "the influences of pain, pain relief, and intrapartum medical interventions on subsequent satisfaction are neither as obvious, as direct, nor as powerful as the influences of the attitudes and behaviors of the caregivers" (Hodnett 2002: 171–172). Attitudes and behaviors stem from particular philosophies, or paradigms, that form the template for the caregiver's beliefs about birth. In other words, it's the model behind the "model that works" that most determines the kind of care a practitioner will provide.

In this volume, we have taken an educated tour of birth models that work whose practitioners are providing optimal maternity care. It is readily apparent that all of the models that work presented here share a common ideology based on the fundamental notions that birth is normal and that women are its protagonists. What should we call this shared ideology? It has received various names over time. It was first described in print by sociologist Barbara Katz Rothman (1982) as the "midwifery model of care"—this label has since become internationally recognized as a useful signature by which to differentiate the philosophy and ideology of midwifery from that of obstetrics. Recognition of the difference between the two professions—midwives focus on normalcy, obstetricians on pathology—goes back centuries; serious discussions about the implications of those differences have been taking place since that time. Because midwives are the most numerous primary maternity care practitioners and have long engaged in discussion and reflection with each other and with social scientists about what it is that they do that works and doesn't work, they have continued to articulate and refine "the midwifery model of care" (e.g., Rooks 1999). In many midwifery educational programs around the world, this model is held out as an ideal for midwifery practice; in others, it is actively taught as the standard for midwifery care. Others have suggested other names for this model, in part to avoid identifying it with a particular profession and to acknowledge that many midwives over-medicalize their treatment of birth even as some physicians work very hard to practice "the midwifery model." To date there is no international consensus on the most appropriate name for the ideology and practice of supporting normal birth.

In *Birth as an American Rite of Passage* (2004), Robbie Davis-Floyd expanded on Rothman's discussion of the differences between the "medical" and "midwifery" models of care, using the labels "the technocratic model of birth" and "the holistic model of birth" to name these contrasting paradigms (see Appendix C.1). Some years later, Davis-Floyd expanded her understanding of the dominant paradigms operative in global maternity care to include a third paradigm, the humanistic model, which stretches across the divide between the technocratic and holistic models (see Appendix C.2). As Davis-Floyd notes, humanists wish simply to humanize technomedicine—that is, to make it relational, partnership oriented, individually responsive, and compassionate: "Humanism counterbalances technomedicine with a softer approach, which can be anything from a superficial overlay to profoundly alternative methods. It is superficially humanistic to decorate a technocratic labor room so the machines don't stand out so much; it is deeply humanistic to provide women with flexible spaces in which they have room to move around as much as they like, to be in water if they wish, to labor as they choose" (Davis-Floyd 2001: 15).

Birth activists in all Spanish-speaking countries appear to have reached consensus around the term "humanization"—they speak of *la humanización del parto y nacimiento* (the humanization of birth), *parto humanizado* (humanized birth), and so on. But to focus reform efforts on the humanization of birth can be a relevant strategy only when birth is *dehumanized,* as indeed it is in many large Latin American hospitals, but not, generally speaking, in hospitals in the United States and Canada, where the technocratic approach still prevails and yet women are humanistically treated—that is, with compassion and respect, and support from companions they choose— the essential ingredients of a humanistic approach. And therein lies the rub: the humanistic paradigm is highly co-optable—we have witnessed some Latin American hospitals suddenly start calling their maternity care "humanistic" simply because they decided to allow a partner to accompany the mother during labor or to allow mothers to stay with their babies in the freshly painted postpartum ward while many unnecessary interventions are still routinely performed. If "humanistic" is to become as widely used in other countries as it is in the Hispanic world, we must be careful to distinguish the *superficial humanism* of the respectful and caring unnecessary cesarean from the *deep humanism* that acknowledges and facilitates the deep physiology and emotionality of birth, for example, through freedom of movement, upright positions for birth, and full emotional support and physical support.

As Davis-Floyd (2001) explains, the technocratic model of birth constitutes the hegemonic paradigm influencing the attitudes and behaviors of biomedically oriented birth practitioners. This technocratic model views the mind as separate from the body, and defines the body as a machine and the patient as an object ("the cesarean in room 112")—definitions that facilitate the distancing of practitioner from patient, the supervaluation of mechanical diagnoses via ultrasound and electronic fetal monitoring (EFM), and the overuse of technological intervention designed to improve or correct the malfunctions of the maternal body-machine. In contrast, the humanistic model of birth places supreme importance on mind-body connection (the influence of mental and emotional states on the body, and vice versa), defines the body not as a machine but as an organism, and stresses the importance of the caregiver-patient relationship. The essence of a humanistic approach to birth, according to Davis-Floyd, is relationship, communication, and caring between patient and practitioner—a supervaluation of the needs of the individual instead of those of the institution. The distinction we have mentioned between superficial and deep humanism is key: superficial humanism involves beautifying the environment of birth, making the mother more comfortable, and treating her kindly and respectfully—an approach that can easily include respectful and caring administration of multiple technological interventions. In contrast, deep humanism goes much further, involving a profound understanding of the normal physiology of birth and how to facilitate it, and including an understanding of the power of the mother's emotions to affect the progress of labor. The *holistic model of birth* goes beyond the definition of the body as an organism and views the body as an energy field in interaction with other energy fields (see Appendix C.2). In the holistic view—one incorporated by many midwives and some obstetricians such as Ricardo Jones—practitioners can preclude the need for technological interventions by intervening at the level of energy, changing or focusing the "energy of birth" to facilitate optimal outcomes, as Jones describes in Chapter 10.

All of the birth models that work described in this volume incorporate aspects of both the humanistic and holistic paradigms of birth (see Appendix C.2). Some of the developers and practitioners of these models think of them in these specific terms, while others do not. Thus, naming the paradigm under which all these models operate proves a challenging undertaking, given the lack of international consensus on a single name. In *Pursuing the Birth Machine* (1994), Marsden Wagner contrasted the medical model with the "social model" of birth—terminology followed by Lesley Barclay in her discussions of midwives in Samoa, one that emphasizes the sociality of birth. Dutch midwives speak of the "physiologic" model because their focus is on understanding and facilitating the deep physiology of birth. Yet a focus on physiology can appear to minimize birth's social aspects, while a focus on sociality can seem to minimize the importance of physiology. Coming from France is the term *naissance respecté* (respected childbirth)—a highly humanistic focus. U.S. activists struggle with "natural" versus "normal" birth as their conceptual standard because both of these terms are problematic: nearly all human births are culturally shaped, and "normal" is hard to define, especially when interventions are "the norm" in hospitals. Anthropologist Brigitte Jordan (1993) used a "biocultural" approach in her analysis of birth in four cultures—and yet birth is more than a combination of biology and culture.

An international collaboration between the World Health Organization (WHO) and the United Nations Children's Fund (UNICEF) resulted in the creation of the Baby-friendly Hospital Initiative, the focus of which is on facilitating successful breastfeeding. The Coalition for Improving Maternity Care (CIMS) in the United States developed a national initiative based on a mother-friendly model of care (see www.mother-friendly.org); its daughter organization, the International MotherBaby Childbirth Organization (IMBCO), has recently launched the International MotherBaby Childbirth Initiative (IMBCI): 10 Steps to Optimal Maternity Services (IMBCO 2008). This initiative organizes itself around what its proponents have labeled the MotherBaby Model of Care, acknowledging its basis in the midwifery model. Two of its principles are these:

> The MotherBaby Model of Care promotes the health and well-being of all women and babies during pregnancy, birth, and breastfeeding, setting the gold standard for excellence and superior outcomes in maternity care. All maternity service providers should be educated in, provide, and support the MotherBaby Model of Care.
>
> Midwives, who are the primary care providers for millions of birthing women in most countries, have developed a model of care based on the normal physiology, sociology, and psychology of pregnancy, labour, birth, and the postpartum period. The International MotherBaby Childbirth Initiative draws on the midwifery model of care and affirms that midwifery knowledge, skills, and behavior are essential for optimal MotherBaby care. (IMBCO 2008: 3)

Wanting to name and describe the model that underlies our birth models that work, we note that by definition, midwives are or should be the primary guides and guardians of normal pregnancy and birth, while obstetricians, by definition, are or should be the backup providers dealing with conditions of actual danger or risk (with family physicians somewhere in between). Midwives are indeed primary practitioners in all the models described in this book, and "the midwifery model" seems to us at this point the most appropriate term to use. The midwifery model as we define it here combines all elements of humanism with many elements of holism (see Appendices C.2 and C.3). Although the midwives in the practices described in these pages do practice according to the midwifery model, many thousands of midwives around the world are technocratically trained and do not. Nurses serve as primary birth attendants in some places. In almost every country, one can find committed obstetricians and family practice physicians who apply the midwifery model daily in their practices. And any primary maternity care practitioner can apply the group-oriented Centering model of pregnancy care described in Chapter 13. Thus we use the term "midwifery model of care practitioners" or "MMOC practitioners" to categorize those care providers who practice according to the ideology we describe in the following section.

THE MIDWIFERY (HUMANISTIC/HOLISTIC) MODEL OF CARE

The midwifery model of care comes from a woman-centered perspective, defines women as active agents in pregnancy and birth, sees the female body as normal in its own terms, and understands pregnancy and birth as healthy, normal parts of women's lives. It takes a holistic, integrating approach, defining the body not as a machine but as an organism and an energy field in constant interaction with other energy fields (Davis-Floyd 2001; Davis-Floyd and St John 1998), and viewing mind and body as one and mother and baby as an inseparable unit—the use of the term "MotherBaby" in the International MotherBaby Childbirth Initiative indicates its authors' understanding of how profoundly the treatment of one affects the other. The safety and emotional needs of the mother and baby are the same; what is good for the mother is good for the child. As Rothman put it: "The medical model dichotomizes not only mind and body, but also mother and infant. Mother/fetus are seen in the medical model as a conflicting dyad rather than an integral unit. In the midwifery model, mother and fetus are genuinely one, and what meets the needs of the one meets the needs of the other. Emotional, physical, maternal, and infant needs are not, in the midwifery model, at odds" (1982: 48). The family, not the institution, constitutes the most significant social unit, and the mother, not the practitioner, is the most significant birthing agent.

Birth as Normal

Fundamentally, nature works well the vast majority of the time—birth outcomes are better when labor and birth are nurtured and supported but not interfered with. MMOC practitioners understand the deep physiology of birth. They know that labor allowed to flow has its own rhythms—it can start and stop, speed up or slow down, take a few hours or a few days. Facilitation is appropriate; intervention is usually inappropriate. MMOC practitioners use specific technologies (e.g., artifacts that facilitate upright positions, including birthing balls and chairs) and modalities (such as acupressure and visualization) that work to support normal birth but generally minimize medical interventions, relying on a physiologically and emotionally supportive range of strategies and watchful vigilance. They read and understand the scientific evidence showing that laboring women should be encouraged to do as they please—to eat, drink, move about, rest. The first line of care for minor delays and complications is with low-tech interventions such as position changes, emotional support, massage, immersion in warm water, aromatherapy, herbs, homeopathy, hand maneuvers, and most fundamentally "changing the energy" by working to create a more positive and trust-based atmosphere; higher-tech interventions are reserved for cases of true need. It is time that such modalities move into the mainstream.

MMOC practitioners see that labor pain is normal and that a woman's ability to bear it can be greatly increased by nurturant care and a supportive environmental ambience permeating what Ricardo Jones (Chapter 10) calls the "psychosphere" of labor and birth. Patience is the most essential attribute of the MMOC practitioner. In their discussion of Japanese maternity homes, Matsuoka and Hinokuma (Chapter 8) explain midwives' emphasis on "the importance of waiting": "Waiting does not mean so much time wasted or the time of just enduring pain for a birthing woman.

It is a meaningful time, shared by the birthing woman, her family, and the midwife together." These midwives consider labor pain to be "metamorphic"—"a necessary process for a birthing woman as she grows into motherhood—to face her own self through the experience of pain." They believe that the comforting presence of the midwife and family members is enough to support the woman to experience this pain in a positive way, because the pain is in fact positive: it is *productive* of the baby's birth and of the woman's birth as a mother. They also see it as a way for the entire family and friends attending the birth to bond and thus recognize the actual benefit of long hours of labor. MMOC practitioners are not afraid of labor pain or of watching women experience it; they know that their own calmness facilitates the woman's ability to move through the pain without producing the anxiety that increases it.

The Importance of Emotions and Intuition

The uterus responds to the mother's emotional state; thus, the best care is based not only on measurements and information but also on body knowledge and intuition (Davis-Floyd and Davis 1997). In the midwifery model, experiential and emotional knowledge count as much as or more than technical knowledge. Essential attributes of maternity care include empathy, compassion, caring, and loving touch. MMOC practitioners know the importance of "*presence:* the ability to *be* fully with another person, completely attentive and focused, listening with an open heart" (Houston et al. n.d. p. 32). The women who experience the Centering model receive this kind of care not only from their practitioner but also from each other. Denis Walsh's chapter on the Lichfield Maternity Unit describes the effect of this open-hearted approach on a mother's severe abdominal pain an hour after the birth, which seemed to have no clinical cause: "Judith managed it by just sort of cradling the woman in her arms, resting her head on her lap and holding it gently and massaging her hair and scalp in a very sort of motherly, maternal way. And she did that for a long time, 20–30 minutes. Just sort of held her safe I suppose." The mother later said, "She [midwife] was great afterwards because it was like having my Mum there. I remember having my head on her lap and she was just stroking the back of my head saying you will be all right. Just kind of nursing you which was invaluable. It was like you were her daughter" (Chapter 6).

Reflective Practice and Preservation of Knowledge

MMOC practitioners value and work hard to achieve cultural appropriateness and sensitivity, treating women as they wish to be treated and upholding their rights. They rely on introspection and case review with colleagues to reflect on what they are doing and make efforts at improvement on an ongoing basis. They are aware of the *de-skilling* of obstetricians—who are increasingly taught simply to perform a cesarean for any complication—so they consciously work to learn and preserve the myriad of skills that some midwives and obstetricians have learned and recorded over time that can keep birth normal: massage; external cephalic version; positions and hand maneuvers for breech and twin delivery; variations on upright positions; stair climbing or using a *rebozo* (shawl) to shake loose a stuck baby; and non-medical means of stopping hemorrhage (drugs are not always available). Such skills and more have long been part of the repertoire of traditional midwives in many regions and are consciously sought out by MMOC practitioners. For example, professional midwives in Samoa (Chapter 4), the CASA students in San Miguel (Chapter 11), the licensed midwives working with Mercy in Action in the Philippines (Chapter 12), and the nurse-midwives teaching traditional midwives in the Brazilian Amazon (Chapter 14) all describe in these pages skills and attitudes they learn from traditional midwives. In models that work, this is always a two-way exchange—each group learns from and teaches the other, with mutual attitudes of respect.

Relationships of Midwives and Obstetricians: Collaboration as Key

As we noted above, the midwifery model positions the midwife as the guide and guardian of the normal birth process; her skills should be used to keep birth normal in the vast majority of cases and to identify and treat complications herself if she is qualified, or to seek appropriate medical help when she is not. (Globally, approximately 1% of midwives are male. We note with humor that our use of the word "she" to apply to midwives in general is generally supported by male midwives themselves, who often tell us that they are very comfortable with developing "their feminine side.") Humanistic obstetricians work respectfully and collaboratively with midwives, and provide appropriate services for high-risk and emergency births. As American midwife Judith Rooks explains, "Midwifery and medical obstetrics are separate but complementary professions with different philosophies and overlapping but distinct purposes and bodies of knowledge. Physicians are experts in pathology and should have primary responsibility for the care of pregnant women who have recognized diseases or serious complications. Midwives are experts in normal pregnancy and in meeting the other needs of pregnant women—the needs that are not related to pathology" (1999: 370).

If obstetricians who practice according to the midwifery model, such as those of the Netherlands and Ontario, receive a client referred by a midwife for a risk or complication that later resolves, they will then *reclassify her as normal and refer her back to midwifery care* because they understand that normal birth is the midwife's specialty, while complicated conditions are theirs. Obstetricians are trained in how to manage complication and pathology; midwives are (or should be) trained in how to facilitate normal birth. Yet obstetricians in most countries increasingly seek to claim normal birth as their (lucrative) territory, and often use their legal claims on medical interventions and technologies to impede midwives' ability to provide care. For example, Japanese independent midwives have been placed in a catch-22 position: they are not legally allowed to perform episiotomies or administer pitocin without permission from their backup physician, but a recent change in the law requires that backup to be an obstetrician, and most obstetricians refuse to provide that service. This new situation reflects the power of income generation and the incentive physicians have to increase or retain their incomes, and it works to consolidate the hegemony of Japanese obstetrics and threaten the survival of the maternity homes, in spite of their excellent records—revealing the extreme fragility of birth models that work for mothers and babies but go against cultural trends.

Community-Based, Caseload, and One-to-One Midwifery: The Importance of Continuity of Care

As illustrated in all the chapters in this volume, MMOC practitioners are more likely to be community-based, even if they use hospitals for birth. Their woman-centered ideology is reflected in the priority they place on continuity of care. When continuity of care is reflected in employment models, these may be described as "team," "caseload," or "one-to-one" midwifery. The more common practice of hospital-based "shift midwifery" interferes with full provision of the humanistic model—midwives leave after eight or ten hours no matter where the mother is in labor, a situation that can feel disruptive to the laboring mother. This situation can also produce anxiety for the midwife, especially when the midwife who is leaving was providing the midwifery model of care and knows that the midwife replacing her will not, and that the mother will find the sudden switch to technocratic care an unpleasant shock that may interfere with her ability to give birth successfully. But even shift midwifery can constitute a model that works when all staff midwives practice the MMOC, as is demonstrated at the Lichfield Maternity Unit described in Chapter 6, where the departing midwife knows that her client will continue to receive the same kind of nurturant care that she was providing.

The Albany Midwifery Practice (Chapter 5) provides an excellent example of a caseload model of care, in which several midwives see the mother prenatally, getting to know her, and one of them is guaranteed to be present throughout her labor and birth. The Albany Practice offers continuity of midwifery care with two known midwives for each woman, providing antenatal, intrapartum, and postnatal care, as described in Chapter 5:

> Each whole caseload midwife looks after thirty-six women per year as a primary midwife and a further thirty-six women per year as a second midwife; each of the two half-caseload midwives looks after eighteen "primaries" and eighteen "seconds." We are on call for our own caseload at all times unless we are on vacation. . . . The primary midwife is responsible for the woman's midwifery care and provides an overview of her individual situation. . . . The second midwife also builds up a relationship with the woman, sharing her antenatal care. . . . Both of the woman's named midwives plan to attend the birth, the primary midwife calling the second when the birth is near or at any time she feels in need of support. . . . We are on call for the women up to twenty-eight days postnatally, and arrange to visit them at home when appropriate during this time.

It is important to note that this kind of research is coming out of the United Kingdom—a country that traditionally embraced continuity of carer by midwives until modern obstetrics took over, and is now struggling to return to some of its earlier, community-based practices.

As at St George Hospital in Sydney, a number of midwives have found that caseload midwifery is not only better for the mother but also for the midwife—there is less burnout than is found in the team model of care, in which a group of midwives share the care of a large number of women. Women in the team system are less likely to build close, continuous relationships with a particular midwife, and more likely to have midwives they do not know at their birth. The team model provides less continuity of carer and is associated with high levels of burnout for midwives.

One-to-one midwifery care means that the same midwife attends a pregnant woman throughout her prenatal, labor, and postpartum care. This ideal, however, is very difficult to achieve—midwives have families and busy lives and cannot always be present to one mother; caseload midwifery is the next best thing. As the Albany Practice demonstrates, in the great majority of cases, caseload midwifery does result in one-to-one care from a known midwife. The practitioners described in our book who attend births at home—including almost all midwives of the Netherlands and Ontario, a significant number in New Zealand, the traditional midwives of Samoa, the professional midwives of the United States, and those of CASA in Mexico— all often provide one-to-one care, as do most of the midwives (most of the time) who work in the freestanding birth centers described in these pages: the maternity homes of Japan, the Northern New Mexico Birth Center in Taos, and the Mercy in Action birth centers in the Philippines. A salient example of complete continuity of care is the obstetrician–midwife–doula practice in Porto Alegre, Brazil, in which the whole team stays with the mother for any kind of birth.

The phrase "the midwife follows the mother" means that the mother is free to choose her place of birth—home, freestanding birth center, or hospital—and the midwife will attend her there. This principle represents an evidence-based ideal that has always been the norm in the Netherlands and was one of the founding principles of the midwifery renaissance in New Zealand and Ontario, and of the Albany Practice in the United Kingdom. Various chapters in this book make it clear that homes and freestanding birth centers are the places where the MMOC can be most fully applied, and the excellent outcomes of these models as described in each chapter firmly demonstrate the safety of the practices of the skilled attendants who offer out-of-hospital care. And yet our chapters on hospital-based practices—St George in Sydney and the CASA hospital in Mexico—and the application of the humanistic model by midwives attending hospital births in the Netherlands, New Zealand, Ontario, Samoa, and the United States make it clear that the humanistic/midwifery approach can thrive in highly biomedical environments as well. Again, as Hodnett (2001, 2002) showed, *it is the ideology of the practitioner, not of the society, that has the greatest effect on an individual birth.*

Mutual Accommodation

"Mutual accommodation," a phrase coined by Brigitte Jordan (1993) to describe ideal relationships between medical practitioners and traditional midwives, also encapsulates the ideal relationship and position of the midwife vis-à-vis other systems and institutions: one where negotiation and respect govern the interactions that occur not only between colleagues who work around birth but also with community organizations and support systems that should form part of the family or women's networks. For example, the Taos midwives created a number of support groups for various types of women that later became community sponsored, facilitating the integration of the Taos model with the full community.

Mutually accommodative interactions are vital at both organizational and individual levels, and they must include out-of-hospital practitioners, who need not only effective forms of communication with biomedical systems but also efficient and inexpensive transport to hospitals in cases of need, and respectful and accommodative treatment upon arrival. As in Samoa and at the CASA Hospital in Mexico, traditional midwives who transport should continue to be included in their client's care to incorporate the information they bring and to provide continuity of emotional and social support.

A milestone in mutual accommodation occurred in 2004 when the International Federation of Gynecology and Obstetrics (FIGO), recognizing that midwifery has added important philosophical and practical elements to pregnancy and birthing practice, hired its first midwife. Maternal mortality concerns were driving the FIGO initiative, and Betty-Anne was taken on as project manager for their Safe Motherhood Program, a move regarded within FIGO as "glue" in the official relationship between FIGO and the International Confederation of Midwives (ICM). In addition, the hiring recognized not only that obstetrics and midwifery have an important relationship, but also that midwives have something to offer obstetricians, particularly regarding an evidence-based and humanistic approach to pregnancy and childbirth. A major part of Betty-Anne's work was to ensure that the proposals being submitted to FIGO for funding had the involvement of four key players: the country's obstetric society, its midwifery association(s), the Ministry of Health, and civil society. It has become an important step to ensure that midwives and obstetricians work together as a team for the empowerment of women and engage national ministries of health in the process.

Practitioner Education

Health care practitioners tend to practice as they were taught, so much so that when new information is presented, many long-time practitioners refuse to integrate or implement it because they are so habituated to doing things the way their teachers did (Davis-Floyd and St John 1998). A primary key to the creation and maintenance of birth models that work is the reform of professional education so that instead of being educated in the technology- and pathology-oriented biomedical approach to birth, student doctors, nurses, and midwives are educated in the humanistic and normality-oriented midwifery model of birth. Such education is exemplified in medical, midwifery, and nursing training in the Netherlands; in midwifery education in New Zealand and Ontario; at the CASA School in Mexico and in many U.S. midwifery programs (see Chapters 9 and 15); and in Samoa, where the best features of both traditional and professional midwifery are incorporated into an integrated, university-based degree that involves traditional midwives as teachers in the program.

In most of the other models that work described in this volume, the practitioners were educated in more biomedical and technocratic approaches but overcame these strong influences through exposure to a different model in the settings where they came to work. The British midwives presently working in the Albany Practice and the Lichfield Birth Center, and the Australian midwives at St George. were originally trained in the standard British and Australian midwifery systems, which have traditionally been known to be rigid, hierarchical, and very medically oriented. Yet they still found within themselves the knowledge and ability to re-socialize themselves into a much more humanistic approach, as did Brazilian obstetrician

Ricardo Jones and the Japanese midwives who have left the medical system to practice independently in maternity homes.

Sustainability: The Importance of Effective Leadership

Sustainability depends in large part on economic stability. For small-scale birth models that work, financial viability and sustainability can be extremely difficult to achieve. They must include a cost-effective mix of skills, technology use, setting, and sufficient salaries for staff. Having enough money to operate is an ongoing problem for the Northern New Mexico Women's Health and Birth Center in Taos, and the continued success of the CASA School and Mercy in Action depends on ongoing fundraising. Brazilian obstetrician Ricardo Jones accepts much lower fees for the home births he attends than his hospital-based obstetrical colleagues would dream of doing, and his volume of births is much lower than theirs because attending home birth takes much more time, limiting the number of clients he can accept—a situation equally true for the home birth midwives of the United States. Around the world, dozens if not hundreds of small-scale models that work have operated for a while and then ceased to exist because of financial non-viability. The second volume in this series will examine some of these.

In dramatic contrast, large-scale national systems like those of the Netherlands, New Zealand, and Samoa, and the provincial system of Ontario, are government funded and thus financially secure, as are some of the small-scale models in our book such as the Albany Practice. Full government funding of maternity care precludes the opportunity for private practitioners to make large incomes. In contrast, the chapters on Brazil show us the dramatic dichotomy that results when both public- and private-sector maternity services are available, and it also points up the tension within the humanistic paradigm between superficial and deep humanism: public-sector mothers may be treated in dehumanizing ways in Brazil's large public hospitals yet have normal vaginal births, and private-sector mothers usually receive nonindicated yet caring cesareans.

Sustainability also depends on staff and organizational structure. In all cases, effective leadership is key. None of the models that work presented in these pages would exist without strong leaders, who hold a vision and work hard to generate a cultural space for its existence. Even the long-established Dutch midwives need such leadership: conditions of overwork and underpay and a falling home birth rate led them to galvanize themselves during the 1990s to revitalize their system—a successful effort in which Chapter 1 co-author Beatrijs Smulders played a key role. At St George in Sydney, a few determined leaders, including chapter authors Pat Brodie and Caroline Homer, were able to effect significant and long-term change through consistent efforts and team building. Lesley Barclay, working in collaboration with strong local midwives, was instrumental in creating effective systems of communication and referral among the traditional and professional midwives of Samoa. Vicki Penwell brought mother- and baby-friendly birth centers to the Philippines. Nadine Goodman dreamed and then created the CASA Hospital and school. One new director at the Lichfield Maternity Unit was primary in effecting the needed culture change.

Of course, none of these leaders acted alone. In all our models, we note that the kind of leadership employed so effectively is what Denis Walsh describes in Chapter 6 as "a postmodern leadership style":

> Prior to [Helen's] coming, the staff structure was very hierarchical and relationships with the women and each other were formal and deferential. Anita . . . addressed staff by their first names . . . introduced informal visits for women considering booking at the center. . . . She relaxed the institutional feel of the center by deregulating visiting times and abandoning maternal postnatal observations and morning routines like bed making. She brought in midwifery-led care by negotiating the withdrawal of GPs from intrapartum care and the setting up of an antenatal clinic at the unit, run by the midwives. She continued the refurbishment of the unit and deregulated staff work patterns. In all of these initiatives, she used a variety of methods in bringing about change. She worked with a supportive GP who mediated the changes in GP practice. For clinical changes, she used a combination of explaining her rationale and leading by example. Other staff were especially interested in upgrading the décor, and she gave them the freedom to lead this initiative. She built a team ethos by organizing regular social outings and shared, fund-raising activities. She eschewed role demarcations by encouraging all staff to be involved in the upkeep and cleanliness of the facility. . . . "She would never say to us, could you make them a cup of tea? She would clean the kitchen out just like the rest of us." . . . Over time, older members of staff who did not like the changes Anita instituted left to be replaced with new ones who were inducted into the new philosophy.

Walsh notes that characteristics of this postmodern leadership style include flexibility, an integrated and team-based approach, a value placed on diversity, empowerment of others, change as a constant, and a focus on people and relationships instead of places and things. His findings resonate with Davis-Floyd's description of the "postmodern midwife":

> With this term, I am trying to highlight the qualities that emerge from the practice, the discourse, and the political engagement of a certain kind of contemporary midwife—one who often constructs a radical critique of unexamined conventions and univariate assumptions. Postmodern midwives as I define them are relativistic, articulate, organized, political, and highly conscious of both their cultural uniqueness and their global importance. . . . Postmodern midwives are scientifically informed: they know the limitations and strengths of the biomedical system and of their own, and they can move fluidly between them. These midwives play with the paradigms, working to ensure that the

uniquely woman-centered dimensions of midwifery are not subsumed by bio-medicine. They are shape-shifters, knowing how to subvert the medical system while appearing to comply with it, bridge-builders, making alliances with bio-medicine where possible, and networkers . . . [with a sense of mission around preserving and growing midwifery], and an understanding that *for a midwife, the professional is always political:* midwives and their colleagues must have an organized political voice if they are to survive. So postmodern midwives work to build organizations in their communities, join national and international midwifery organizations, and work within them for policies and legislation that support midwives and the mothers they attend. (Davis-Floyd 2005)

Postmodern midwifery and postmodern leadership as Robbie and Denis describe them are profoundly characteristic of birth models that work. This brand of postmodernism, eschewing hierarchy in favor of relationship and rigidity in favor of flexibility, encourages the levels of creativity, generativity, and out-of-box thinking that are essential to transcending the limits of the technocratic medical model in favor of what really works.

Those who have been part of reform understand this well and are politi-cally astute observers of the environment, trying to "risk proof" their new models as much as is possible. In Chapter 2, Chris Hendry describes how the members of the College of Midwives in New Zealand have preserved and protected their gains over a decade in efforts to stay ahead strategi-cally in a volatile policy environment, as have Nadine Goodman, founder of CASA; Vicki Penwell, founder of Mercy in Action; and all the rest of our chapter authors. No founder of a model that works can bury her head in the sand just because it is working at present; birth practices are heavily influenced by hegemonic forces, and counteracting those forces requires patience, vigilance, and constant, proactive effort.

In such work, the participation of consumers is extraordinarily impor-tant. When the Lichfield unit was scheduled to be closed, it was the large numbers of orange-ballooned consumers who saved the day. Consumer involvement in the New Zealand College of Midwives and consumer sup-port for the Ontario midwives, Dutch midwives, the Japanese maternity homes, the CASA hospital and midwifery school, and the Taos practice have played a large role in their success. And the American midwives described in Chapter 15, who are generally marginal in the country as a whole and have to work hard to preserve any gains they achieve, have frequently benefited from and depend heavily on consumer activism and support.

SUMMARY

The birth models that work presented in this volume are (1) ideologi-cally and practically based on the midwifery (humanistic/holistic) model of care—a model that can be adopted and applied by any and all birth practitioners; and (2) are possible, sustainable, replicable, and fragile. They produce far better outcomes for mothers and babies than standard, hegemonic technocratic practices. Their fragility highlights the need for more attention to and valuation of such models. We urge further study of these and other models that work, their replication, and the designing and dissemination of similar models that work.

Birth models that work improve the physiological, psychological, and social outcomes of pregnancy and birth and save money for systems and families. They expose the need for the total reform of existing dysfunctional, hegemonic models. They issue a clarion call to global health organizations, nongovernmental organizations, and individuals to replace birth models that don't work with those that do, at local, regional, and global levels, in order to reduce maternal and perinatal mortality and morbidity, empower women and their families, and facilitate healthy birth and breastfeeding. The end game is healthy mothers and babies who can generate a more conscious and sustainable future for our human family. The models that we have presented in this volume are paving and lighting the way toward this goal.

APPENDIX C.1. THE MEDICAL (TECHNOCRATIC)
AND MIDWIFERY (HUMANISTIC AND HOLISTIC)
MODELS OF BIRTH

The technocratic model of birth	*The holistic model of birth*
male perspective	female perspective
male-centered	female-centered
woman = object	woman = subject
male body = norm	female body = norm
female = defective male	female normal in own terms
classifying, separating approach	holistic, integrating approach
mind is above, separate from body	mind and body are one
body = machine	body = organism, energy field
female body = defective machine	female body = healthy organism
female reproductive processes dysfunctional	female reproductive processes normal, healthy
pregnancy and birth inherently pathological	pregnancy and birth inherently healthy, normal
doctor = technician	midwife = nurturer, guide
hospital = factory	nurturing psychosphere essential for birth
baby = product	mother/baby inseparable unit
baby grows itself through mechanical process	intimate connection between growth of baby and state of mother
fetus is separate from mother	baby and mother are one
safety of fetus pitted against emotional needs of mother	safety and emotional needs of mother and baby are the same
best interests of mother and fetus antagonistic	good for mother = good for child
supremacy of technology	sufficiency of nature
importance of science, things	importance of people
institution = significant social unit	family = essential social unit
action based on facts, measurements	action also based on body knowledge and intuition
only technical knowledge is valued	experiential and emotional knowledge valued as highly as or more than technical knowledge

(continued)

APPENDIX C.1. *(continued)*

The technocratic model of birth	*The holistic model of birth*
appropriate prenatal care is objective, scientific	best prenatal care stresses subjective empathy, caring
health of baby during pregnancy ensured through drugs, tests, techniques	health of baby ensured through physical and emotional health of mother, attunement to baby
labor = a mechanical process	labor = a flow of experience
uterus = an involuntary muscle	uterus = responsive part of whole
adherence to time charts	flow of experience
birth must happen within a specified period	labors can be short or can take several days
once labor begins, it should progress steadily; if it doesn't, intervention necessary	labor can stop and start, follow its own rhythms of speeding up and slowing down
some medical intervention necessary in all births	facilitation (proper food, effective positioning, support) is appropriate; medical intervention usually inappropriate
environmental ambience is not relevant	environmental ambience— the psychosphere—is the key to safe birth
woman in bed hooked up to machines with frequent exams by staff is appropriate	woman doing what she feels like—movement, sexual play, eating, sleeping—is appropriate
labor pain is problematic, unacceptable	labor pain is acceptable, normal, valuable
analgesia and anesthesia for pain during labor	mind/body integration, labor support for pain
iatrogenic pain and damage are acceptable	practitioner must strive not to cause pain or damage to the woman
unusual presentations, such as breech, require severe intervention, usually cesarean	midwifery techniques for unusual presentations (e.g., external version or delivery on hands and knees for breech)

APPENDIX C.1. *(continued)*

The technocratic model of birth	*The holistic model of birth*
birth = a service medicine owns and supplies to society	birth = an activity a woman does that brings new life
tradition-based practice	evidence-based practice
segmentation of care	continuity of care
lack of learning from reflection	focus on reflection that encourages change
hierarchy, dominance of biomedicine	flexibility and mutual accommodation between practitioners and systems of knowledge
obstetrician = supervisor/ manager/skilled technician	midwife = skillful guide
doctor controls	midwife supports, assists
doctor delivers the baby	mother gives birth to the baby
biomedicine counts	all knowledge systems count and are taken into account from a position of informed relativism
biomedical dominance	effective, mutually respectful collaboration
practice to maximize profit	income important but the needs of the mother and baby come first
practitioner socialization and education in traditional medicine	practitioner socialization and education in the MMOC
hegemonic and thus easily sustainable	counterhegemonic, fragile
the system sustains itself	effective leadership and team commitment to the MMOC can generate sustainable models as long as the team remains committed, the outcomes are good, and the leaders retain effectiveness
some degree of financial viability within the system	financial viability an ongoing challenge
unquestionably modernist orientation	relativistic, postmodern orientation

(continued)

APPENDIX C.1. *(continued)*

The technocratic model of birth	*The holistic model of birth*
only biomedical knowledge counts	multiple knowledge systems count, including the best of biomedicine, evidence-based care, professional midwifery knowledge, and alternative and indigenous knowledge systems
there is power in organization	there is power in organization and networks that can challenge accepted practice and support the MMOC
consumer participation is irrelevant	consumer participation is essential to the promotion of the MMOC
professionalization is key	professionalization is essential but so is generating a movement with consumer participation
social power and its preservation lie in the political realm	power and its preservation lie in the political realm

Source: Adapted and expanded from *Birth as an American Rite of Passage* by Robbie Davis-Floyd (1992), 140–41.

APPENDIX C.2. THE TECHNOCRATIC, HUMANISTIC, AND HOLISTIC MODELS OF MEDICINE

The technocratic model of medicine	*The humanistic (biopsychosocial) model of medicine*	*The holistic model of medicine*
1. Mind/body separation	1. Mind-body connection	1. Oneness of body-mind-spirit
2. The body as machine	2. The body as an organism	2. The body as an energy system interlinked with other energy systems
3. The patient as object	3. The patient as relational subject	3. Healing the whole person in whole-life context
4. Alienation of practitioner from patient	4. Connection and mutual respect between practitioner and patient	4. Essential unity of practitioner and client
5. Diagnosis and treatment from the outside in (curing disease, repairing dysfunction)	5. Diagnosis and healing from the outside in and from the inside out	5. Diagnosis and healing from the inside out
6. Hierarchical organization and standardization of care	6. Balance between the needs of the institution and those of the individual	6. Individualization of care and lateral, webbed organizational structure
7. Authority and responsibility inherent in practitioner, not patient	7. Information, decision making, and responsibility shared between patient and practitioner	7. Authority and responsibility inherent in each individual
8. Supervaluation of science and technology	8. Science and technology counterbalanced with humanism	8. Science and technology placed at the service of the individual
9. Aggressive intervention with emphasis on short-term results	9. Focus on disease prevention	9. A long-term focus on creating and maintaining health and well-being
10. Death as defeat	10. Death as an acceptable outcome	10. Death as a step in a process
11. Insistence on the superiority of technomedicine and intolerance of other modalities	11. Technomedicine as the baseline, with open-mindedness toward other modalities	11. Healing as the focus
12. A profit-driven system	12. Compassion-driven care	12. Embrace of multiple healing modalities
Basic underlying principle: Separation	Basic underlying principles: Balance and connection	Basic underlying principles: Connection and integration
Type of thinking: Unimodal, left-brained, linear	*Type of thinking: Bimodal*	*Type of thinking: Fluid, multimodal, right-brained*

Source: Adapted from *From Doctor to Healer: The Transformative Journey,* by Robbie Davis-Floyd and Gloria St John (1998), 142–43.

APPENDIX C.3. THE MEDICAL SPECTRUM

Technocratic Model	>>>>><<<<	Humanistic Model	>>>><<<<	Holistic Model

REFERENCES

Davis-Floyd, R. 2001. "The Technocratic, Humanistic, and Holistic Models of Birth." *International Journal of Gynecology and Obstetrics* 75, Suppl. no. 1:S5–S23.

———. 2003. "Home Birth Emergencies in the U.S. and Mexico: The Trouble with Transport." *Social Science and Medicine* 56.9: 1913–31.

———. 2004 [1992]. *Birth as an American Rite of Passage*. Berkeley and London: University of California Press.

———. 2005. "Daughter of Time: The Postmodern Midwife." *MIDIRS Midwifery Digest* 15.1:32–39.

Davis-Floyd, R., and E. Davis. 1997. "Intuition as Authoritative Knowledge in Midwifery and Home Birth." In *Childbirth and Authoritative Knowledge: Cross-Cultural Perspectives*, edited by R. Davis-Floyd and C. Sargent, 315–49. Berkeley and London: University of California Press.

Davis-Floyd, R., and G. St John. 1998. *From Doctor to Healer: The Transformative Journey*. New Brunswick, NJ: Rutgers University Press.

Hodnett, Ellen D. 2001. "Caregiver Support for Women During Childbirth." *Cochrane Library*, Issue 4. Cochrane Database Syst Rev. 2002;(1):CD000199.

———. 2002. "Pain and Women's Satisfaction with the Experience of Childbirth: A Systematic Review." *American Journal of Obstetrics and Gynecology* 186.5: S160–S172.

Houston, J., J. Foster, A. Davenport, A. Anderson, A. Romano, V. Lamprecht, and G. Frenkel. N.d. "Weaving Traditional and Professional Midwifery: Midwives for Midwives in Guatemala." Unpublished manuscript.

International MotherBaby Childbirth Organization (IMBCO). 2008. *The International MotherBaby Childbirth Initiative: 10 Steps to Optimal MotherBaby Maternity Services*. Chapel Hill, NC: IMBCO. http://www.imbci.org/USERIMAGES/File/IMBCI%20%20%2004-05-08.pdf. Accessed November 17, 2008.

Jordan, B. 1993. *Birth in Four Cultures*. Prospect Heights, Ohio: Waveland Press.

Rooks, J. 1999. "The Midwifery Model of Care." *Journal of Nurse-Midwifery* 44.4: 370–74.

Rothman, B. K. 1982. *In Labor: Women and Power in the Birthplace*. New York: W. W. Norton.

Sandall, J. 1997. "Midwives' Burnout and Continuity of Care." *British Journal of Midwifery* 5.2:106–11.

Wagner, M. 1994. *Pursuing the Birth Machine*. Australia: Ace Graphics.

Witz, A. 1992. *Professions and Patriarchy*. London: Routledge.

EDITORS

Robbie Davis-Floyd, PhD, senior research fellow, Department of Anthropology, University of Texas–Austin, and Fellow of the Society for Applied Anthropology, is a medical anthropologist specializing in the anthropology of reproduction. An international speaker and researcher, she is author of over eighty articles and of *Birth as an American Rite of Passage* (1992, 2004); co-author of *From Doctor to Healer: The Transformative Journey* (1998); and co-editor of eight collections, including *Childbirth and Authoritative Knowledge: Cross-Cultural Perspectives* (1997); *Cyborg Babies: From Techno-Sex to Techno-Tots* (1998); and *Mainstreaming Midwives: The Politics of Change* (2006). Her research on global trends and transformations in childbirth, obstetrics, and midwifery is ongoing. She speaks regularly at universities and conferences around the world. She currently serves as senior advisor to the Council on Anthropology and Reproduction and editor for the International MotherBaby Childbirth Initiative. E-mail: davis-floyd@mail.utexas.edu.

Lesley Barclay, RM, PhD, is a midwife who has worked as a clinician, midwife educator, and researcher. She serves as foundation director and professor at the Centre for Family Health and Midwifery at the University of Technology–Sydney. Her work focuses on improving knowledge, services, and policy supporting the health and parenting experiences of women and their families. She does this as a researcher and through educating others, as well as through policy leadership and systems improvement. Her research has been supported by twenty-eight grants in the past fifteen years, many from prestigious granting bodies. Lesley also provides research-oriented consultancies for national and international governments; she leads "development" projects for the World Health Organization, AusAID, and the World Bank. With her students and others, she has published twenty-five refereed journal articles and fourteen major reports for governments in the past five years and has co-authored a number of books, including *Samoan Nursing: The Story of Women Developing a Profession* (1998); *Constructing Fatherhood: Discourses and Experiences* (1997); and *Midwifery: Trends and Practices in Australia* (1996). Her most recent co-authored book is *Midwives' Tales: Stories of Social and Professional Birthing in Samoa* (2005). E-mail: lesley.barclay@cdu.edu.au.

Betty-Anne Daviss, RM, MA, BJ, is a midwife who has worked on five continents in over thirty years. As adjunct professor at the Pauline Jewett Institute of Women's Studies, Carleton University, Ottawa, Canada, she teaches social movement theory and midwifery history. She was involved with midwifery legislation in Canada, particularly in Quebec and Ontario, after three years of work as a midwife in Alabama, giving her a unique Canadian and American perspective. Her ethnographic work is mixed with strategizing for change among the Inuit in northern Canada, the traditional midwives in Guatemala and Afghanistan, and the Eastern European midwives, particularly in Hungary. Among her epidemiologic investigations, she considers the largest prospective home birth study ever to be published (*British Medical Journal* 2005) one of her proudest achievements. She is chair of the International Bureau of the Canadian Association of Midwives and was the first midwife to be hired by the International Federation of Gynecology and Obstetrics, serving as project manager for its Safe Motherhood Program. E-mail: betty-anne@rogers.com.

Jan Tritten is founder and editor-in-chief of *Midwifery Today* magazine and *The BirthKit* newsletter, author of over one hundred articles and editorials, and co-editor of *Getting an Education: Paths to Becoming a Midwife* (1998, 2003). She became a home birth midwife twenty-seven years ago. She hosts two to three *Midwifery Today* conferences per year in cities around the world, maintains an international networking midwifery database, gives frequent talks, and is internationally renowned as a unifying figure in midwifery and a key organizer of the global development of midwifery as both social movement and profession. She is founder of the International Alliance of Midwives (IAM), an online organization for networking and support that maintains a list of country contacts for fifty-six different countries with links to birth websites in those countries. The quarterly electronic newsletter for this organization can be accessed at www.midwiferytoday.com/iam. Jan has organized forty-five Midwifery Today conferences in over twelve different countries from 1992 through the present, many on international issues and all with international classes. E-mail: jan@midwiferytoday.com.

CONTRIBUTORS

Isa Paula Hamouche Abreu, MD, specializes in public health and Chinese traditional medicine. From 2000 to 2007 she was responsible for the program Working with Traditional Midwives through the Women's Health Program, Ministry of Health, Brazil. She was also one of the instructors of the seminars.

Maria José de Oliveira Araújo, MD, is resident in general pediatrics and neonatology at the Instituto Fernandes Figueira of the Oswaldo Cruz Foundation. She specialized in maternal and child health at the University of Paris–Sorbonne. She served as transmissible diseases epidemiologist in maternal and child health at the Institute Pasteur, Paris, and as primary health care gynecologist at the Dispensaire des Femmes, Geneva, Switzerland. She is the founder of the Latin American and Caribbean Network of Women's Health (Red de Salud de las Mujeres Llatinoamericanas e del Caribe) (RSMLAC) and of the Brazilian Feminist Network for Sexual and Reproductive Rights (Rede Nacional Feminista de Saude Direitos Sexuais e Direitos Reprodutivos). From 2003 to May 2007, she was the national coordinator of the Women's Health Program of the Ministry of Health, Brazil, when the seminar project was launched.

Ivy Lynn Bourgeault, PhD, is associate professor (sociology/health, aging, and society) and Canada Research Chair in Comparative Health Labour Policy at McMaster University. As a medical sociologist, Ivy specializes in the study of health professions and health policy from a gender perspective, as well as women's health, carework, complementary and alternative health care, and qualitative health research. Her doctoral research examined the integration of midwifery in the province of Ontario, which she followed with an examination of this policy's impact in Ontario and British Columbia for her postdoctoral fellowship. Ivy has published extensively in national and international journals on midwifery and maternity care in Canada as well as in the United States, contributing to two chapters in the international edited volume *Birth by Design,* co-editing *Reconceiving Midwifery* with Cecilia Benoit and Robbie Davis-Floyd, and publishing her own book, *Push! The Struggle to Integrate Midwifery in Ontario* (2006). Ivy is a member of the board of the International Sociology Association Research Committees on Medical Sociology and Professional Groups, serves on the National Steering Committee on Rural and Remote Women's Health, and is the scientific officer of the Canadian Institutes of Health Research Gender, Sex and Health Peer Review Committee. E-mail: bourgea@mcmaster.ca.

Pat Brodie, RN, RM, MN, DM, is professor of midwifery practice development and research in the Sydney South West Area Health Service and the University of Technology–Sydney, which sees her engaged in multiple strategies of practice and policy reform that aim to increase the involvement of midwives as primary carers and enhance continuity of care. Pat is passionately committed to strengthening midwifery through improved education, regulation, and the use of collaborative models of care that place women at the center. She is the current national president of the Australian College of Midwives and has been engaged in midwifery practice, education, management, and research for over twenty-five years. E-mail: p.brodie@bigpond.com.

Raymond De Vries, PhD, is a member of the Bioethics Program, the Department of Obstetrics and Gynecology, and the Department of Medical Education at the Medical School, University of Michigan. He is the author of *A Pleasing Birth: Midwifery and Maternity Care in the Netherlands* (2005), and co-editor of *The View from Here: Bioethics and the Social Sciences* (2007). His current research is focused on the regulation of science; clinical trials of genetic therapies and deep brain stimulation; international research ethics; and the social, ethical, and policy issues associated with voluntary cesarean section. E-mail: devries@med.umn.edu.

Adson Roberto França Santos, MD, MA, is an obstetrician and gynecologist, with the World Health Organization (WHO). He has specialized in sexology with the Latin American Society of Sexology and Sexual Education; in ultrasound with the Brazilian Medical Association and Brazilian College of Radiology; in obstetrics and neonatal pediatrics with the Institute of Perinatology of Bahia (IPERBA); in fetal medicine at the Kings College School, United Kingdom; in gynecological surgery at the Saint Antoine School of Medicine, France; in high-risk gestation and image diagnosis at the School of Medicine of Valencia, Spain; in gynecological microsurgery, endoscopy, and laser at the Hospital Gineco-Obstétrico Ramon Gonzalez Covo, Havana, Cuba; in diagnosis and treatment of uterine cervix pre-malignant lesions at the Hospital Materno Infantil 10 de octubre, Havana, Cuba; and in risk approach in perinatal health at the Hospital Gineco-Obstétrico America Arias, Havana, Cuba. Adson França has worked for ten years as researcher and consultant on women's health for the WHO Committee of Studies in Women's Health. He also was the substitute director of the Department of Programmatic and Strategic Actions of the Brazilian Ministry of Health and currently is the national coordinator of the Brazilian Pact for the Reduction of the Maternal and Neonatal Deaths. He has helped to shape the strategy of the seminars and has been one of the instructors.

Elizabeth Gilmore was born in New York and raised in Mexico. She planned to be a teacher for Spanish-speaking children who needed to learn

English. Pregnancy changed her life when she tried to obtain the home birth in Massachusetts in 1970 that she could have gotten in Mexico. Doctors told her she was either suicidal or hated her baby: "We don't squat in some field in the USA; we go to nice, clean hospitals to have our babies with expert doctors." This attitude sent her on a journey to find a cheerful, friendly, gentle birth at home for herself and friends, and finally for all the mothers in Taos where she moved in 1977. During her journey over the last forty years, she started a birth center, a midwifery college, and an accrediting agency for midwifery schools while providing clinical midwifery care in mothers' homes and in the birth center. In addition, she has been a community leader in the field of maternal and child health through her continual service on the local coalitions for health organizations in Taos. Her experiences have been characterized by the constant challenge to change, to be flexible and creative in order to successfully address the complex needs of mothers, babies, and their families. Her story of models that work reflects an astonishing capacity for trying and accomplishing many approaches for helping families and midwives. E-mail: bettygilmore@gmail.com.

Chris Hendry, PhD, NZRN, RM, BA (Canterbury), MPH (Otago), DMid (Sydney), has been a midwife in New Zealand for over thirty years, working in a variety of roles and settings. Career highlights include establishing one of the first stand-alone diploma in midwifery (pre-registration) programs in New Zealand in 1991; setting up one of the first hospital-based continuity of midwifery care services in 1994; completion of a midwifery doctorate focusing on the organization of maternity services by midwives; completion of maternity service reviews and development of strategic plans for maternity services for district health boards; and taking responsibility for the strategic national development of the Midwifery and Maternity Provider Organisation (MMPO) in 2002 for the New Zealand College of Midwives. This organization provides self-employed midwives throughout the country with access to reliable practice management services (www.mmpo.org.nz). Chris works in a number of roles as a consultant and advisor in maternity service development throughout New Zealand. Currently, she serves as executive director of the MMPO and acting midwifery advisor for the MidCentral District Health Board, having facilitated a strategic review of maternity services in the region (www.midcentral.co.nz). E-mail: hendry@netaccess.co.nz.

Fumiko Hinokuma, RN, RM, MsocSc, is professor of Midwifery at the Graduate School of Health Sciences in the Research Institute of Health and Welfare Science, Tochigi, Japan. She is currently undertaking qualitative research on intersubjectivity in Japanese maternity homes and is the organizer of the Normal Childbirth Conference held every two years in Japan, with the aim of reevaluating normal childbirth. She hopes to establish a midwife-led care system within Japanese perinatal care. She is co-author of *Umu, Umanai, Umenai* [Can't Have, Won't Have, Will Have a Baby] (2007). E-mail: Bhnkm@iuhw.ac.jp.

Caroline Homer, RM, PhD, is professor of midwifery at the University of Technology–Sydney. She was previously the midwifery consultant in practice development at St George Hospital. Caroline has been researching the effectiveness of midwifery continuity of care for some years. She continues to provide continuity of care to a small group of women through St George Hospital. E-mail: Caroline.Homer@uts.edu.au.

Rima Jolivet, CNM, MPH, worked as a childbirth educator, a doula, and an interpreter for non-English-speaking women in labor; a breastfeeding counselor; and then a lactation consultant before becoming a midwife. She has practiced in a variety of settings, including federally qualified health centers, private and hospital-based practices, birth centers, a home birth practice, and a large government teaching hospital, where she was interim patient safety director. She received a master's degree in public health in 2005 and is currently working to complete her doctorate. Rima joined Childbirth Connection as associate director of programs in 2007. Prior to that, she was senior technical advisor in the Department of Professional Services at the American College of Nurse-Midwives, specializing in the areas of quality improvement and patient safety. She is on the teaching faculty of the Centering Healthcare Institute and leads training workshops in the CenteringPregnancy® model of group prenatal care around the USA. Rima lives in the suburban Washington, D.C., area with her teenage son, Lucas. E-mail: rima.jolivet@usa.net.

Ricardo Herbert Jones, MD, specializes in gynecology, obstetrics, and homeopathy and is an international speaker on the humanization of birth. He graduated in medicine from the Universidade Federal do Rio Grande do Sul (Federal University of Rio Grande do Sul) in 1985 and completed his medical residency in obstetrics and gynecology in 1987. He obtained postgraduate education in homeopathy in 1994. He has served as a board member of the Brazilian Humanization of Childbirth Network (ReHuNa), vice president of the Homeopathic League of Rio Grande do Sul, medical advisor to HumPar (the Portuguese Association for the Humanization of Birth) and to ANDO (National Association of Doulas), the representative of IMBCO (International MotherBaby Friendly Organization) to Brazil, and collaborator in the development of the International MotherBaby Childbirth Initiative. In his book *Memoirs of the Man Made of Glass* (2004), which was written in Portuguese and has been translated into Spanish, English, and German, he describes his personal transformative journey into a feminine approach to birth and discusses the foundations of technocracy in the Western world. He lives and attends births with his wife, Zeza, a nurse-midwife, in Porto Alegre in the south of Brazil. They have two children— Lucas (age twenty-four) and Isabel (age twenty). E-mail: rhjones@superig. com.br.

Holly Powell Kennedy, PhD, entered the U.S. Army Nurse Corps in 1972, retiring as a colonel after thirty-one years of active and reserve service. Her experience as a student in obstetrical nursing was during an era when women received shaves, preps, enemas, and mind-numbing drugs, and it was never a specialty she contemplated. However, during her education as a family nurse practitioner at the Medical College of Georgia, she completed an internship at the Frontier School of Midwifery and Family Nursing (FSMFN). It was there that she first saw midwives in practice and realized that this was her future. She completed her midwifery education at FSMFN and has practiced in Kentucky, Vermont, Massachusetts, Rhode Island, and California. She has dedicated her career to midwifery practice, education, and research for the past twenty-two years. Dr. Kennedy helped establish the graduate program in nurse-midwifery at the University of Rhode Island in 1993, where she completed her PhD in nursing. She established a faculty practice at Memorial Hospital in Pawtucket, Rhode Island, and received a Governor's Citation for her service in primary care in that state. She is currently an associate professor at the University of California– San Francisco, where she is the co-director of the nurse-midwifery educational program. Dr. Kennedy is best known for her research linking midwifery practice to outcomes and for her leadership in the profession of midwifery. Her model of midwifery care is used by many educational programs, and she is recognized internationally for her support of normal birth. E-mail: holly.kennedy@nursing.ucsf.edu.

Margaret E. MacDonald, PhD, is assistant professor of anthropology at York University. She is a medical anthropologist specializing in gender and health with particular interests in women's reproductive health. Her new book *At Work in the Field of Birth: Midwifery Narratives of Nature, Tradition and Home* (2007) is an ethnographic account of contemporary midwifery in Ontario in the wake of its historic transition from the margins as a grassroots social movement to a profession within the public health care system. She is also engaged in a study on the impact of international maternal and infant health policy and programs on traditional birth attendants and birthing women in Africa. E-mail: maggie@yorku.ca.

Etsuko Matsuoka, PhD, is associate professor of anthropology at Asahikawa Medical College. She has conducted anthropological fieldwork in Europe and Asia, focusing on traditional reproductive customs, birth attendants, and cultural aspects of modern hospital births. She is currently undertaking comparative research on reproductive changes in rapidly modernizing Asian countries, and is especially interested in postpartum blues and depression and the effect sleep patterns have on them. E-mail: matsuoka@asahikawa-med.ac.jp.

Lisa Mills, PhD, is assistant professor in the School of Public Policy and Administration, Carleton University, Ottawa, Canada. She is currently working on a book-length manuscript on local midwifery advocacy, maternal health, and the politics of health sector reform in Mexico. E-mail: lisa_mills@carleton.ca.

Vicki Penwell, CPM, MS, has been a midwife for twenty-seven years. Originally self-taught in Alaska, she went on to earn a master's degree in midwifery and state licenses in Alaska and New Mexico, as well as becoming a certified professional midwife (CPM). Vicki and her husband, Scott, founded Mercy in Action, a nonprofit, Christian charity, and live in the Philippines as medical missionaries working on projects to bring humanitarian aid in the area of maternal and child health. She has established five birth centers in the Philippines and helped deliver more than 12,000 babies free of charge for the poorest of the poor. Scott and Vicki have three grown sons, who are all training in different branches of medicine with visions to care for the poor, and two daughters-in-law who are midwives. Vicki continues to train midwives, attend births, and speak all over the world about social justice and maternal/child health care while working on her doctorate in midwifery. E-mail: vickipenwell@ gmail.com.

Daphne Rattner, MD, MPH, PhD in epidemiology at the University of North Carolina, specialized in public health and tropical diseases at the University of São Paulo; in hospital and health services administration at the Fundação Getúlio Vargas; in community-oriented primary health care at Hebrew University, Israel; and in primary health care, policy, planning and politics of health in development at the University of Sussex, United Kingdom. She served as national coordinator of the Rede Nacional pela Humanização do Parto e Nascimento (Brazilian Network for the Humanization of Childbirth) (ReHuNa) from 2000 to 2004. Daphne organized the book *Humanizando Nascimentos e Partos* (2005). She currently works for the Brazilian Ministry of Health in the Women's Health, and served as one of the instructors in the Seminars described in her chapter. E-mail: daphne@isaude.sp.gov.br.

Rebecca (Becky) Reed, BA (Hons), SRN, RM, works as an individual caseload midwife in the Albany Midwifery Practice, South East London, England. Continuity of carer is her passion, as well as keeping birth normal, home birth, and water birth. She helped to set up the South East London Midwifery Group Practice in 1994, and has worked in the Albany Practice since it started in 1997. Becky writes regularly for *The Practising Midwife* (UK) and has contributed to other midwifery publications. She is currently working on "The 2000 Women Study," looking at outcomes for mothers and babies from the Albany Practice. She lectures on the Albany Practice model both nationally and internationally. Becky has four children and two grandchildren; both of the latter were born at home in a pool with their Grandma as their midwife. E-mail: rebecca-reed@hotmail.co.uk.

Sharon Schindler Rising is a certified nurse-midwife who graduated from the Yale School of Nursing, taught on the faculty there, and then established the graduate nurse-midwifery program and the Childbearing Childrearing Center at the University of Minnesota. In 1993–94 she developed and piloted the CenteringPregnancy® Program in Waterbury, Connecticut, and began doing instructional workshops nationally and internationally. She is the executive director of the Centering Pregnancy and Parenting Association (CPPA), a nonprofit organization dedicated to the promotion of the Centering model of group care to providers and parents. She also is on the clinical nursing faculty at the Yale School of Nursing. Sharon has had over thirty years' experience in providing midwifery care to pregnant women and their families. She has led prenatal education groups, mother/baby groups, and parenting groups. Listening to the stories of the women and realizing the common themes helped her to change the care paradigm to one in which women, rather than the provider, became the major support for each other. The CenteringPregnancy® model is one of community building and empowerment, a powerful way to give and receive care for women/couples and for providers. E-mail: rising@centeringpregnancy.org.

Beatrijs Smulders has been a practicing independent midwife in the Netherlands since 1978 and has played a leading role in the development of modern obstetrics in that country. In 1983 she co-designed Birth-Mate, a popular, lightweight plastic birthing stool as part of a campaign to promote active birth in the Netherlands. She has co-produced numerous films about the Dutch obstetrical system and home birth, and has served as keynote speaker at many national and international conferences. From 1988 to 1991, she served as vice president of the Dutch Association of Midwives and became known as their spokeswoman. In 1992 she founded the Birthcenter Amsterdam and currently serves as its managing director. This multifunctional, client-focused center helps strengthen the position of the Dutch midwife and serves as a leader in finding new ways to help protect the Dutch obstetrical system against unnecessary medicalization. In 1992 and 1995, she gave birth herself to her two sons, Mees and Stijn. She is co-author of several Dutch bestsellers on pregnancy, birth, and the year after birth. She works to inspire women and midwives to empower themselves and to treasure the enormous, creative womanpower that is concealed in pregnancy, birth, and motherhood. She is convinced that this is what the modern, male-dominated world is in need of today. E-mail: info@beatrijssmulders.nl.

Edwin van Teijlingen, PhD, is a medical sociologist based at the University of Aberdeen in Scotland. He is involved in a range of studies in the field of maternity care in the United Kingdom, the Netherlands, and Nepal. He has published widely on the organization of maternity care in Scotland and the Netherlands. His co-edited books include *Birth by Design* (2001) and *Midwifery and the Medicalization of Childbirth* (2004). E-mail: van.teijlingen@abdn.ac.uk.

Denis Walsh, RM, RGN, DPSM, PG DipEd, MA, PhD, trained as a midwife in Leicester, United Kingdom, and has worked in a variety of midwifery environments. He is now reader in normal birth at the University of Central Lancashire and an independent midwifery consultant, teaching on evidence and normal birth across Europe and Australia. He publishes widely on normal birth and recently completed his PhD on the birth center model, findings from which help inform Chapter 6 in this volume. E-mail: denis.walsh@ntlworld.com.

Cathy Walton was a founder member of the South East London Midwifery Group Practice in 1994, becoming an original member of the Albany Midwifery Practice in 1997. She continued working as a midwife with the practice until 2004, when she moved away from London for family reasons. She is now a consultant midwife at King's College Hospital in London. Her areas of midwifery interest are home birth, normality in birth, vaginal birth after cesarean section, and supporting and enabling choice in childbirth. She has an MSc in advancing midwifery practice from King's College, London. She has two children, both of whom were born at home. E-mail: cathy@coomasaru-walton.com.

Therese A. Wiegers, PhD, is a senior researcher at the NIVEL (Netherlands Institute for Health Services Research). She uses her training in psychology and epidemiology to study the social and professional context of maternity care, including midwives, general practitioners, gynecologists/obstetricians, and maternity care assistants. E-mail: t.wiegers@nivel.nl.

INDEX

Note: Page numbers followed by *f* indicate a figure; page numbers followed by *n* indicate a note; page numbers followed by *t* indicate a table.

Text: 10/12 Baskerville
Display: Baskerville
Compositor: Publication Services
Printer and binder: Maple-Vail Book Manufacturing Group

Lightning Source UK Ltd.
Milton Keynes UK
UKHW011904030323
418007UK00001B/6